NUTRITION 98/99

Tenth Edition

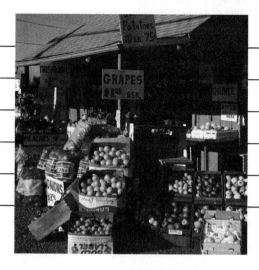

Editor

Charlotte C. Cook-Fuller
Towson University

Charlotte Cook-Fuller has a Ph.D. in community health education and graduate and undergraduate degrees in nutrition. She has worked for several years in public health services and has also been involved with the federally funded WIC (Women, Infants, and Children) program. Now as a professor, she teaches nutrition within both professional and consumer contexts, as well as courses for health education students. She has coauthored a nutrition curriculum for grades K–12 and is currently involved in a multidisciplinary effort to provide strategies to public school teachers for teaching about global issues such as hunger.

Editorial Consultant

Stephen Barrett, M.D.
Editor, *Nutrition Forum*

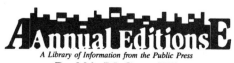

Annual Editions
A Library of Information from the Public Press
Dushkin/McGraw-Hill
Sluice Dock, Guilford, Connecticut 06437

Visit us on the Internet—http://www.dushkin.com/

The Annual Editions Series

ANNUAL EDITIONS, including GLOBAL STUDIES, consist of over 70 volumes designed to provide the reader with convenient, low-cost access to a wide range of current, carefully selected articles from some of the most important magazines, newspapers, and journals published today. ANNUAL EDITIONS are updated on an annual basis through a continuous monitoring of over 300 periodical sources. All ANNUAL EDITIONS have a number of features that are designed to make them particularly useful, including topic guides, annotated tables of contents, unit overviews, and indexes. For the teacher using ANNUAL EDITIONS in the classroom, an Instructor's Resource Guide with test questions is available for each volume. GLOBAL STUDIES titles provide comprehensive background information and selected world press articles on the regions and countries of the world.

VOLUMES AVAILABLE

ANNUAL EDITIONS

Abnormal Psychology
Accounting
Adolescent Psychology
Aging
American Foreign Policy
American Government
American History, Pre-Civil War
American History, Post-Civil War
American Public Policy
Anthropology
Archaeology
Astronomy
Biopsychology
Business Ethics
Canadian Politics
Child Growth and Development
Comparative Politics
Computers in Education
Computers in Society
Criminal Justice
Criminology
Developing World
Deviant Behavior
Drugs, Society, and Behavior
Dying, Death, and Bereavement

Early Childhood Education
Economics
Educating Exceptional Children
Education
Educational Psychology
Environment
Geography
Geology
Global Issues
Health
Human Development
Human Resources
Human Sexuality
International Business
Macroeconomics
Management
Marketing
Marriage and Family
Mass Media
Microeconomics
Multicultural Education
Nutrition
Personal Growth and Behavior
Physical Anthropology
Psychology
Public Administration
Race and Ethnic Relations

Social Problems
Social Psychology
Sociology
State and Local Government
Teaching English as a Second
    Language
Urban Society
Violence and Terrorism
Western Civilization, Pre-Reformation
Western Civilization, Post-Reformation
Women's Health
World History, Pre-Modern
World History, Modern
World Politics

GLOBAL STUDIES

Africa
China
India and South Asia
Japan and the Pacific Rim
Latin America
Middle East
Russia, the Eurasian Republics, and
    Central/Eastern Europe
Western Europe

Cataloging in Publication Data
Main entry under title: Annual editions: Nutrition. 1998/99.
    1. Nutrition—Periodicals. 2. Diet—Periodicals. I. Cook-Fuller, Charlotte C., *comp*. II. Title: Nutrition.
ISBN 0–697–39176–0   613.2'.05   91–641611   ISSN 1055–6990

Tenth Edition

Cover image © 1998 PhotoDisc, Inc.

Printed in the United States of America   1234567890BAHBAH901234098   Printed on Recycled Paper

Editors/Advisory Board

Members of the Advisory Board are instrumental in the final selection of articles for each edition of ANNUAL EDITIONS. Their review of articles for content, level, currentness, and appropriateness provides critical direction to the editor and staff. We think that you will find their careful consideration well reflected in this volume.

EDITORS

Charlotte C. Cook-Fuller
Towson University

with Stephen Barrett, M.D.
Editor, Nutrition Forum

ADVISORY BOARD

Staff

To the Reader

You may agree with Pudd'nhead Wilson (a character created by Mark Twain) who said, "The only way to keep your health is to eat what you don't want, drink what you don't like, and do what you'd rather not." Nutritionists would argue that you can't achieve or maintain good health on a diet of soft drinks and vending machine foods. But you might be surprised to learn that many of your favorite foods can fit into a good diet. In making food choices, remember that variety and moderation are two key words that will assist you in achieving positive health outcomes and avoiding the negative results of excesses or deficiencies.

An array of resources is available to help you make decisions, including popular publications, the news media, scientific journals, and people from many educational backgrounds. Your dilemma is to select reliable sources that will supply factual information based on science rather than exaggerations based on bias. It is important to avoid overreacting to nutrition- and food-related news items or promotional materials, especially if they sound sensational or have shock value. The exaggeration and the myth are what much of the public grasps and, in large measure, reacts to. My challenge to you is to use *Annual Editions: Nutrition 98/99,* preferably with a standard nutrition text, as an invitation to learning. Become a discriminating learner. Compare what you hear and read to the accepted body of knowledge. If this volume provides you with useful information, challenges your thinking, broadens your understanding, or motivates you to take some useful action, it will have fulfilled its purpose.

While this entire volume is essentially one of current events and current thinking, the first unit focuses on trends that give a preview of the future and that relate to characteristics of today's food consumer, the food industry, and views of foods and food components. The next three units are devoted to nutrients, diet and disease, and weight control. All are topics that directly relate to our health, and the dynamic state of knowledge on these subjects requires each of us to be constantly learning and adjusting. Units on food safety and health claims follow, areas in which consumers are especially vulnerable to media and promotional hype and misinformation. The last unit addresses hunger and malnutrition as social and political issues as well as one requiring scientific knowledge for solution. Originally, this unit was intended as a forum for global concerns, but it has become abundantly clear that hunger is also a national issue.

Although the units in this book are distinct, many of the articles have broader significance. The *topic guide* will help you to find other articles on a given subject. You also will find that many of the articles contain at least some element of controversy, the origin of which may be incomplete knowledge, questionable policy, pseudoscience, or competing needs. Sometimes these are difficult issues to resolve, and frequently any resolution creates further dilemmas. But creatively solving problems is our challenge. We take the world as it is and use it as the foundation for tomorrow's discoveries and solutions.

New to this edition are *World Wide Web* sites that can be used to further explore the topics. These sites are cross-referenced by number in the topic guide.

Annual Editions: Nutrition 98/99 is an anthology, and any anthology can be improved, including this one. You can influence the content of future editions by returning the postage-paid article rating form on the last page of this book with your comments and suggestions.

Charlotte C. Cook-Fuller

Charlotte C. Cook-Fuller
Editor

Contents

UNIT 1

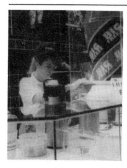

Trends Today and Tomorrow

Nine articles examine the eating patterns of people today. Some of the topics considered include nutrients in our diet, eating trends, food labeling, and self-service outlets.

The concepts in bold italics are developed in the article. For further expansion please refer to the Topic Guide, the Glossary, and the Index.

UNIT 2

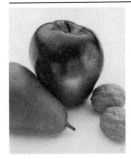

Nutrients

Ten articles discuss the importance of nutrients and fiber in our diet. Topics include dietary standards, carbohydrates, fiber, vitamins, supplements, and minerals.

The concepts in bold italics are developed in the article. For further expansion please refer to the Topic Guide, the Glossary, and the Index.

vi

UNIT 3

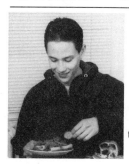

Through the Life Span: Diet and Disease

Eleven articles examine our health as it is affected by diet throughout our lives. Some topics include the links between diet and disease, cholesterol, and eating habits.

The concepts in bold italics are developed in the article. For further expansion please refer to the Topic Guide, the Glossary, and the Index.

UNIT 4

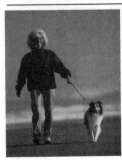

Fat and Weight Control

Seven articles examine weight management. Topics include the relationship between dieting and exercise, the effects of various diet plans, and the relationship between being overweight and fit.

The concepts in bold italics are developed in the article. For further expansion please refer to the Topic Guide, the Glossary, and the Index.

UNIT 5

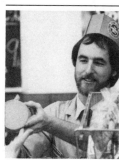

Food Safety

Five articles discuss the safety of food. Topics include food-borne illness, pesticide residues, naturally occurring toxins, and food preservatives.

The concepts in bold italics are developed in the article. For further expansion please refer to the Topic Guide, the Glossary, and the Index.

UNIT 6

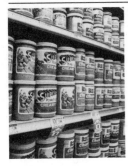

Health Claims

Ten articles examine some of the health claims made by today's "specialists." Topics include quacks, fad diets, and nutrition myths and misinformation.

The concepts in bold italics are developed in the article. For further expansion please refer to the Topic Guide, the Glossary, and the Index.

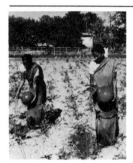

UNIT 7

Hunger and Global Issues

Five articles discuss the world's food supply. Topics include global malnutrition, water quality, agriculture, and famine.

The concepts in bold italics are developed in the article. For further expansion please refer to the Topic Guide, the Glossary, and the Index.

Topic Guide

This topic guide suggests how the selections in this book relate to topics of traditional concern to students and professionals involved with the study of nutrition. It is useful for locating articles that relate to each other for reading and research. The guide is arranged alphabetically according to topic. Articles may, of course, treat topics that do not appear in the topic guide. In turn, entries in the topic guide do not necessarily constitute a comprehensive listing of all the contents of each selection. **In addition, relevant Web sites, which are annotated on pages 4 and 5, are noted in bold italics under the topic articles.**

TOPIC AREA	TREATED IN	TOPIC AREA	TREATED IN
Additives	18. Fluoridation 21. Most Frequently Asked Questions... about Diet and Cancer 41. How Much Are Pesticides Hurting Your Health? *(3, 11, 12, 13, 14, 26)*	Coronary Heart Disease (cont.)	25. Triglycerides Turn Troublesome 30. Alcohol: Benefits and Risks *(5, 8, 9, 12, 14, 16, 23, 24, 25)*
Alcohol	30. Alcohol: Benefits and Risks *(5, 9, 18)*	Cultural Influence	29. Nutritional Implications of Ethnic and Cultural Diversity *(6, 17)*
Antioxidants	6. Phytochemicals: Drugstore in a Salad? 16. Trials of Beta-Carotene 21. Most Frequently Asked Questions... about Diet and Cancer *(5, 6, 8, 9, 10, 11)*	Diet/Disease	6. Phytochemicals: Drugstore in a Salad? 10. Type of Fat We May Need More Of 11. Facts about Fats 13. 'Bran-New' Look at Dietary Fiber 17. Too Little Sun? 18. Fluoridation 20. Beating the Odds 21. Most Frequently Asked Questions... about Diet and Cancer 22. Diet and Hypertension 24. Deciphering Blood Cholesterol 25. Triglycerides Turn Troublesome *(6, 8, 9, 10, 11, 12, 13, 14, 15, 16, 17, 18, 20, 21)*
Athletes	52. Don't Buy Phony 'Ergogenic Aids' *(30)*		
Attitudes/ Knowledge	1. "What We Eat in America" Survey 9. Coming Boom(er) Market *(5, 6, 7, 8, 9, 10, 12)*		
Biotechnology	54. Will the World Starve? 56. Crop Gurus Sow Some Seeds of Hope *(31, 32, 33, 34)*	Dieting	28. When Eating Goes Awry 32. History of Dieting and Its Effectiveness 33. Diet Pills 36. Dysfunctional Eating 37. Reduced-Fat Foods *(21, 22, 23, 24, 25)*
Cancer	6. Phytochemicals: Drugstore in a Salad? 16. Trials of Beta-Carotene 17. Too Little Sun? 20. Beating the Odds 21. Most Frequently asked Questions... about Diet and Cancer 30. Alcohol: Benefits and Risks *(5, 9, 11, 12, 13, 14, 15, 17, 20)*	Eating Disorders	28. When Eating Goes Awry 36. Dysfunctional Eating *(23, 24, 25)*
		Elderly	23. Boning Up on Osteoporosis *(20)*
Children/Infants	10. Type of Fat We May Need More Of 26. Breast-Feeding Best Bet for Babies 31. Three Major U.S. Studies Describe Trends 35. Diet and Exercise *(11, 12, 13, 14, 24, 25)*	Fats/Substitutes	5. Meat Meets Its Match? 10. Type of Fat We May Need More Of 11. Facts about Fats 37. Reduced-Fat Foods *(8, 9, 10, 11, 12, 13, 14)*
Controversies	3. Health Claims under the Nutrition Labeling and Education Act 7. Food Police 22. Diet and Hypertension 30. Alcohol: Benefits and Risks 32. History of Dieting and Its Effectiveness 33. Diet Pills 37. Reduced-Fat Foods 48. Vitamin and Nutritional Supplements 49. Nutrition Shortcut in a Can? 50. 'Dietary Supplement' Mess 54. Will the World Starve? *(5, 8, 9, 12, 17, 28, 29, 30)*	Fiber	13. 'Bran-New' Look at Dietary Fiber 21. Most Frequently Asked Questions... about Diet and Cancer *(11, 12, 13, 14, 17, 18, 21)*
		Food and Drug Administration (FDA)	33. Diet Pills 50. 'Dietary Supplement' Mess *(24, 25)*
		Food Industry	8. High Price of Shelf Space 9. Coming Boom(er) Market
Coronary Heart Disease	6. Phytochemicals: Drugstore in a Salad? 10. Type of Fat We May Need More Of 11. Facts about Fats 24. Deciphering Blood Cholesterol	Food Safety	39. For Safety's Sake: Scrub Your Produce 40. New Risks in Ground Beef Revealed 41. How Much Are Pesticides Hurting Your Health? 50. 'Dietary Supplement' Mess *(26, 27)*

Selected World Wide Web Sites for
Annual Editions: Nutrition

All of these Web sites are hot-linked through the *Annual Editions* home page:
http://www.dushkin.com/annualeditions (just click on this book's title). In addition, these sites are referenced by number and appear where relevant in the Topic Guide on the previous two pages.

Some Web sites are continually changing their structure and content, so the information listed may not always be available.

General Sources

1. American Medical Association—*http://www.ama-assn.org/*—The venerable AMA offers this site for consumers and health practitioners to find up-to-date nutritional and medical information, discussions of such topics as women's health, and important publications such as the *Journal of the American Medical Association.*

2. Health Links—*http://www.hslib.washington.edu/*—Open this site to find links to sites of interest to people with knowledge of nutrition and other health sciences. There are links to international health statistics, journals, public health topics, library services, and so on.

3. University of Pennsylvania School of Medicine Nutrition Education and Prevention Program—*http://www.med.upenn.edu/~nutrimed/*—The aim of the Nutrition Education and Prevention Program is to engage medical students in active learning about nutrition and medicine through interdisciplinary study. This home page provides links to many related Web sites.

4. U.S. National Institutes of Health—*http://www.nih.gov/*—Consult this site for links to extensive health information and scientific resources. Comprised of 24 separate institutes, centers, and divisions—including the Institute of Mental Health—the NIH is one of eight health agencies of the Public Health Service, which, in turn, is part of the U.S. Department of Health and Human Services.

Trends Today and Tomorrow

5. Center for Science in the Public Interest—*http://www.cspinet.org/*—Search the links of this page of CSPI's Web site for information on food allergies, improving one's diet, Olestra, alcohol, food safety, and other topics. CSPI is a nonprofit education and advocacy organization that focuses on educating the public about nutrition and alcohol.

6. The Gallup Organization—*http://www.gallup.com/*—Open this Gallup Organization page for links to an extensive archive of public opinion poll results and special reports on a huge variety of topics. It will help in gaining understanding of people's food choices.

7. The Society of Behavioral Medicine—*http://socbehmed.org/sbm/sisterorg.htm*—This site of the Society of Behavioral Medicine provides listings of major, general health institutes and organizations as well as discipline-specific links and resources in medicine, psychology, and public health.

8. U.S. Department of Agriculture—*http://www.usda.gov/news/news.htm*—Visit this site of the USDA to keep up with nutritional news and information. The site provides links to publications, educational resources, and related congressional news.

9. U.S. Food and Drug Administration—*http://www.fda.gov/fdahomepage.html*—This is the home page of the FDA, which describes itself as the United States' "foremost consumer protection agency." Visit this site and its links to learn about food safety, food and nutrition labeling, and other topics of importance in the study of nutrition.

10. Vegetarian Pages—*http://www.veg.org/veg/*—The Vegetarian Pages are intended to be an independent, definitive Internet guide for vegetarians, vegans, and others. The index and listings will lead you to information about all things vegetarian.

Nutrients

11. Encyclopedia Britannica—*http://www.ebig.com/*—This huge "Britannica Internet Guide" will lead you to a cornucopia of informational sites and reference sources in nutritional health. This is a good starting point for research into vitamins and other nutrients.

12. Food and Nutrition Information Center—*http://www.nal.usda.gov/fnic/*—Use this site to find dietary and nutrition information provided by various USDA agencies, to find links to food and nutrition resources on the Internet, and to access FNIC publications and databases.

13. Nutrient Data Laboratory—*http://www.nal.usda.gov/fnic/foodcomp/*—This USDA Agricultural Research Service site provides information about the USDA Nutrient Database. Search here for answers to FAQs, a glossary of terms, facts about food composition, and useful links.

14. U.S. National Library of Medicine—*http://www.nlm.nih.gov/*—This huge site permits you to search a number of databases and electronic information sources such as MEDLINE, learn about research projects and programs, keep up on recent nutrition-related news, and peruse the national network of medical libraries.

Through the Life Span: Diet and Disease

15. American Cancer Society—*http://www.cancer.org/frames.html*—Open this site and its various links to learn the concerns—and lifestyle advice—of the American Cancer Society. It provides information on tobacco, alternative therapies, other Web resources, and more.

16. American Heart Association—*http://www.amhrt.org/*—The AMA offers this site to provide the most comprehensive information on heart disease and stroke as well as late-breaking news. The site presents facts on the warning signs of heart disease and stroke, a reference guide, explanations of diseases and treatments, and so on.

17. American Studies Web—*http://www.georgetown.edu/crossroads/asw/*—This eclectic site provides links to a wealth of resources on the Internet related to American studies, from gender studies, to environment, to race and ethnicity. It is of great help when doing research in demography and population studies and in topics such as health differentials between races or ethnic groups.

18. Columbia University Health Services—*http://www.columbia.edu/cu/healthwise/about.html*—This interactive site provides discussion and insight into a number of personal issues of interest to college-age people—and those younger and older. Many questions about physical and emotional health and well-being in the modern world are answered.

19. Dr. Ivan's Depression Central—*http://www.psycom.net/depression. central.html*—This extensive site describes itself as the "Internet's central clearinghouse for information on all types of depressive disorders and on the most effective treatments" for these disorders—and it lives up to the billing. The site provides extensive information about eating disorders.

20. National Institute on Aging—*http://www.nih.gov/nia/*—The NIA, one of the institutes of the U.S. National Institutes of Health, presents this home page to lead you to a variety of resources on health and lifestyle issues that are of interest to people as they grow older.

21. Sympatico: Healthy Way: Health Links—*http://www.ab.sympatico. ca/Contents/Health/GENERAL/sitemap.html*—This Canadian site meant for consumers will lead you to many links addressing human sexuality over the life span, general health, and reproductive health.

Fat and Weight Control

22. American Society of Exercise Physiologists—*http://www.css.edu/ users/tboone2/asep/toc.htm*—ASEP is devoted to promoting people's health and physical fitness. This extensive site provides links to journals and other publications related to exercise, career opportunities in exercise physiology, and the process of professionalization of the field.

23. The Blonz Guide to Nutrition—*http://www.wenet.net/blonz/*—The categories in this valuable site report news in the fields of nutrition, food science, foods, fitness, and health. There is also an excellent selection of search engines and other important links.

24. Healthfinder—*http://www.os.healthfinder.gov/*—This U.S. Department of Health and Human Services consumer site has extensive links to information on such topics as the health benefits of exercise, weight control, and prudent lifestyle choices. Bibliographies on a multitude of health topics can be accessed here.

25. MedWeb: Nutrition—*http://www.gen.emory.edu/ MEDWEB/keyword/nutrition.html*—The links in this massive Emory University site will take you to information and resources on virtually all topics in nutritional health, from dietary supplements to eating disorders. This site is useful for research into other topics of concern to students of health sciences, such as weight control.

Food Safety

26. Centers for Disease Control and Prevention—*http://www.cdc.gov/*—The CDC—which calls itself "The Nation's Prevention Agency," offers this home page, from which you can learn information about travelers' health, data and statistics related to disease control and prevention, general nutritional and health information, publications, and more.

27. Food Safety and Inspection Service—*http://www.usda.gov/agency/ fsis/homepage.htm*—The FSIS, part of the U.S. Department of Agriculture, is the government agency "responsible for ensuring that the nation's commercial supply of meat, poultry, and egg products is safe, wholesome, and correctly labeled and packaged." This is its home page.

Health Claims

28. Agency for Health Care Policy and Research—*http://www.ahcpr. gov/*—The aim of the AHCPR is to improve health care quality through education and research. Open this site to find information on consumer health, U.S. health care policy and trends, clinical research, and data and surveys.

29. Alt-MEDMarket—*http://alt.medmarket.com/indexes/indexmfr.html*—This commercial site bills itself as "the Internet guide to alternative therapies and products." Click on the "Alternative Health E-Mall" for an alternative medicine directory and herbal information center; alternative medicine providers, listed by geographic area and specialty; a listing of articles; herbs with their corresponding treatments; and other information.

30. Science News Digest for Physicians and Scientists—*http://genome. eerie.fr/bioscience/news/scientis/obesity2.htm*—This site provides information about neuropeptide Y and its known and suspected functions in regulation of body weight and circadian rhythms, sexual functioning, and anxiety and stress response. A bibliography is included.

Hunger and Global Issues

31. Penn Library: Nutrition—*http://www.library.upenn.edu/resources/ healthscience/disciplines/nutrition.html*—This site is rich in links to information about virtually every subject you can think of in nutrition. From here, click to Penn Library's other health study sites and its extensive population and demography resources, which address such concerns as family planning and nutrition in various world regions.

32. World Health Organization—*http://www.who.ch/Welcome.html*—This home page of the World Health Organization will provide you with links to a wealth of statistical and analytical information about health and nutrition around the world.

33. World Hunger Year—*http://www.iglou.com/why/ria.htm*—WHY offers this site as part of its program called Reinvesting in America, its effort to help people fight hunger and poverty in their communities. Various resources and models for grassroots action are included here.

34. WWW Virtual Library: Demography & Population Studies—*http:// coombs.anu.edu.au/ResFacilities/DemographyPage.html*—This is a definitive guide to demography and population studies. A multitude of important links to information about global poverty and hunger can be found here.

We highly recommend that you review our Web site for expanded information and our other product lines. We are continually updating and adding links to our Web site in order to offer you the most usable and useful information that will support and expand the value of your Annual Editions. You can reach us at: *http://www. dushkin.com/annualeditions/.*

Trends Today and Tomorrow

It is change, continuing change, inevitable change, that is the dominant factor in society today. No sensible decision can be made any longer without taking into account not only the world as it is, but the world as it will be.
—Isaac Asimov 1981

The average consumer is a phantom, constantly reshaping and reemerging under the influences of the food industry, the media, activist organizations, and whatever health messages are currently most persuasive. Years ago, for the sake of heart health, we were persuaded to switch from butter and lard to vegetable oil and margarine. Later, we obediently avoided tropical oils. More recently we were told to beware of trans-fatty acids produced in the manufacture of solid margarines. Thus, for the last half century, Americans have been constantly bombarded by health and nutrition messages and admonitions at an increasingly rapid rate, many of which have been misleading and contradictory. It is no wonder that consumers have become more and more confused and have grown disenchanted with conventional sources of advice. Respondents frequently report being unhappy with conflicting information, and many say they'd rather get information *after* nutrition and health professionals have reached consensus. As more and more people access the Internet, this problem may be exacerbated rather than lessened.

All of this does not mean that Americans are unconcerned or disinterested in their dietary habits, although one survey finds that fewer are doing all they can to eat a balanced diet. Other surveys repeatedly show that the average consumer is knowledgeable and very interested in the health effects of nutrition. The average consumer is also confused and holds many misconceptions, believing that foods can be divided into categories of good and bad foods, that tasty foods are not nutritious, and that it is simply too time-consuming to eat well. The first article in this book provides new data showing the correlation between people's attitudes and knowledge about nutrition and their nutrient intakes and food choices. Overall, fat consumption has dropped slightly, with about one-third of Americans meeting the guideline of less than 30 percent of calories coming from fat. At the same time, *total* calorie consumption is 9 percent *higher* than 20 years ago, and this in spite of the many reduced-fat and fat-free products available. Issues of fat content in food products are addressed in "Meat Meets Its Match?"

Today's sophisticated consumer is desirous of information about diets and food. Responses have come from government agencies and the food industry as well as professionals and voluntary associations. A revision of the Recommended Dietary Allowance (RDA) is not yet published, although we await it eagerly and expect at least some changes in the recommendations. The 1995 Dietary Guidelines, however, are available. Issued jointly by the U.S. Departments of Agriculture and Health and Human Services, their purpose is to provide advice to healthy Americans about the relationship between food choices and health. They reflect a clear linkage to the popular Food Pyramid and the Nutrition Facts Label. A review of these guidelines is mandatory every 5 years, and publication of a new edition follows a lengthy process of literature review; solicitation of written comments from health professionals, trade organizations, and the public; and public hearings.

One way to achieve a diet that conforms to the 1995 Dietary Guidelines and the Food Pyramid is to eat a minimum of three vegetables and two fruits daily, a subject discussed in "Fruits & Vegetables: Eating Your Way to 5 a Day." According to data reported by the National Cancer Institute, the average American now approaches this goal, having actually consumed 4.4 servings daily in 1994. Other surveys, however, indicate that potatoes may account for half the vegetables eaten and that less than one-third of the daily serving comes from the dark green and yellow vegetables that are so rich in vitamin A. Children are the most likely to have eaten french fries or possibly tomatoes in a pasta sauce. Even less popular than vegetables, fruits averaged two servings only because of the apples in apple pie. Again, children consume lots of boxed juices, but most of them are juice drinks, not 100 percent fruit juice. Clearly variety seems limited, and consumers would benefit from eating more of the 350 to 400 fresh products available in most supermarkets.

In this unit, two articles address the subject of consumer information on labels and, more recently, in restaurants. In both instances, this information is an application of the Nutrition Labeling and Education Act of 1990. Well-substantiated health claims indicating the benefits of specific foods or food substances are permitted on labels and can be useful to the consumer in making food choices. Examples of permitted claims are the relationship between dietary fat and heart disease and between folic acid and neural tube defects. A very recent addition to the list of permitted claims states that diets both high in oat bran or oatmeal and low in fat may be protective against heart disease. Regulations now also require restaurants to sup-

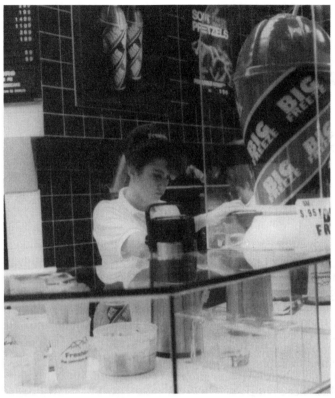

ply verifying information if menu items claim to have specific nutritional content or health benefits. The consumer must ask for this information, and it may be produced in almost any form. Some analysts predict that the process will be too cumbersome and that claims on menus will disappear. However, 57 percent of the population eats out daily, and that represents a lot of people who might find the information useful.

Another trend worthy of note is the increased interest in food chemicals other than nutrients, the topic in the article "Phytochemicals: Drugstore in a Salad?" Phytochemicals represent an expanded knowledge of the chemical composition of normal plant foods and the potential for promoting good health and preventing diseases such as cancer and heart disease. More and more frequently we read about the possible advantages of isoflavones, saponins, flavinoids, phytoestrogens, and many others. The promises are great but are mostly unproven, making the balance between developing this new market and maintaining public health and safety a challenge. The best current wisdom dictates eating a wide variety of foods with emphasis on fruits, vegetables, and whole grains rather than on supplements or manufactured foods.

Manufacturers and market forces are accused of dictating food choices and programming consumers, and there is evidence to this effect. In "High Price of Shelf Space," for example, Sean Somerville confirms what you may have suspected about grocery stores—that the placement of foods and the amount of space allotted sometimes fol-

lows a hidden plan. It is equally true that markets respond to consumer demands. Baby boomers (see "The Coming Boom(er)"), now entering their 50s, have sufficient numbers to influence the food industry. Although boomers will have the same nutritional needs as their forebears, they will live longer, and they will demand foods that are more convenient and that specifically address medical and weight-loss needs. Current trends in this direction seem well established. Of the nearly 17,000 new products introduced in 1995, over a tenth were low-fat items.

Leading opponents of the fat substitute Olestra, fast foods, high-fat items, and a good many other products are the Center for Science in the Public Interest (CSPI) and its director, Michael Jacobson. Otherwise known as the food police, they have alerted the public to many problems of the average American diet. Critics claim that CSPI exaggerates facts out of proportion to reality. Thus, truth blurs with fiction, making it difficult for the consumer to draw a reasonable conclusion. Minna Morse explores these issues in "The Food Police," allowing the reader to decide.

In other news, Campbell's is bidding for an increased market share by adding more chicken to a favorite, chicken noodle soup, and is introducing new lines of frozen soups, nearly fat-free cream soups, and soups in glass jars. Rice cakes have made a comeback since their manufacturer added chocolate and popcorn flavors, thus conceding that taste is the most important issue. H. J. Heinz will capitalize on the consumer's fixation with organic products and will offer organic baby foods, at a significantly higher price, of course. And KFC, which sells half the fried chicken in the United States, boosted its stagnant sales by adding roast chicken as well as chicken pot pies. Thus we end another year.

Cultural change clearly is occurring in our lifetimes. An orange was a treat in the toe of my mother's Christmas stocking. As a child I had fresh oranges and orange juice in cans. For my daughters, frozen orange juice was commonplace. My grandchildren enjoy drinking it from sealed cartons and fortified with calcium, although all of the previous options remain. Which of the new food experiences being planned for us will we like, and which will retreat into oblivion? Perhaps all we can say with certainty is that there will be change.

Looking Ahead: Challenge Questions

What current consumer trends and trends in the food industry will and will not support healthier lifestyles?

What demands do you think your generation will place on the food industry two or three decades from now?

What do you think is the role of a consumer watchdog organization such as CSPI? Would you change its approach, and if so, how?

Does change always equal progress? Why or why not? Give examples from the nutrition field.

"What We Eat in America" Survey

Highlights from USDA's 1994 Continuing Survey of Food Intakes by Individuals and 1994 Diet and Health Knowledge Survey[a]

Results of the first year of the USDA's 10th Nationwide Food Consumption Survey has been released in a set of 14 tables. Information from the table recording the mean nutrient intake per individual by age and sex for 1 day in 1994 is presented in Table 1. The complete set of data tables can be accessed on the Internet at http://www.barc.usda.gov/bhnrc/food survey/csfii94.htm.

These surveys are being conducted by the Agricultural Research Service (ARS) of the US Department of Agriculture (USDA). The CSFII 1994–96, popularly known as "What we Eat in America", is the third in a series of continuing surveys conducted since 1985. The Diet and Health Knowledge Survey (DHKS), which is a telephone follow-up to CSFII, was initiated in 1989. Both surveys were uniquely designed so that individuals' attitudes and knowledge about healthy eating could be linked with their food choices and nutrient intakes.

OBJECTIVES AND SCOPE

The objectives of the surveys are to:

- **Measure the kinds and amounts of food eaten by Americans.** This objective addresses the requirements of the National Nutrition Monitoring and Related Research Act of 1990 (P.L. 101-445) for continuous monitoring of the nutritional status of the American population, including the low-income population.
- **Measure attitudes and knowledge about diet and health among Americans.**

Following a pilot study of the data collection methods, data collection for the full survey began in January 1994. In each of the 3 survey years, a nationally representative sample of approximately 5000 individuals is asked to provide, through in-person interviews, food intake for 2 nonconsecutive days and socioeconomic and health-related information. About 2 weeks after the CSFII, 2000 selected individuals from the survey households are asked to answer a series of questions in a telephone about knowledge and attitudes toward dietary guidance and health. The number of CSFII respondents is anticipated to be between 15,000 and 16,000 over 3 years. The number of DHKS respondents is expected to be between 4,000 and 5,000 over 3 years. The results of the 2nd and 3rd years will be released in subsequent reports.

CHANGES

The CSFII/DHKS 1994–96 differs from the 1989–91 surveys in several important ways. Compared with earlier surveys, the 1994–96 surveys include:

[a]Highlights presented were based on information provided by L. E. Cleveland, J. D. Goldman, and L. G. Borrund. Data tables: Results from USDA's Continuing Survey of Food Intakes by Individuals and 1994 Diet and Health Knowledge Survey. Agricultural Research Service, US Department of Agriculture, Riverdale, MD 20737.

Table 1
Mean Nutrient Intake per Individual by Age and Sex for 1 Day[a]

Sex and Age (yr)	Percentage of population	Food energy (kcal)	Protein (g)	Total fat (g)	Saturated fatty acids (g)	Mono-unsaturated fatty acids (g)	Poly-unsaturated fatty acids (g)	Cholesterol (mg)	Carbohydrate (g)	Dietary fiber (g)	Vitamin A[b] (μg)	Carotenes[b] (μg)	Vitamin E[c] (mg)	Vitamin C (mg)	Thiamin (mg)	Riboflavin (mg)	Niacin (mg)	Vitamin B-6 (mg)	Folate (μg)	Vitamin B-12 (μg)	Calcium (mg)	Phosphorus (mg)	Magnesium (mg)	Iron (mg)	Zinc (mg)	Copper (mg)	Sodium (mg)	Potassium (mg)
Males and females:																												
>1	1.0	840	22.8	37.4	15.8	10.5	82	66	104.3	3.1	993	194	13.6	96	.90	1.40	10.9	0.63	113	3.72	671	536	94	16.0	5.7	.8	507	1084
1-2	3.2	1322	50.0	48.0	19.6	17.6	72	185	177.4	8.8	741	273	4.6	98	1.11	1.67	13.0	1.31	176	3.34	823	952	185	10.9	7.2	.7	1988	2000
3-5	4.7	1552	55.0	58.0	219	2Z2	9.8	183	208.8	10.2	758	244	5.6	93	1.29	1.75	15.6	1.40	206	3.49	796	1010	196	11.9	7.9	.8	2419	1999
≥5	8.9	1392	49.7	52.1	20.3	19.3	8.7	171	186.1	8.9	776	249	6.1	95	1.18	1.68	14.2	1.29	185	3.46	792	938	181	12.0	7.4	.8	2056	1900
Males																												
6-11	4.6	1980	70.4	73.8	27.4	28S	12.5	234	266.1	13.3	1061	354	6.9	96	1.76	2.29	21.3	1.86	288	4.83	972	1251	243	15.9	10.5	1.0	3067	2409
12-19	5.7	2760	97.4	00.6	35.4	39.2	18.4	327	372.1	17.4	1010	297	9.7	122	2.10	2.57	28.0	2.21	328	5.86	1,125	1619	311	19.2	14.2	1.4	4223	3023
20-29	7.0	2943	110.8	108.9	37.6	42.2	20.6	375	344.9	18.6	953	428	10.1	121	2.06	2.50	32.9	2.47	321	5.97	1,025	1691	350	19.3	15.1	1.6	4574	3337
30-39	8.8	2614	100.3	100.8	33.9	39.0	20.2	351	316.8	19.2	1087	482	12.2	113	2.07	2.36	29.6	2.37	325	6.14	943	1546	341	19.4	15.0	1.6	4317	3326
40-49	6.7	2448	100.1	93.6	31.2	36.2	18.7	343	288.7	18.6	1161	543	10.0	104	1.96	2.23	28.7	2.16	297	5.98	895	1527	344	17.9	13.4	15	4197	3346
50-59	4.7	2160	85.0	82.2	26.1	31.9	17.8	295	262.7	17.5	1038	528	9.3	100	1.78	1.99	26.3	2.04	281	5.48	728	1300	302	16.0	12.6	1.4	3746	2987
60-69	3.5	2079	83.7	80.5	26.4	31.0	16.6	302	250.1	18.6	1244	641	9.2	100	1.70	2.03	25.1	2.01	279	6.04	766	1308	310	17.5	12.6	1.4	3549	3054
≥70	3.3	1873	74.0	71.1	24.0	27.4	14.0	275	234.8	18.2	1560	641	9.6	100	1.69	2.10	22.5	1.98	297	7.42	750	1217	288	17.1	12.3	1.4	3234	2799
≥20	34.0	2460	96.1	93.6	31.4	36.2	18.7	334	294.9	18.6	1129	521	10.4	109	1.93	2.25	28.5	2.23	305	6.10	884	1482	330	18.2	13.9	1.5	4048	3207
Females																												
6-11	4.4	1747	61.1	64.8	23.8	24.8	11.4	195	237.2	11.6	792	246	6.4	98	1.45	1.92	17.7	1.48	237	3.74	859	1121	217	13.0	9.0	.9	2724	2113
12-19	5.5	1898	67.5	69.4	24.8	26.6	12.7	220	257.7	13.1	884	373	6.8	96	1.47	1.82	18.8	1.54	236	4.12	809	1148	225	13.8	10.2	1.0	3081	2279
20-29	7.1	1791	65.9	66.1	22.8	25.0	13.3	225	228.5	12.4	764	340	7.2	89	1.34	1.65	19.0	1.52	224	3.94	725	1098	223	12.7	9.5	1.1	2917	2208
30-39	8.9	1648	64.0	60.4	19.9	23.1	12.6	209	210.7	13.4	982	521	7.0	79	1.33	1.60	19.0	1.54	228	4.19	638	1031	231	12.8	9.6	1.0	2850	2253
40-49	6.7	1663	65.3	61.6	20.2	23.5	13.1	213	214.0	14.4	952	570	8.2	94	1.34	1.58	19.5	1.49	227	3.85	663	1029	244	13.2	9.5	1.1	2833	2477
50-59	52	1559	629	59.4	19.3	22.	13.2	217	192.5	14.0	943	513	7.2	93	1.27	1.50	18.7	1.51	218	4.40	607	1001	237	11.9	8.4	1.0	2702	2399
60-69	4.3	1507	61.0	56.4	18.6	212	12.0	215	191.8	15.3	1115	586	6.8	103	1.29	1.55	18.0	1.48	224	5.25	602	968	236	12.8	8.7	1.1	2718	2415
≥70	4.7	1363	56.4	47.9	15.7	18.0	10.3	188	182.1	14.0	1049	509	6.0	87	1.24	1.50	17.6	1.48	229	4.62	547	893	217	12.0	8.3	1.0	2413	2177
≥20	36.9	1613	63.2	59.5	19.8	22.5	12.6	212	206.4	13.8	953	500	7.0	89	1.31	1.57	18.8	1.15	225	4.29	639	1015	231	12.6	9.1	1.1	2768	2315
All	100.0	1985	75.6	74.2	2S.4	28.4	14.6	257	251.0	15.0	994	448	8.2	99	1.59	1.93	22.3	1.79	259	4.91	798	1224	264	15.1	11.0	1.2	3264	2615
Individuals																												

[a] Excludes breast-fed children.
[b] Retinol equivalents.
[c] Tocopherol equivalents.

- A target population of noninstitutionalized individuals in all 50 states rather than the 48 coterminous states.
- The collection of 2 nonconsecutive days of food intake through in-person interviews rather than 3 consecutive days of food intake using a 1-day recall and a 2-day record.
- Oversampling of the low-income population, rather than a separate low-income survey.
- A larger sample in selected age-sex categories, specifically young children and elderly.
- Subsampling within households, rather than the collection of information from all members of a household.
- Collection of DHKS data from adults 20 years of age and older, rather from only main meal-planners/-preparers.
- Additional questions on attitudes and knowledge about using food labels, and
- Tighter management controls to minimize nonresponse.

The tables provide national probability estimates for the US population. The results are weighted to adjust for differential rates of selection and nonresponse and to calibrate the sample to match population characteristics that are correlated with eating behavior. Sample sizes on which estimates are based are provided in an Appendix. In general, the sample sizes for each sex-age group provide a sufficient level of precision to ensure statistical reliability of the estimates. The one exception is the sample size for children less than 1 year of age. Estimates for that group should be used with caution. Statistical issues are discussed in another Appendix.

SELECTED HIGHLIGHTS FROM TABLE 1: NUTRIENT INTAKE OF INDIVIDUALS

Among adults 20 years of age and older:

- Men consume an average of about 2500 calories per day. Women consume an average of about 1600 calories/day.
- The average cholesterol intake by men (334 mg/day) exceeds

the recommendation to consume no more than 300 mg/day. Women's average intake (212 mg/day) meets the recommendation.

- Average daily sodium intakes from foods alone are over 4000 mg for men and almost 3000 mg for women. Total intakes of sodium are even higher, because these values do not include sodium from salt added to foods at the table. These intakes exceed the recommendation to consume no more than 2400 mg/day.
- Men consume an average of 19 g of dietary fiber/day, and women consume an average of 14 g. The National Cancer Institute recommends that people consume 20 to 30 g of dietary fiber daily.
- Although Americans have a wide variety of nutritious foods from which to choose, some people choose diets that put them at risk for nutrient shortfalls. Average intakes of women 20 years of age and older are below Recommended Dietary Allowances (RDAs) for six nutrients—vitamin E, vitamin B-6, calcium, magnesium, iron, and zinc. Average intakes of men are below RDAs for zinc and magnesium. The farther that average intakes fall below the RDAs, the greater the likelihood that some people have inadequate intakes.

Highlights from Data on Percentage of Individuals Meeting 100% of the 1989 RDAs by Sex and Age, 2-Day Average, 1994.
Interpreting the data in this table: "The RDAs provide a safety factor appropriate to each nutrient, and exceed the actual requirements of most individuals." Thus, individuals with intakes below the RDA do not necessarily have inadequate intakes. However, as the percentage of the population with intakes below 100% of a given RDA increases, so does the likelihood that some individuals in the population are at nutritional risk.

Selected Highlights.

- Less than one fourth of women 20 years of age and older have

diets that provide 100% of the RDAs for calcium (21%), magnesium (22%), and zinc (17%).
- Less than one half the men of the same age, 45%, 37%, and 35%, have diets providing 100% of the RDA for these nutrients, respectively.

Intakes for Total Fat, Saturated Fat, and Cholesterol, 2-Day Average, 1994. *Selected Highlights.* The 1995 Dietary Guidelines for Americans recommend that people 2 years of age and older choose a diet with no more than 30% of calories from total fat, less than 10% of calories from saturated fat, and no more than 300 mg/day from cholesterol. Among individuals 20 years of age and older:

- 35% of women and 29% of men meet the recommendation for total fat of 30% or less of calories
- 41% of women and 34% of men meet the recommendation for saturated fat of less than 10% of calories.
- 78% of women and 56% of men meet the recommendation for cholesterol of 300 mg or less.

On the basis of 1-day intake:

- Women consume 32% of calories from fat and 11% from saturated fat
- Men consume 34% of calories from fat and 11% from saturated fat
- Intake of alcohol for men and women 20 years of age and older represented 2.8% and 1.3%, respectively, of total calories.
- Male and female respondents 20 to 29 years of age consumed 4.3% and 1.9% of calories from alcohol, respectively, for men and women.

Food eaten away from home:

- About one fourth of calories consumed by both men and women 20 years of age and older are from foods obtained and eaten away from home.
- Among adults, calories from foods obtained and eaten away from home are highest among those 20 to 29 years of age and

lowest among those 70 years of age and older.

- Nutrients contributed by foods eaten at breakfast:

- Men consume an average of 17% of calories, 16% of total fat, and 18% of cholesterol at breakfast.
- Women have similar percentages.
- Percentage of calories and total fat contributed by foods eaten at breakfast increase with age for men.
- Women consume only 18% of their calories at breakfast, but about 23% to 24% of their calcium, iron, and magnesium and 22% to 26% of riboflavin, folate, vitamins A and C, and thiamin, nutrients often low in the diets of women.

Highlights of Nutrient Intakes Contributed by Foods Eaten as Snacks. In this table, "snack" refers to any eating occasion designated by the respondent as a food and/or beverage break, including the snack, alcoholic beverage, and other beverage categories.

- Americans consume an average of 17% of their calories and 15% of their total fat intake as snacks.
- Adolescents consume about 21% of their calories and about 20% of both total fat and saturated fat from snacks.
- Girls obtain over 20% of their intake of vitamins A and E and calcium from snacks.

Selected Highlights about Quantities of Food Consumed by Individuals. The 1995 Dietary Guidelines for Americans advise people to choose a diet with most of the calories from grain products, vegetables, fruits, low-fat milk products, lean meats, fish, poultry, and dry beans and choose fewer calories from fats and sweets. They place special emphasis on grain products, vegetables, and fruits as key parts of a varied diet.

- Americans consume an average of 300 g of grain products each day. More than one third (112 g) is consumed as grain mixtures— such as lasagna and pizza. Yeast

breads and rolls and cereals, rice, and pasta are also substantial contributors.

- Americans consume low levels of nutrient-packed dark green and deep yellow vegetables, despite guidance to do otherwise. Men 20 years of age and older consume an average of 21 g of dark green and deep yellow vegetables/day, and women consume an average of 24 g.
- More than half of the white potatoes eaten by children 6 to 19 years old are in the form of fried potatoes.
- Adolescent boys consume about 1¼ cups (305 g) of fluid milk/ day; adolescent girls consume less than 1 cup. For both, about one third is whole milk and about two thirds is low-fat or skim milk. By contrast, adolescent boys consumed about 2⅔ (658 g) of carbonated soft drinks; adolescent girls, about 1½ cups (381 g).
- On any given day, only about half (54%) of Americans eat fruit, and only about three fourths (79%) consume milk or milk products.
- One fourth of all Americans eat fried potatoes on any given day.
- One half of all Americans drink carbonated soft drinks on any given day.

Perceived Diet Quality by Self-Assessment. Respondents were asked: *Compared with what is healthy, do you think your diet is too low, too high, or about right in (NU-TRIENT/FOOD COMPONENT)?*

The question covers the following nutrients and food components: calories, calcium, iron, vitamin C, protein, fat, saturated fat, cholesterol, salt or sodium, fiber, and sugar and sweets.

Selected Highlights. Among adults 20 years of age and older:

- 36% of men and 43% of women think their diets are *too high* in calories.
- 48% of men and women think their diets are *too high* in fat.
- 29% of men and 24% of women think their diets are *too high* in salt or sodium.
- 42% of women think their diets

are *too low* in calcium.
- 36% of women think their diets are *too low* in iron.

Respondents were asked the following question: *To you, personally, is it very important, somewhat important, not too important, or not at all important to (statement)?*

Each statement covers one of the Dietary Guidelines for Americans.

Guidelines published in 1995 advise Americans to:

- Eat a variety of foods
- Balance the food you eat with physical activity—maintain or improve your weight
- Choose a diet with plenty of grain products, vegetables, and fruits
- Choose a diet low in fat, saturated fat, and cholesterol
- Choose a diet moderate in sugars
- Choose a diet moderate in salt and sodium
- If you drink alcoholic beverages, do so in moderation

Selected Highlights of Respondents Perception of the Importance of Dietary Guidance.

Among adults 20 years of age and older:

- Most say it is important to them to maintain a healthy weight. In fact, 70% of men and 79% of women say it is very important.
- Many also say it is very important to them to choose a diet with plenty of fruits and vegetables—61% of men and 73% of women.
- However, only 30% of men and 37% of women say choosing a diet with plenty of breads, cereals, rice, and pasta is very important despite the emphasis on these foods in the Dietary Guidelines

Individuals who wish to conduct their own analyses can order the macro data on CD-ROM ($50) or magnetic tape ($240) from National Technical Information Service at 5285, Port Royal Road, Springfield, VA 22161 (703-487-4650).

Fruits &
Eating Your Way to 5 A Day
Vegetables

by Paula Kurtzweil

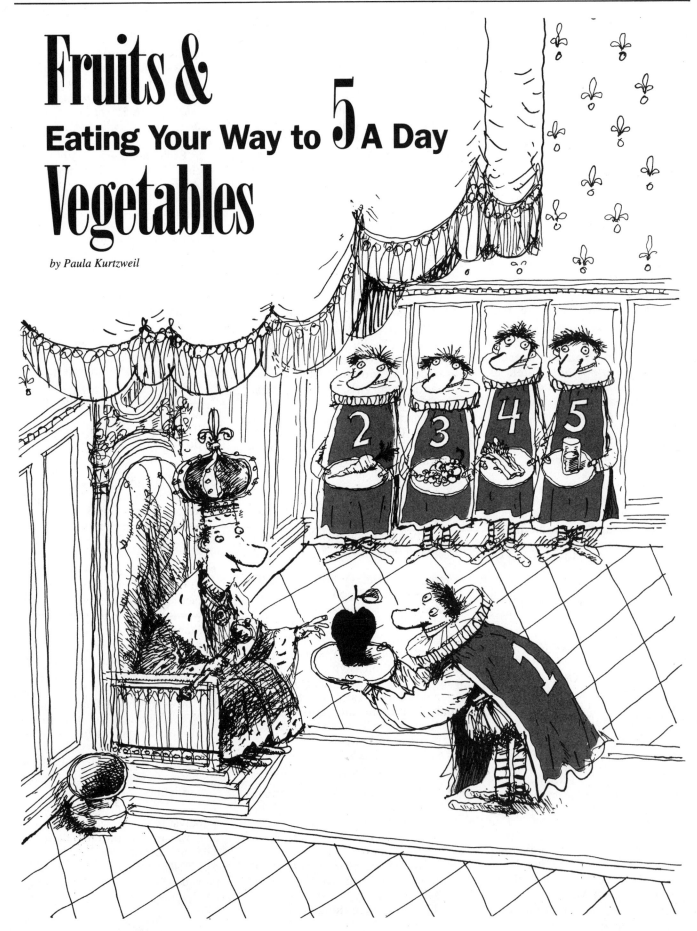

Are you taking the 5 A Day challenge? You may be if you find yourself:
• snacking on raw vegetables instead of potato chips
• adding fruit to your cereal at breakfast
• using the salad bar when you go out for lunch or to the grocery store
• loading up on juice instead of a usual coffee, tea or soda.

The challenge, offered by the National Cancer Institute—a branch of the National Institutes of Health—is to eat at least five servings of fruits and vegetables a day, and these are some ways consumers are rising to the occasion.

They're taking advantage of the healthful benefits of fruits and vegetables. Studies by the U.S. Department of Health and Human Services, U.S. Department of Agriculture, and the National Academy of Sciences suggest that the nutritional goodness of fruits and vegetables, with a diet that is low in fat, saturated fat and cholesterol and that contains plenty of whole-grain breads and cereals, may decrease the risk of heart disease and cancer.

Fruits' and vegetables' potential to help improve the health of Americans led NCI to begin a multi-year public education campaign in 1992. Its goal is to increase consumers' awareness of the importance of fruits and vegetables and to give consumers ideas on how they can increase their intake. With its partner, the Produce for Better Health (PBH) Foundation—a nonprofit consumer education foundation funded by the produce industry—NCI has taken the "5 A Day for Better Health" message to grocery stores, classrooms, television, work sites, churches, and elsewhere.

Food labeling of fresh, frozen and canned fruits and vegetables may carry the message, too. And if you need more specific nutrition information about a particular item, you can find it in the labeling of most products, as well. The Food and Drug Administration regulates this information, which corresponds to NCI's Five A Day guidance and the government's Dietary Guidelines for Americans.

Emphasis on More

A 1991 NCI and PBH survey, which has the best available, most up-to-date information on consumers' consumption of fruits and vegetables, found that the average American consumer eats only about three servings of fruits and vegetables a day. Forty-two percent eat less than two servings a day. Compare those figures with the five to nine servings a day recommended by the Dietary Guidelines for Americans and you can see that many of us have a way to go.

A major reason to eat more fruits and vegetables is their nutritiousness. Unless baked in a pie or dripping in butter, most are low in fat and calories—except avocados, coconut and olives, all of which contain fat naturally. Many are excellent sources of the important vitamins A and C and provide ample fiber.

In addition, many fruits and vegetables, particularly dried beans and peas, are significant sources of folate, a B vitamin that can help reduce the risk of certain serious and common birth defects. (See "How Folate Can Help Prevent Birth Defects" in the September 1996 *FDA Consumer*.)

Produce has other positive qualities. Many items, such as raisins, grapes, cherry tomatoes, and bananas, can be eaten on the spot, with minimal preparation. (Fresh produce in which the peel will be eaten should be rinsed with water beforehand to remove any surface dirt and bacteria.) NCI campaign literature refers to fruits and vegetables as the "original fast food."

"They're easy to pick up and eat," said Daria Chapelsky, state coordinator for NCI's 5 A Day Program. "Just as easy as picking up fast food."

And, unlike other types of foods (such as those high in fat that many of us eat too much of), plain fruits and vegetables are items we don't need to restrict. Genda Potter, a registered dietitian for cardiac patients at Memorial Medical Center in Springfield, Ill., said that factor was a major reason she began a regular 5 A Day class for outpatients.

"I wanted to emphasize something positive," she said. "People often look on dietitians as people 'out-to-ruin-my-enjoyment-of-food.' But fruits and vegetables are foods they can add to their diet rather than something they're going to be told to take away."

No Excuses

Still, for any number of reasons, consumers often find it difficult to eat more fruits and vegetables. They may avoid them because they believe they are too expensive or take too long to prepare. These and other perceived problems became evident to NCI in 1991, when it asked members of small group studies to come up with reasons people may not want to or might be unable to eat at least five servings of fruits and vegetables a day.

Their responses led NCI to develop ideas to help consumers overcome reported difficulties in meeting the 5 A Day goal. Some of those ideas follow, along with other information from nutritionists and food safety experts to help

What's a Serving Size?

Here's what the National Cancer Institute recommends as a serving of fruit and vegetables:

1 medium fruit or 1/2 cup of small or cut-up fruit
3/4 cup (180 milliliters) of 100 percent juice
1/4 cup dried fruit
1/2 cup raw non-leafy or cooked vegetables
1 cup raw leafy vegetables (such as lettuce)
1/2 cup cooked beans or peas (such as lentils, pinto beans, and kidney beans)

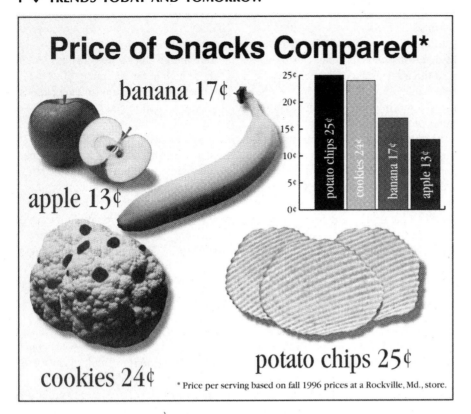

Price of Snacks Compared*

banana 17¢

apple 13¢

cookies 24¢

potato chips 25¢

* Price per serving based on fall 1996 prices at a Rockville, Md., store.

consumers overcome any reluctance they may have to eating fruits and vegetables.

Perceived Problem: Fruits and vegetables cost too much.
Possible Solutions:

It may help to realize, according to dietitians, that fruits and vegetables are actually good buys, if you consider that they are nutrient-dense, containing many of the vitamins and minerals we need more of—for example, vitamins A and C. But the foods we often buy in place of them—cookies and chips, for example—usually offer more of the nutrients—fat and sodium, for example—that most of us should eat less of. And the cookies and chips aren't cheap. For example, based on prices at a Rockville, Md., grocery store, a serving of potato chips costs about 25 cents and a serving of packaged chocolate chip cookies about 24 cents. A banana, on the other hand, sold for 17 cents, and the price of an apple ran as low as 13 cents.

"Compared to packaged foods, fruits and vegetables are not expensive," says Diane Quagliani, a registered dietitian and spokeswoman for the American Dietetic Association.

And there are ways to reduce the costs of fruits and vegetables even further:
• Buy fresh fruits and vegetables in season. Not only will they be cheaper but they also will be at their flavor and nutritional peaks, Quagliani says.
• Clip coupons for money off on your favorite canned and frozen fruits and vegetables and juices.
• Watch local grocery advertisements for reduced prices on your favorite fruits and vegetables.
• If you're not partial to a particular brand, compare prices of different brands of canned and frozen fruits and vegetables and juices and buy the cheapest.

Perceived Problem: Fruits and vegetables take too long to prepare.
Possible Solutions:
• Take advantage of grocery store salad bars, which offer ready-to-eat raw vegetables and fruits and prepared salads made with fruits and vegetables.
• Shop for precut and cleaned fruits and vegetables. Many grocery stores now

carry packaged precut fruits, such as melons and pineapple; cleaned and cut-up salad greens and stir-fry vegetables; and cleaned, peeled baby carrots.
• Keep on hand canned and frozen fruit, canned and bottled juices, and dried fruits. Just open and use.
• Stock up on frozen vegetables for easy cooking in the microwave oven.
• Prepare fruits and vegetables ahead of time; for example, wash and, if feasible, cut up fresh produce and store it in the refrigerator for handy, immediate use.

Perceived Problem: Fresh fruits and vegetables spoil too quickly.
Possible Solutions:
• If you shop once a week or less often, buy both fresh and processed—that is, canned or frozen—fruits and vegetables, and juices. Use the fresh first; save the processed items for use later.
• Buy both ripe and not-so-ripe fresh fruits and vegetables—for example, yellow and green bananas—so that the not-so-ripe items will last a few days longer and be ready for eating after you've finished the ripe ones.
• Keep fruits and vegetables where you can see them often—on the top shelf of the refrigerator, or, for fruits that don't need refrigeration (such as bananas and apples), on the table or counter or another easy-to-spot-place. The more often you see the fruits and vegetables, the more likely you may be to eat them.

Perceived Problem: Fruits and vegetables contain harmful pesticides.
Possible Solutions:

It is a fact that pesticides are used in the production of most fruits and vegetables sold in this country. They help protect crops from insects, diseases, weeds, and mold, thus helping to increase crop yield. "They allow for production of a plentiful and affordable food supply," said John Jones, Ph.D., pesticides and chemical contaminants strategic manager in FDA's Center for Food Safety and Applied Nutrition.

"They are not contaminants. They are substances applied intentionally for a specific purpose and therefore are subject to very rigorous regulatory control," he said. "A new pesticide law enacted in

1996 puts even tighter controls on the use of pesticides."

Several federal agencies share responsibility for pesticide oversight. The Environmental Protection Agency registers pesticides for food use and sets tolerance levels—the upper permitted limit for pesticide residues in individual foods. FDA enforces these limits for all foods except meat and poultry, which fall under USDA's jurisdiction.

FDA collects and analyzes almost 10,000 samples of fruits and vegetables yearly for pesticide residues. Since 1987, when the agency began reporting the results of its monitoring program annually, more than 99 percent of domestic fruit and vegetable samples and more than 95 percent of imported samples have been found free of illegal pesticide residues or had low-level residues that fell within established tolerances. Violations mainly occurred because low-level pesticide residues not approved for a particular product were identified in that food. However, most of the pesticides causing these violations were approved for use on many other foods, Jones said.

"Most violations are not due to the presence of banned pesticides, such as DDT, chlordane and heptachlor, or to very high levels of residues," he said. "Most are due to very low-level residues on the wrong commodity."

So, FDA's position is that the U.S. fruit and vegetable supply does not contain excessive pesticide residues and that the benefits of eating fresh produce far exceeds any risk from residues, Jones said.

However, if you're still concerned, here are some steps you can take to reduce your risk further:
• Wash fruits and vegetables with water and scrub with a dish brush when appropriate: for example, before eating apples, cucumbers, potatoes, or other produce in which the outer skin or peeling is consumed.
• Throw away the outer leaves of leafy vegetables, such as lettuce and cabbage.
• Peel and cook when appropriate, although some nutrients and fiber may be lost when produce is peeled.

What to Eat

For the most part, any fruit or vegetable will do in helping consumers reach their 5 A Day goal. But certain types of fruits and vegetables should be selected regularly because of their nutritional value. These include those that are good sources of vitamins A and C and fiber.

Variety also is important because fruits and vegetables provide other nutrients, such as folate, potassium, calcium, and iron. Varying choices increases the likelihood of getting all the nutritional advantages of fruits and vegetables.

Also, nutrition experts advise against replacing all fruits and vegetables in the diet with dietary supplements because supplements often do not contain all the known—and perhaps unknown—nutritional benefits of fruits and vegetables.

Preparation presents another nutritional concern. Since a reduced-fat, reduced-saturated-fat intake is important to a healthful diet, it's important not to overindulge in fruits and vegetables prepared with high-fat ingredients. Some dishes to look out for include fried vegetables, such as french fries; cooked vegetables in cheese or cream sauces or with added bacon or butter; fruit pies or fruit served with whipped cream; and dips for raw vegetables. Some of these high-fat foods now have reduced-fat versions, such as low-fat dips and whipped toppings.

A Label with a Lot

You can determine the nutritional value of fruits and vegetables by looking at the Nutrition Facts panel on the side or back of labels of frozen and canned items. Nutrition information also is available for many fresh items, under FDA's voluntary point-of-purchase nutrition information program for raw foods. This information may appear on the labels of packaged fresh fruits and vegetables or on posters or brochures at or near the point of purchase.

The nutrition information lists the kinds and amounts of important nutrients in a serving of the fruit or vegetable and gives the Percent Daily Value, which shows how much those amounts contribute to the daily diet.

Some information is required: for example, the amount of fat, fiber, vitamins A and C, and iron and calcium, even if there is none. Some labels will carry ad-

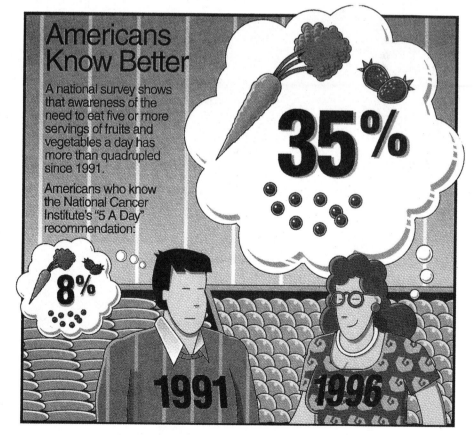

Americans Know Better

A national survey shows that awareness of the need to eat five or more servings of fruits and vegetables a day has more than quadrupled since 1991.

Americans who know the National Cancer Institute's "5 A Day" recommendation:

35%

8%

1991   1996

Source: National Cancer Institute

A National Cancer Institute Graphic

A High Five

In selecting your daily intake of fruits and vegetables,
- At least one serving of a vitamin A-rich fruit or vegetable a day.
- At least one serving of a vitamin C-rich fruit or vegetable a day.
- At least one serving of a high-fiber fruit or vegetable a day.
- Several servings of cruciferous vegetables a week. Studies suggest that these vegetables may offer additional protection against certain cancers, although further research is needed.

High in Vitamin A*	High in Vitamin C*	High in Fiber or Good Source of Fiber*	Cruciferous Vegetables
apricots	apricots	apple	bok choy
cantaloupe	broccoli	banana	broccoli
carrots	brussels sprouts	blackberries	brussels sprouts
kale, collards	cabbage	blueberries	cabbage
leaf lettuce	cantaloupe	brussels sprouts	cauliflower
mango	cauliflower	carrots	
mustard greens	chili peppers	cherries	
pumpkin	collards	cooked beans and peas	
romaine lettuce	grapefruit	(kidney, navy, lima,	
spinach	honeydew melon	and pinto beans, lentils,	
sweet potato	kiwi fruit	black-eyed peas)	
winter squash	mango	dates	
(acorn, hubbard)	mustard greens	figs	
	orange	grapefruit	
	orange juice	kiwi fruit	
	pineapple	orange	
	plum	pear	
	potato with skin	prunes	
	spinach	raspberries	
	strawberries	spinach	
	bell peppers	strawberries	
	tangerine	sweet potato	
	tomatoes		
	watermelon		

eat fruits & vegetables

5 a Day–for Better Health!

*Based on FDA's food labeling regulations

(Source: National Cancer Institute)

pertain to fruits and vegetables. These claims can describe how:

• fruits and vegetables may help lower the risk of some cancers

• fruits, vegetables and grain products that contain fiber, particularly soluble fiber, may help reduce the risk of coronary heart disease

• fiber-containing grain products, fruits and vegetables may help reduce the risk of some cancers.

In addition, in spring 1996, FDA approved a claim stating that a diet with adequate folic acid may reduce the risk of certain birth defects. This claim might appear, for example, on labels of dried beans, brussels sprouts, asparagus, tomato juice, and orange juice—foods that are excellent or good sources of folate.

A Campaign Continues

Are consumers paying attention to all this information?

In a way, yes, according to a 1996 NCI/PBH survey. That survey found that the percentage of consumers who were aware of the need to eat at least five servings of fruits and vegetables a day rose from 8 percent in 1991 to 35 percent in September 1996.

But whether the information has helped increase Americans' consumption of fruits and vegetables remains to be seen. Late last year, NCI planned to analyze national food consumption data—the most recent of which was collected in 1994—to determine whether fruit and vegetable intake had increased since the 1991 survey. According to Gloria Stables, a registered dietitian and NCI's 5 A Day Program director, NCI plans to release the results this year.

Meanwhile, NCI, the produce industry, state health departments, and other groups will continue the 5 A Day campaign through at least the year 2000. Said Stables, "This is the largest national public-private nutrition education program ever launched."

Paula Kurtzweil is a member of FDA's public affairs staff.

Health Claims Under the Nutrition Labeling and Education Act

By **Johanna Dwyer** • D.Sc., R.D. • Professor of Medicine and Nutrition • Schools of Medicine and Nutrition • Tufts University; and **Donna Porter** • Ph.D., R.D. • Specialist in Life Sciences • Congressional Research Service • Library of Congress

Note: The comments in this article represent those of the authors and not those of their respective institutions.

Overview

Health messages and the benefits of specific foods can be communicated via health claims and nutritional labeling, advertising, and the media. Each communication vehicle is regulated to a different degree. The closer the proximity of the health message to the food, the more specific the claim, the higher is the degree of regulatory oversight. Information on labels is the most product specific and most highly regulated form of nutrition information.

What Are Health Claims?

The *Nutrition Labeling and Education Act of 1990* (NLEA) was a giant step forward in fostering consumer awareness of the nutrients in food. Labeling formats became more informative and regulated, and some authorized health claims were permitted. Health claims are statements that describe a relationship between a food or a substance in food and a disease or condition. Table 1 presents the current status of the diet-disease risk reduction relationships that FDA evaluated. Of the 10 proposed claims, eight have been approved.

Why Are Health Claims Important?

The prevalence of certain chronic degenerative diseases can be reduced and the quality of life improved with changes in diet and other lifestyle habits. Information on the nutrient composition and health impact of foods can influence eating decisions. Therefore, communication of the relationships between diet and health is important to the public's health.

When information appears on food labels, it can influence consumer purchasing decisions, benefitting both industry and consumers. The results of a recent study with respect to fat, saturated fat and cholesterol consumption suggest that as the regulatory environment governing diet-disease claims was relaxed to make it easier to make explicit health claims, consumption of lipids fell faster than it had in the prior period, and corresponding diet–disease knowledge rose.[1]

Because sanctioned health claims may affect the public health, they cannot be misleading and must be closely regulated. Ultimately, recommendations for public policy regarding health claims should promote the consumption of foods that advance health and the development of foods that will do so.

Rules for Making Health Claims

First there is a process for establishing the scientific basis for the proposed health claim which is accomplished by applying the standard of "significant scientific agreement" among experts qualified by scientific training and experience to evaluate the relationship. The evidence cited comes from epidemiological, mechanistic, and intervention studies. The research is evaluated to assess the potential validity of the diet/food disease relationship. The criteria include: the consistency, strength and quali-

From *Nutrition & the M.D.*, April 1997, pp. 1-5. © 1997 by Lippincott-Raven Publishers. Reprinted by permission.

ty of the evidence; biological plausibility; dose-response character; temporal relationships; and specificity. Because diet-disease relationships often take many years to develop, surrogate markers or intermediate endpoints often have to be employed. Recognized markers include total cholesterol and high- and low-density lipoprotein levels as markers of heart disease, and bone density as a predictor of osteoporotic fracture. Next it is important to identify an effective level of the nutrient, and whether the substance is safe at this level and at somewhat higher intake levels.

Given the significant scientific agreement standard, a high level of confidence can be placed in the diet-disease relationships stated by the health claims on the food label. A current question is whether this standard is so strict as to prevent authorization of a number of supportable health claims.

The food vehicle containing the substance must also qualify, or meet certain nutrient standards before it can be considered for a health claim. Issues relating to health claims arise in determining the best way to communicate scientifically valid, nonmisleading health claims that are understandable to consumers.

Some foods consumed regularly contribute little to a healthful diet and would be inappropriate candidates for bearing a health claim. For example, vitamin-fortified jelly beans might fall in such a category. There are a number of qualification and disqualification rules for food products that are permitted to bear a health claim. Although these provisions are controversial, they do address and correct previous abuses.

Current regulations under NLEA establish levels of four nutrients (fat, saturated fat, cholesterol, sodium) that have been found to increase the risk of chronic disease. Foods that bear the descriptor "healthy" must not have levels of total fat, saturated fat, cholesterol or sodium exceeding certain limits. They must also exceed at least 10% of the daily value for one of six nutrients (i.e., must satisfy the "jelly bean" rule).

Foods must also have some minimum nutritional value prior to fortification. Current regulations require that the food bearing the claim has a minimum level of one or more of six nutrients (vitamins A and C, iron, calcium, protein and fiber). This rule excludes some grains, fruits, and vegetables from bearing claims. However, more frequent consumption of these foods is encouraged by the USDA's Food Guide Pyramid and the Dietary Guidelines for Americans. Some groups, such as the National Food Processors Association advocate preserving the spirit of the law while permitting some exemptions for vegetables, fruits or grains.

Finally FDA has rules about the foods for which nutrient content claims may be used on the label. Usually these claims can be made even if a possible risk-increasing nutrient is present in the food, as long as its presence is disclosed on the label.

The final issue concerns the best way to word health claims. Surprisingly, there is relatively little scientific information about the most compelling ways of providing NLEA health claims involving foods to consumers, or how consumers interpret these health claims.

Recent Developments

The first group of health claims approved under NLEA involved those that applied to large populations and were based on a great deal of evidence that had accumulated over many years (Table 1).

The second wave of proposed health claims is likely to involve issues that apply to smaller populations, with less evidence, but balancing risks and benefits. Claims for foods rather than for specific substances in food may increase.

In mid-1995, FDA granted a request from the National Food Processors Association to determine whether some of the required elements in health claims and nutrient content claims should be eliminated or made optional. It concluded that modifications might further the purposes of the NLEA.

Emerging Issues

Several issues are presently being actively debated:

1. What messages are most important and how should they be stated? The challenge is to assure that consumers are accurately informed to make wise food choices.

2. Incentives for reformulating existing products or developing new ones.

3. How should claims for new and potentially helpful food substances be assessed?

4. Communicating emerging scientific information about diet-disease relationships. Is rational decision making on the part of consumers best made by permitting manufacturers to disseminate such information on labels and in advertising?

5. Harmonization of labeling and advertising

Table 1
Ten Original Health Claims Evaluated Under NLEA

Food Substance/ Disease Relationship	Example of Acceptable Health Claim
Fat and cancer	Development of cancer depends on many factors. A diet low in total fat may reduce the risk of some cancers.
Fiber and cancer	Lowfat diets rich in fiber-containing grain products, fruits and vegetables may reduce the risk of some types of cancer, a disease associated with many factors.
Fat and heart disease	While many factors affect heart disease, diets low in saturated fat and cholesterol may reduce the risk of the disease.
Fiber and heart disease	Diets low in saturated fat and cholesterol and rich in fruits, vegetables, and grain products that contain some types of dietary fiber, particularly soluble fiber, may reduce the risk of heart disease.
Sodium and hypertension	Diets low in sodium may reduce the risk of high blood pressure, a disease associated with many factors.
Calcium and osteoporosis	Regular exercise and a healthy diet with enough calcium helps teens and young adult white and Asian women maintain good bone health, and may reduce their high risk of osteoporosis.
Antioxidant vitamins and cancer	Evidence judged insufficient, but permitted identification of fruits and vegetables that were related to reductions in cancer risk: Development of cancer depends on many factors. Eating a diet low in fat and high in fruits and vegetables, foods that are low in fat and may contain vitamin A, vitamin C and dietary fiber may reduce your risk of some cancers. Oranges, a food low in fat, are good sources of fiber and vitamin C.
Folic acid and neural tube defects	Health claim was not initially approved, but after seeking advice of Folic Acid Advisory Subcommittee, the FDA published regulations authorizing a folic acid health claim for conventional foods and dietary supplements and required fortification of enriched cereal-grain products with 140 micrograms of folic acid per 100 grams.[2] Until the proposed rule for conventional foods is finalized, FDA permits the health claim on foods naturally rich in folic acid and foods with a history of fortification consistent with current fortification guidelines.
Zinc and immune function in elderly persons	Insufficient data to establish significant scientific agreement.
Omega-3 fatty acids and heart disease	Insufficient data to establish significant scientific agreement.

policies for authorized health claims and nutrient content claims, e.g., among FDA, USDA and FTC.

Conclusion

Representatives of private, public and voluntary organizations all agree that health claim messages should be scientifically valid, nonmisleading, and compelling. The problem for regulators is how best to strike an appropriate balance between effective communication of health information to consumers, and the prevention of misleading claims about the effects of food on health. The nutrition education goal is to protect consumers from harm and empower consumers to choose foods that contribute to a healthful diet.

References

1. Ippolito,P.M. and Mathios,A.D. Information and Advertising Policy: A Study of Fat and Cholesterol Consumption in the United States, 1977-1990 Bureau of Economics Staff Report, Federal Trade Commission September 1996 Washington DC.

2. DHHS,FDA. Food labeling: Health claims and label statements: folate and neural tube defects, and food standards: Amendments of standards of identity for enriched grain products to require addition of folic acid, final rules. *Fed. Reg.* , v. 61, no. 44, part III, Mar. 5, 1996; pp 8749-8807.

About the Author

Dr. **Johanna Dwyer** is Director of the Frances Stern Nutrition Center at New England Medical Center, Professor of Medicine and Community Health at the Tufts University School of Medicine, and Professor of Nutrition at Tufts University School of Nutrition. Her work centers on life-cycle related concerns such as preventing diet-related disease in children and adolescents and maximizing quality of life and health in the elderly. She is the immediate past president of the American Institute of Nutrition, past secretary of the American Society for Clinical Nutrition and past president and current fellow for the Society for Nutrition Education.

Today's ♡ Special
NUTRITION Information

by Paula Kurtzweil

Although nutrition information is not required to appear on the menu, it must be made available to consumers when they request it.

Remember the dieter's plate? For many years, it was the only menu item that really catered to the health conscious among us. It usually came with cottage cheese, several pieces of fruit, and a few crackers neatly arranged atop a lettuce leaf. If you looked carefully, you could usually spot it on the menu between other such fine restaurant fare as gelatin cubes and fruit cocktail in syrup.

These days, restaurants have a lot more to offer consumers concerned about calories and cholesterol, fat, and other nutrients that may help reduce their risk of certain diseases. Menus now may carry items ranging from low-fat, low-calorie tostados to full-course meals featuring seafood or chicken dishes that are low in sodium and fat and high in fiber and vitamins A and C. And restaurants boast about their nutritionally modified dishes with symbols, such as a big red heart signifying that the dish fits in with a diet that is consistent with general dietary recommendations or with claims such as "low fat," "light," or "heart healthy."

But the question is: Are these claims accurate and can they be trusted?

Regulations from the Food and Drug Administration effective May 2 are de-signed to ensure that the answer is "yes." The regulations, published in the Aug. 2, 1996, *Federal Register,* apply the Nutrition Labeling and Education Act (NLEA) of 1990 to restaurant menu items that carry a claim about the food's nutritional content or health benefits.

Under NLEA, FDA established regulations mandating specific nutrition information on the labels of most store-bought products and set up criteria under which nutrient and health claims can be used in food labeling. Claims like these that appear on signs or placards in most restaurants have been covered by the requirements of the food labeling regulations since 1994.

The new menu regulations affect all eating establishments—whether a small-town corner tavern or a big-city four-star restaurant, a grocery store deli or a deli that delivers. All will have to follow requirements for nutrition and health claims for menu items that bear a claim and give customers the appropriate nutrition information for these items when requested.

"The idea is for the claims to mean the same thing wherever they show up—on food labels in the store or on menus in a

From *FDA Consumer,* May/June 1997, pp. 21-23, 25. Reprinted by permission of *FDA Consumer,* the magazine of the U.S. Food and Drug Administration.

restaurant," said Michelle Smith, a food technologist in FDA's Office of Food Labeling.

Eating Out in the 1990s

According to Smith, nutrition and health claims on menus can help people better understand the role of diet in health and choose restaurant foods that contribute to a healthy diet.

This is important, considering that more and more Americans are eating their meals outside the home. According to the National Restaurant Association, Americans spent 44 percent of their food dollars outside the home in 1996, up from 25 percent in 1955.

According to the association's report, *Tableservice Trends—1995,* more than half of consumers 35 and older and 2 out of 5 consumers 18 to 34 look for lower fat menu options when eating out. Also, restaurateurs report that their customers are increasingly requesting meatless dishes.

The frequency with which eating establishments have been catering to these preferences by making claims about menu items is not well known. In its final rule on claims for restaurant foods, FDA cited information from the National Restaurant Association's annual menu contest, in which the group found that 89 percent of all printed menu entries had at least one nutritional or health claim. But it is not known how representative this number is for menu practices across the country.

In 1996, after a federal district court ordered FDA to include menu claims under food labeling regulations, Bruce Silverglade, legal director for the Center for Science in the Public Interest, said in a press statement: "For years, many restaurant menus have made misleading health and nutrition claims from 'low fat' claims for high-fat desserts to claims that foods flavored with Chinese herbs

will lower blood pressure and improve vision. A restaurant menu should not be a work of fiction." (CSPI and another public advocacy group, Public Citizen, filed suit in 1993 against the government for excluding menu claims from the labeling regulations.)

There are indications that interest in healthier restaurant fare is growing. Heart Smart Restaurants, an Arizona-based company that helps restaurants, food processors, and vending companies develop and promote products suitable for nutrition and health claims, has seen a steady rise in the number of its restaurant clients since the early 1990s. Judy Peters, director of customer relations for the company, reports that the company's restaurant clients now number in the hundreds and offer from one to many Heart Smart dishes. The clients are located across the country and include both single restaurants and national chains, ranging from juice bars to steakhouses and ethnic restaurants.

Heart Smart is among a number of companies, health professionals, and other consultants that offer such services to restaurants, usually for a fee. Their services are not endorsed by FDA because, as a federal agency, FDA cannot endorse any particular third-party certification programs.

On a smaller scale, the health, fitness and nutrition program of Suburban Hospital in Bethesda, Md., a suburb of Washington, D.C., found considerable interest from area restaurateurs in its Heart Healthy Restaurant Program. This program, which helps chefs create and promote heart-healthy foods on their menus, signed up 20 fine-dining restaurants within a county-wide area in the first six months of its operation, according to Linda Dolan, a registered dietitian and director of Suburban's Well Works program. Many of the participating restaurants offer Italian and French cuisine.

Look to the Menu

FDA's regulations permit restaurants to promote their healthier menu fare using the following:

• *Specific claims about a menu item's nutrient content:* for example, low fat or high fiber. These are known as nutrient claims.

• *Claims about the relationship between a nutrient or food and a disease or health condition:* for example, a dish that is low in fat, saturated fat, and cholesterol might be able to carry a claim about how diets low in saturated fat and cholesterol may reduce the risk of heart disease. These are known as health claims, and they may initially appear on the menu in simple terms, such as "heart healthy." More information about the claim should be available on the menu or in other labeling—for example, with the accompanying nutrition information that must be provided on request.

Consumers can use these claims to spot foods that may be more healthful for them. They also can look for statements giving what FDA considers general dietary guidance. For example, the salad section may start with the message "Eating five fruits and vegetables a day is an important part of a healthy diet." This statement would refer to the National Cancer Institute's recommendation that Americans eat more fruits and vegetables to help reduce their risk of cancer and heart disease.

Restaurants do not have to provide nutrition information about foods that do not bear nutrient content or health claims or that are referred to in general dietary guidance messages. However, restaurateurs need to be careful that the general guidance they provide on the menu doesn't turn into a claim, such as "Fruits and vegetables can help reduce the risk of cancer." This, then, would require the item to meet FDA's nutrition information and claims' requirements.

"The idea is for the claims to mean the same thing wherever they show up—on food labels in the store or on menus in a restaurant."

—Michelle Smith, food technologist in FDA's Office of Food Labeling

Claims that promote a nutrient or health benefit must meet certain criteria established by FDA and the U.S. Department of Agriculture; for example, the food must provide a requisite amount of the nutrient or nutrients referred to in the claim. In addition, a menu item carrying a health claim must provide significant amounts of one or more of six key nutrients, such as vitamin C, iron or fiber, and cannot contain a food substance at a level that increases the risk of a disease or health condition. For example, a restaurant meal that contains 26 grams of fat (40 percent of the Daily Value for fat) or 960 milligrams of sodium (40 percent of the Daily Value for sodium) is disqualified from making a heart-healthy claim.

These same rules apply to claims used in the labeling of commercial food products. But the requirements for further information differ between restaurant and commercially manufactured foods.

To meet FDA's criteria, food manufacturers may choose to do chemical analyses to determine the nutritional value of their products. But the criteria for menu items are more flexible, and, under FDA's requirements, restaurants may back up their claims with any "reasonable" base, such as databases, cookbooks, or other secondhand sources that provide nutrition information.

Also, restaurants do not have to provide the standard nutrition information profile and more exacting nutrient content values required in the Nutrition Facts panel of packaged foods. Instead, restaurants can present the information in any format desired, and they have to provide only information about the nutrient or nutrients that the claim is referring to. They can say simply that the amount of the nutrient in question does not exceed the limit imposed by FDA—for example, "This low-fat restaurant

dish provides no more than 5 grams of fat per serving."

"It should be accurate," FDA's Smith said, "but not necessarily precise."

Although nutrition information is not required to appear on the menu, it must be made available to consumers when they request it. Restaurants can present it in a printed format—such as a notebook—or by having the staff recite it.

FDA is granting restaurants more flexibility because they don't produce foods according to the more exacting standards that food manufacturers follow, Smith said. She notes that restaurants change their menus frequently and produce smaller quantities than commercial food operations. And restaurant products often vary, depending on the type of ingredients available.

"A commercial operation has more stability than a restaurant," she said. "It would be an unreasonable burden to re-

A Roundabout Route To MENU Regulation

1990: Congress passes the Nutrition Labeling and Education Act (NLEA), which makes nutrition information mandatory for most foods. Among the few foods exempted were restaurant items—unless they carried a nutrient or health claim.

January 1993: FDA issues regulations under NLEA that require restaurants to comply with regulations for nutrient and health claims that appear on signs and placards. Menu claims are exempt.

March 1993: Two consumer advocacy groups, Public Citizen Inc. and Center for Science in the Public Interest, file suit against the Department of Health and Human Services and FDA, charging that the menu exemption violates NLEA and the Administrative Procedure Act.

June 1993: FDA proposes to require that menu items about which claims are made be subject to the nutrient and health claims' regulations.

June 1996: Because FDA failed to finalize its June 1993 proposal, the U.S. District Court in Washington, D.C., rules that Congress intended restaurant menus to be covered by NLEA and orders FDA to amend its nutrition labeling and claims' regulations to include menu items about which claims are made.

August 1996: FDA issues a final rule removing the restaurant menu exemption and establishing criteria under which restaurants must provide nutrition information for menu items.

May 2, 1997: FDA's regulations for nutrition labeling of restaurant menu items that bear a claim take effect.

—P.K.

quire restaurants to follow the same labeling regulations for packaged foods."

Much of the enforcement of the menu claims' regulations will likely be provided by state and local public health departments. The reason, Smith said, is that state and local health departments have direct jurisdiction over restaurants, including monitoring their food safety and sanitation practices, and regularly visit them to ensure compliance with various federal and state laws. Also, she said, FDA doesn't have the resources.

Whether restaurants will continue to make claims on menus now that they will be more closely monitored remains to be seen. "We're not sure what the result will be," said Bob Harrington, vice president of technical services for the National Restaurant Association. "Our fear is that the rules are so complex and compliance so confusing that [restaurants] will quit giving claims at all."

Healthful Foods with Flair

But some restaurants that have added healthier menu choices highlighted with claims report that those dishes sell well. Barbara Hartman, head chef for Geppetto, an Italian restaurant in Bethesda, Md., and a participant in Suburban Hospital's Heart Healthy Restaurant Program, said the restaurant's "Healthy Menu" items account for 5 to 10 percent of daily sales. The sandwiches—Tuna Sandwich Dijon, Grilled Vegetable Sub, and others—represent as much as 20 percent of all sandwich sales, she said.

"We've had an excellent response," she said. "Better than we thought we would have."

Although most of the customer feedback has been positive, she noted that customers sometimes complain about the blandness of the food. "There's no salt, no sugar, no oil added," she said. "So I coach the waiters to let customers know that the food may not be as tasty as what they're used to. Then they won't be taken aback by what they're getting."

Healthy menu choices aren't going to appeal to every customer, either. Heart Smart's Peters noted that one previous client, a restaurant that offered only healthy-type foods, went out of business because its selection was too narrow. "People need a choice," she said.

And not every dish is suitable for dietary modification. Some lose their palatability when the fat and sodium contents are reduced to low levels, Peters said, citing fettuccine Alfredo as a prime example. Dishes containing cheese or cream sauces are difficult to modify, dietitian Dolan noted. And chef Hartman said the poached salmon that used to be on her restaurant's Healthy Menu had to be removed because the salmon didn't fit the criteria for a "heart healthy" claim.

But there still are plenty of other dishes that can easily be used or reworked as more healthful food offerings. Among those cited by restaurant menu experts are grilled seafood, chicken, venison, and ostrich; spaghetti with turkey meatballs; several Mexican dishes; salads; and pasta dishes and other entrées traditionally made with wine or herb sauces. Geppetto, for example, offers a single-serving California Bambino Pizza with a whole-wheat crust, fat-reduced mozzarella cheese, tomato basil sauce, roasted garlic, fresh mushrooms, broccoli, and roasted peppers. It provides 506 calories, 10 grams of fat, and 24 milligrams of cholesterol.

Tasty, yet healthful. And, one might add, a far cry from its predecessor, the dieter's plate.

Paula Kurtzweil is a member of FDA's public affairs staff.

Meat meets its match?

New reduced-fat alternatives can help keep burgers and franks on the menu. But beware of the pretenders.

Hot dogs and hamburgers ain't what they used to be. Nowadays, there are turkey burgers and poultry dogs. There are reduced-fat versions of the classic beef and pork originals. And there are dozens of vegetarian varieties, made of everything from beans and bulgur to seaweed and soybeans.

The idea, of course, is to replace the high-fat classics with leaner alternatives. Sometimes, though, the alternatives aren't as lean as you might expect. The table on page 64 compares traditional hamburgers and hot dogs with leading national brands of reduced-fat versions. The report below will help you cut through the fat to find a truly lean choice, whether animal or vegetable.

Burgers: Playing ketchup

Health authorities recommend limiting calories from fat to no more than 30 percent of total calories

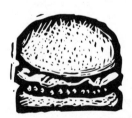

in the diet. For someone consuming 2000 calories a day, that's no more than 600 calories from fat, which translates into a total-fat limit of about 65 grams, since one gram of fat contains nine calories. (To figure the fat limit for a diet that's considerably higher or lower than 2000 calories, see the chart.) Naturally, each food you eat doesn't have to get less than 30 percent of its calories from fat in order for you to keep your *overall diet* below that threshold. But the more fatty foods you consume, the more difficult it will be to stay below your daily fat quota.

As our table shows, a 3-ounce patty of regular ground beef gets 66 percent of its 245 calories from 18 grams of fat—more than one-quarter of the daily allotment of fat for someone on a 2000-calorie diet. A 3-ounce burger made of extra-lean ground beef still delivers a hefty 14 grams of fat, which accounts for 58 percent of its 215 calories—and about one-fifth of the day's allotment.

Note that the standard 3-ounce portion is a pretty modest patty. While a bigger burger would get the same *proportion* of calories from fat, it would pack more fat grams and more calories—potentially much more. Ground turkey can be considerably leaner than extra-lean ground beef—but that depends on the particular blend of light meat, dark meat, and skin. At the high end, *Butterball Seasoned Turkey Burgers* each contain 15 grams of fat, accounting for 64 percent of 210 calories—more fat and a higher proportion of calories from fat than burgers made from extra-lean ground beef. Other brands are considerably leaner.

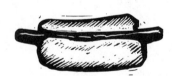

Dietary fat of all kinds packs a caloric wallop and may increase the risk of certain cancers. But it's the saturated-fat portion that can clog your arteries. The standard public-health recommendation calls for limiting saturated fat to less than 10 percent of total calories—or less than 20 grams in a 2000-calorie diet. There are 7 grams of saturated fat in a regular beef burger, and more than 5 grams in extra-lean beef. Among turkey burgers, most deliver no more than about 2 grams of saturated fat—except for *Butterball's* entry, which lives up to its name with three times that amount.

To cut fat to the bone, use ground turkey that

comes entirely from skinless breast: A single patty contains less than a gram of fat and virtually no saturated fat. You can ask the butcher to grind it for you, or look for a brand like *Shady Brook Farms Only One Ground Breast of Turkey*. Since ground turkey breast is so lean, you'll need to give it a bit more care than you might an ordinary burger. Use a fork to mix in seasonings, such as basil, cayenne, oregano, or thyme. Don't overwork the meat while forming patties. Use cooking spray or a small amount of vegetable oil to keep the meat from sticking to the cooking surface. To preserve the little bit of fat in the meat, which adds flavor, don't press down on the patties while cooking. Remove from heat just after the interior is no longer pink (about 165°). And make liberal use of toppings (such as salsa, sprouts, and sliced tomatoes and onions) and sauces (barbecue, hot pepper, soy, or Worcestershire).

To get less fat than you'll find in skinless turkey breast, you need to look lower on the food chain. Some veggie burgers, such as *Boca Burgers* and *Natural Touch Fat Free Vegan Burgers*, use soy protein and other ingredients to mimic beef in taste and texture. Others, such as *Morningstar Farms Garden Vege Patties* and *Wholesome & Hearty Gardenburgers*, don't hide their vegetable heritage—but they can still be served on a hamburger bun with all the fixings. According to tests of a sampling of both types of veggie burgers soon to be published in CONSUMER REPORTS magazine, the current crop is pretty tasty.

Not all those meatless burgers are nearly as lean as skinless ground turkey breast. *Morningstar Farms Grillers*, for example, get 45 percent of their 140 calories from 7 grams of fat. Many other veggie burgers, however, have far less fat—or even none—and most have no saturated fat. (Where would a veggie burger get saturated fat? From soybeans, vegetable oil, and sometimes cheese.)

While it's largely what meatless burgers *don't* have—fat—that makes them healthful, in some cases it's also what they do have—fiber. Several veggie burgers contain at least 5 grams of fiber (20 percent of the recommended daily intake). A few are both fiber-rich and nonfat.

Hot dogs: On a roll

In recent years, hot-dog vendors have had their hands full trying to lighten up that quintessential American delicacy—with mixed success. Not all the "reduced fat" alternatives are lean wieners; some still have more fat than many full-fat meats. That's not to say you can't "pig out intelligently," as meatless *Lightlife Smart Dogs* urge—but you have to be choosy.

A typical beef or mixed-meat dog contains about 13 grams of fat, which accounts for a whopping 80 percent of its 150 calories. (And many people don't stop after just one frank.) A handful of reduced-fat versions of those archetypes, including *Oscar Mayer Free*, have no measurable amount of fat at all. *Oscar Mayer Light* dogs, on the other hand, have 8 grams of fat, which supply 65 percent of their 110 calories—a proportion that's no better than regular ground beef. Other beef and mixed-meat choices hold calories from fat to a more modest 20 to 40 percent.

You might expect hot dogs made from chicken or turkey to be relatively lean. They're not. Aside from *Butterball Fat Free! Franks*, all the brands we found get at least 60 percent of their calories from fat. And as the table shows, poultry dogs tend to have more

Building a better burger

While ground beef will never be lean enough to compete with skinless turkey breast or nonfat meatless burgers, there are a few ways to improve on the real thing yourself. Start by choosing extra-lean meat.

If you plan to use the ground meat in casseroles, chili, spaghetti sauce, or other seasoned dishes, you can literally rinse away as much as three-quarters of the fat: Simply drain the meat after cooking (but before adding other ingredients), then pour hot water over it and drain again.

If you're making burgers, "stretch" them. To each pound of uncooked ground beef, add about a half cup of bread crumbs (softened by soaking briefly in about a half cup of seasoned stock or nonfat milk). Or use a half cup of finely grated raw carrots, potatoes, or cooked and ground soy beans, or one cup of dry breakfast cereal.

If you're feeling more creative, try this recipe.

Recipe adapted from "Slim Cuisine," by Sue Kreitzman and the Editors of Consumer Reports Books, copyright © 1991 by Consumers Union.

◆ **Eggplant hamburgers** (makes 8 patties)

12 oz extra-lean ground beef
1 eggplant (¾ to 1 lb), baked, peeled, and coarsely chopped
1 small onion, finely chopped
1 to 2 cloves garlic, minced
8 tbsp whole-wheat bread crumbs
2 tbsp grated Parmesan cheese
1 tbsp tomato paste
2 tsp nonfat yogurt, plain
salt and fresh ground pepper to taste

• Preheat broiler to its highest temperature.
• Thoroughly mix together all ingredients, reserving half of the bread crumbs. Shape the mixture into eight patties and dredge them on both sides in the reserved crumbs. (At this point, you can freeze any patties you won't be cooking now.)
• Broil on rack (over a foil-lined tray) 4 inches from heat for about three minutes on each side, until crusty on the outside and medium within. (To cook from frozen state, preheat broiler, then broil 2 inches from heat for about five minutes on each side.)
[Each 3½-ounce burger contains about 150 calories, 7 grams of fat, and 3 grams of saturated fat.]

saturated fat and more calories than the reduced-fat beef and mixed-meat alternatives.

Most veggie hot dogs get less than 20 percent of their calories from fat, and none has more than a single gram of saturated fat. Some are fat free.

Hot dogs of all kinds can deliver a heavy dose of sodium. A single link of a meat variety averages nearly 500 mg of sodium—a sizable chunk of the recommended daily limit of 2400 mg. Meatless hot dogs average less than 300 mg of sodium per link. If you're concerned about your sodium intake, you might seek out *Lightlife Tofu Pups* or *Soy Boy Fat Free Leaner Wieners*, which both have 140 mg per link, just qualifying for a "low sodium" claim on the label.

Unlike meatless burgers, veggie franks provide little or no dietary fiber. But you can always look for a whole-grain bun.

Summing up

If you're seeking leaner alternatives to traditional hamburgers and hot dogs, abandon your assumptions and look at the hard data.

■ To compare different options, watch the serving size and total calories, as well as the fat and saturated-fat content.

■ Restrain yourself when forming patties from bulk burger meat. It's easy to exceed the standard 3-ounce portion size. (In general, 4 ounces of uncooked ground beef or poultry cooks down to about a 3-ounce patty.)

■ For the most nutritious burger, look for a vegetarian variety that's nonfat, fiber-rich, and low in calories—such as *Yves Veggie Cuisine Fat Free Garden Vegetable Patties*.

Maximum fat in the daily diet

Daily calories	Total fat (g)	Saturated fat (g)
1500	50	15
2000	65	20
2500	80	25
3000	100	30

Based on a daily diet that gets no more than 30 percent of its calories from total fat and less than 10 percent from saturated fat. (One gram of fat contains 9 calories.)

PHYTOCHEMICALS: DRUGSTORE IN A SALAD?

Researchers have long puzzled over why people who eat lots of fruits, vegetables, beans, and grains have a strikingly lower risk of coronary heart disease and cancer than people who center their diet on meat and dairy products. Part of the benefit undoubtedly stems from the fact that plant foods are low in fat and high in vitamins, minerals, and fiber. But the overall benefit seems greater than the sum of those parts.

Now an emerging body of scientific evidence is pointing to the value of plant chemicals, or phytochemicals, that are neither vitamins nor minerals. Manufacturers eager to capitalize on that research have been flooding the market with phytochemical supplements, accompanied by a host of extravagant claims (see box, "Produce in a Pill?"). Here's a more objective look at the most promising findings so far.

Hormones in grains and beans

Most beans and whole grains are good sources of phytochemicals called **saponins.** Saponins neutralize certain potentially cancer-causing enzymes in the gut; in addition, inactivating those enzymes may indirectly reduce blood-cholesterol levels.

There's stronger evidence on another group of chemicals in beans and grains: **isoflavones** and other **"phytoestrogens,"** which resemble the female hormone estrogen in several ways. For example, human estrogen lowers cholesterol levels; so can a diet rich in soy foods, which are loaded with isoflavones. When researchers remove the phytoestrogens, soy loses most of its cholesterol-cutting power. Some preliminary evidence suggests that isoflavones, like human estrogen, may even help ease hot flashes and slow the bone loss that follows menopause.

In some ways, paradoxically, phytoestrogens may have the opposite effect of human estrogen—and that may also be beneficial. For example, researchers have found that animals fed a high-soy diet and humans who eat a lot of tofu, or soybean curd, have a reduced risk of cancer. Two possible reasons: Isoflavones entering the cells in the breasts or ovaries may crowd out the animal or human estrogen, which is thought to fuel the growth of certain cancers; and one particular isoflavone, called **genistein,** may inhibit the cellular enzymes and suppress the new blood vessels that help cancers multiply.

Garlic and onions: Sulfur power

Allium vegetables—garlic, onions, chives, leeks, and scallions—seem like nutritional weaklings, according to the standard vitamin and mineral tables. But they're rich in beneficial sulfur compounds. For example, **allicin** seems to reduce production of cholesterol in the liver. Consuming just half a clove of garlic per day may indeed cut cholesterol levels, by an average of about 10 percent.

Other sulfur compounds in allium vegetables, particularly **sulfur-allyl cysteine,** help the liver to detoxify chemicals that may cause cancer. A diet that's rich in either garlic or sulfur-allyl cysteine reduces the risk of various cancers in animals. More significant, a five-year retrospective study of some 42,000 women from Iowa found that those who ate garlic at least once a week had one-third less risk of developing colon cancer than those who never ate it. Smaller studies have linked both onions and chives with a comparably reduced risk of colon cancer.

Broccoli, cabbage, and more

There is strong evidence that cruciferous vegetables—including broccoli, Brussels sprouts, cabbage, cauliflower, kale, and turnips—help ward off cancer. In addition to the possibly cancer-fighting antioxidant vitamins, cruciferous vegetables contain at least two potent phytochemical groups.

One is the **indoles,** which help the body convert one type of estrogen into a harmless form of the hormone, rather than into the potentially cancer-fueling

Scientists are unearthing a wealth of obscure, potentially protective chemicals in plant foods.

kind. Indoles sharply retard the growth of malignant breast tumors in animals.

Cruciferous vegetables also contain **isothiocyanates,** yet another group of sulfur compounds. Modest doses of one such chemical, **sulforaphane,** cut the risk of breast cancer in rats by more than half, in theory by boosting the liver's detoxifying power.

Pulp fact

People who eat a lot of oranges and other citrus fruits—or who drink the juice of those fruits—have a clearly reduced risk of cancer. While the vitamin-C content of those fruits may be at least partly responsible, their skin is loaded with apparently potent anticancer chemicals known as **terpenes,** which do end up in the juice. Large doses of one terpene, **limonene,** actually shrink breast cancers in animals; in fact, concentrated limonene may work much like another terpene, the breast-cancer drug tamoxifen (*Nolvadex*).

Antioxidants in a glass

One potent group of phytochemicals—the **flavonoids,** which combat oxidation and blood clots—crops up in lowly or unlikely places. Flavonoids are found in apples, celery, cranberries, grapes, and onions, which are low in most vitamins and minerals. They're particularly abundant in two beverages that contain even fewer nutrients: tea and red wine.

Tea. The "bad" LDL cholesterol seems to clog the arteries only when it has been chemically damaged by oxidation. A two-cup dose of green or black tea temporarily reduces such oxidation. And a retrospective Dutch study of some 800 men found that those who consumed the most flavonoids, mainly from black tea, had two-thirds less risk of coronary disease than those who consumed the least.

Tea flavonoids clearly help ward off cancer in animals, in theory by blocking cancer-causing oxidation of the DNA that controls cell growth. The evidence in humans is mixed, but some studies suggest that regular tea drinkers may have up to 50 percent less risk of certain cancers than other people have.

Red wine. Researchers have shown that moderate consumption of any alcoholic beverage reduces the risk of coronary disease, apparently by boosting levels of the "good" HDL cholesterol and reducing the chance of blood clots. Now some studies are bolstering the suspicion that red wine may protect the heart better than other alcoholic beverages. Several reports have found that red wine but not white wine minimizes both LDL oxidation and blood clotting. One likely reason: Flavonoids are concentrated in grape skins, which are not used in white wine.

Fruit salad, mixed vegetables

Some apparently protective chemicals occur in a wide variety of plant foods. Among the most common are **carotenoids,** which fight disease-causing oxidation. Until recently, researchers have focused almost exclusively on one carotenoid, **beta-carotene.** Last year, Harvard researchers presented the best evidence so far linking carotenoids other than beta-carotene with a reduced risk of disease. Their retrospective study found that people who consume the most **lutein** and **zeaxanthin,** found in green leafy vegetables, had roughly 50 percent less risk of macular degeneration, the leading cause of blindness after age 65, than those who consume the least.

THE FOOD POLICE

**In the name of good nutrition, they've busted
Chinese food, Italian food, movie popcorn,
and now our favorite happy-hour hangouts.
Have they gone too far?** *By Minna Morse*

"I'M THINKING OF HAVING the salad and the baked potato—and the garden burger," the thin man says to his lunch date. "Think that's too much?"

"He eats all the time," she says, talking past him. "Enormous quantities. But healthy food. Only healthy food."

Ordering a meal is a dicey affair when you're known as the country's fussiest eaters—and you're sitting in a restaurant you're about to publicly skewer. The lean and hungry diner is Michael Jacobson, director of the Center for Science in the Public Interest. Seated at the table with him is dietitian Jayne Hurley, mastermind of a three-year campaign to alert Americans to the dangers of restaurant dining.

These are the folks who slammed Chinese meals, proclaiming kung pao chicken "one of the nastiest dishes" served, "with almost as much fat as four McDonald's Quarter Pounders." They're the ones who denounced fetuccine alfredo as "a heart attack on a plate" and revealed that a large tub of movie popcorn delivers more artery-clogging fat than nine hamburgers.

They've lambasted deli sandwiches, Mexican food, and our favorite sugary snacks. Now, in their latest gambit, they're targeting the upscale burger joints and happy-hour havens—Chili's, Houlihan's, Bennigan's, TGIFriday's,

Hard Rock Cafe, Planet Hollywood, Applebees, and others—that occupy urban corners and riddle suburban malls across the country.

Just a few weeks before, comparable dishes ordered to go at each of these chains had arrived at a lab near Baltimore, shipped overnight in foam ice chests from cities as far-flung as Chicago and Los Angeles, to be weighed, picked apart, ground up, combined, and whirred in a blender into a gray brown goop resembling nothing so much as mud. All simply to peg the dishes' average fat, "artery-clogging fat," calorie, and sodium counts.

The three of us are at a TGIFriday's in downtown Washington, D.C. Nearby are clusters of office workers in dark suits and vacationing families in khaki shorts and denim shirts. They're peering at laminated-plastic menus, munching chips.

What's good? "Let's take a look," Hurley says. It's tough going among the appetizers. You wouldn't want to order the stuffed potato skins, which in CSPI's survey averaged 1,120 calories and 79 grams of fat per basket. That's a whole day's fat for an ordinary woman. Nor would the buffalo wings fly.

"No one thinks of buffalo wings as terribly unhealthy," Hurley says. "I mean, it's chicken, right? But it happens to be the fattiest part of the chicken. Then it's

fried. Then it's dipped in blue cheese." The damages: more than 1,000 calories, on average, and around 80 grams of fat, 22 of them saturated.

How about the entrées? Don't pick the mushroom cheeseburger with fries. This dish averaged 1,490 calories, 53 percent from fat—almost 90 grams.

Impatiently, Jacobson and Hurley scan the menu. How about the oriental chicken salad? Their survey results aren't cheerful. "Seven hundred and fifty calories and 49 grams of fat," Hurley says. "We were pretty shocked to learn that this type of salad has twice as much fat as the sirloin steak. Salad dressings can really do you in. Actually, the steak and potato is not that bad a choice. But even better is the grilled chicken and potato."

The results—released in late September—put TGIFriday's and its kin on CSPI's growing roster of eateries where one false move can turn you into a miscreant. At press briefings to trumpet restaurant busts in the past, Jacobson has placed menu items next to big stacks of McDonald's burgers or cylinders full of Crisco to drive home what vast quantities of fat he's talking about.

Jacobson believes the government has not asked Americans to cut back *enough* on the percentage of calories they're getting from fat. "Most experts recommend a 30 percent limit," says a CSPI newsletter. "We say 20 percent." The current average? About 35 percent. Much of that comes from meals eaten in restaurants, Jacobson says, hence the dramatic busts.

"At least 300,000 people a year die from unhealthy diet and sedentary lifestyles," he says. "That's second only to the 400,000 who die from smoking. One in three Americans today is obese. Somebody has to do something."

"We're not out to attack any one chain or restaurant," says Hurley. "We're just trying to provide information on the kinds of selections available on different types of restaurants' menus. We're providing information that cannot be found anywhere else."

"And we're not only trying to change the way people eat," Jacobson says. "We're trying to change an entire industry."

Sure enough, the group's undercover raids convinced movie theaters across the country to switch to unsaturated oils in their popcorn poppers and led Chinese restaurants—where business fell 20 to 35 percent after the exposé—to offer more steamed dishes. But beyond these gains, CSPI's 50 lawyers, scientists, and policy experts can claim a number of victories.

In the 1980s the group pressured fast-food restaurants like Wendy's, Burger King, and McDonald's into cooking their french fries in vegetable oil instead of beef fat, providing nutrition facts to customers, and offering salads and other light choices. They successfully lobbied the Food and Drug Administration to urge pregnant women to avoid caffeine and won a battle to require that alcohol's health risks be printed on the bottles.

What's more, CSPI is credited with leading a coalition—including the American Heart Association and the American Cancer Society—that fought for detailed nutrition labels on all packaged foods. According to William Schultz, the FDA's deputy commissioner, the 1990 law might never have passed without CSPI. "Government gets a lot of pressure from industry," he says. "Jacobson and CSPI are simply pushing from the other side, in the interests of the consumer."

Not without stiff resistance, however. Jacobson and his colleagues have been called "nutritional terrorists," "puritan deniers," "killjoys," and "gastronomical gestapo," not to mention "anorexic left-wing trust-fund East Coast elitist busybodies." Jeff Nedelman, while a vice president at the Grocery Manufacturers of America, accused Jacobson of single-

what's good on the menu?

WHILE SOME RESTAURANTS do offer hints for health-conscious diners, you're on your own most of the time. To help you order wisely, here are lighter options and high-fat pitfalls (based on HEALTH's own research as well as advice offered by the American Heart Association, the Center for Science in the Public Interest, and other organizations). "Best" choices have less than 30 grams of fat, a generous meal's worth for an active, medium-size woman. "Worst" have up to 100.

Fast Food

BEST
Grilled chicken sandwich
Roast beef sandwich
Single hamburger
Salad with light vinaigrette

WORST
Bacon burger
Double cheeseburger
French fries
Onion rings

TIPS Order sandwiches without mayo or "special sauce." Avoid deep-fried items like fish fillets, chicken nuggets, and french fries.

Chinese

BEST
Hot-and-sour soup
Stir-fried vegetables
Shrimp with garlic sauce
Szechuan shrimp
Wonton soup

WORST
Crispy chicken
Kung pao chicken
Moo shu pork
Sweet-and-sour pork

TIPS Share a stir-fry; help yourself to steamed rice. Ask for vegetables steamed or stir-fried with less oil. Order moo shu vegetables instead of pork. Avoid fried rice, breaded dishes, and items loaded with nuts.

Breakfast

BEST
Hot or cold cereal with 2% milk
Pancakes or french toast with syrup
Scrambled eggs with hash browns and plain toast

WORST
Belgian waffle with sausage
Sausage and eggs with biscuits and gravy
Ham and cheese omelette with hash browns and toast

TIPS Ask for whole grain cereal or shredded wheat with 1% milk or whole wheat toast without butter or margarine. Order omelettes without cheese, fried eggs without bacon or sausage.

Italian

BEST
Pasta with red or white clam sauce
Spaghetti with marinara or tomato-and-meat sauce

WORST
Eggplant parmigiana
Fettuccine alfredo
Fried calamari
Lasagna

TIPS Stick with plain bread instead of garlic bread made with butter or oil. Ask for the waiter's help in avoiding cream- or egg-based sauces.

Sandwiches

BEST
Ham and swiss
Roast beef
Turkey

WORST
Tuna salad
Reuben
Submarine

TIPS Ask for mustard, hold the mayo and cheese. See if turkey-ham is available.

Mexican

BEST
Bean burrito (no cheese)
Chicken fajitas

WORST
Beef chimichanga
Chile relleno
Quesadilla
Refried beans

TIPS Choose soft tortillas with fresh salsa, not guacamole. Special-order grilled shrimp, fish, or chicken. Ask for beans made without lard or fat.

Seafood

BEST
Broiled bass, halibut, or snapper
Grilled scallops
Steamed crab or lobster

WORST
Fried seafood platter
Blackened catfish

TIPS Order fish broiled, baked, grilled, or steamed—not panfried or sautéed. Ask for lemon instead of tartar sauce. Avoid creamy and buttery sauces.

handedly taking the fun out of eating, suggesting that as proper punishment he be buried up to his neck in sour cream and guacamole.

Complaints have come from other quarters as well: from food writers who object that CSPI looks at food only as fuel, not as a source of pleasure or as a cultural touchstone; from nutritionists who insist there are no bad foods, only bad diets; and from food packagers and restaurateurs who say CSPI has whipped up a tidal wave of fear and confusion.

But is all that true? Is the group defeating its own purposes, scaring us into buying foods that are low in fat but loaded with calories? Or is it actually protecting us from our own harmful habits?

THEY'VE TURNED US into a nation obsessed with fat," says nutritionist Adam Drewnowski, "as if fat were the only message. The message of responsible nutrition should be balance, moderation, and variety, whereas the message of CSPI seems to be 'Eat it and die.' There's no point in demonizing fettuccine alfredo. You just can't eat it all the time."

Drewnowski, who directs the University of Michigan's human nutrition program, points out that CSPI is attempting to treat public health problems—obesity, high cholesterol, and high blood pressure—that don't afflict all Americans. True, Drewnowski says, a meatless diet with 10 percent of its calories from fat, like that advocated by heart specialist Dean Ornish, can help unclog the arteries of individuals who've led unhealthy lives. But there's no evidence that cut-the-fat advice has saved anyone from a heart attack. And it may even be dangerous.

"Adolescent girls are starving themselves of fat and calories," Drewnowski says, "and I'm not talking about girls with eating disorders, just girls concerned about their weight." For them, he says, eating less than 20 percent of their calories as fat can shortchange their bones and disturb their reproductive hormones.

"All of us need some fat in our diets," he says. "Beta-carotene, for example, needs to be consumed with fat. Without it, carrots are just roughage. I recently saw a very nice study that made just this point, that blood levels of beta-carotene were much higher after a meal that included fat than after an extremely low-fat meal. The fat-carrier the researchers used happened to be Häagen-Dazs ice cream—one of the foods CSPI says you should never, ever eat.

"We're linear thinkers," Drewnowski continues. "CSPI is telling us that a lot of fat is bad. We assume if a lot is bad, and a little is better, then none is better still. People believe that if something is fat-free, it must be good for you, and they gorge on low-fat, high-calorie foods."

In fact, surveys show that in recent years we've added so many calories that while our percentage of calories from fat has dropped, the actual *amount* of fat we're eating is as high as it's ever been. Apparently, we're simply munching all the new fat-free goodies on top of everything else. Among these are the snacks made with Olestra, the chemical fat substitute developed by Proctor & Gamble.

Jacobson and his colleagues are dead set against it, but not because it's highly processed. Eaten in potato chips and crackers, Olestra can have such unsavory side effects as abdominal cramping, diarrhea, and "anal leakage." It also soaks up antioxidants such as lycopene and beta-carotene and carries them away. The FDA requires Frito-Lay—the company now test-marketing Olean brand chips fried in Olestra—to print warnings on the bags.

Yet despite its tell-us-your-side-effects hotline and a write-your-congressman campaign, and despite vocal support from nutrition scientists across the country, CSPI has failed to convince the government to withdraw its approval of Olestra. There is simply too great a demand for low-fat snacks.

That's not the only trap the group may have laid for itself. According to John Stanton, a professor of food marketing at Saint Joseph's University in Philadelphia, a prime eating trend as we head toward the 21st century is a backlash against nutritionally correct "healthy" foods.

"Hamburger consumption is way up," Stanton says. "Steaks ordered in restaurants are up. Pizza Hut just came out with a triple-decker pizza. And McDonald's recently did a multimillion-dollar study to determine what adults want to eat and found that they want a bigger hamburger with bacon and cheese. Voilà: The same year they pull their McLean burger from the market, they introduce the magnificently unhealthy Arch Deluxe. People like what they like. Just giving them facts doesn't necessarily change their behavior."

The backlash may be building, according to a survey by the Food Marketing Institute. Fifty-five percent of consumers say they're tired of experts telling them which foods are good. And 46 percent say there's so much conflicting news they don't know what to eat anymore.

Those attitudes don't surprise Alan Levy, a social psychologist and the director of consumer studies at the FDA. As a source of facts about food and health, he says, CSPI has had a huge impact. But sounding too many alarms, he notes, raises questions in the public's mind: Is this for my benefit or for CSPI's?

"The first restaurant studies—the one on Chinese food, the popcorn study—those were great," Levy says. "The information couldn't be found anywhere else, and it was a shock to everyone. But now they've carried it to such an extent that they're seen as the food police. It doesn't do wonders for their credibility—or their ability to change how people eat."

What about the 97 percent of consumers who say they're trying to eat better? Surely the warnings have convinced *some* people. "Actually," says Levy, "the best study I've seen on that was CSPI's own—on their milk campaign in West Virginia. A completely controlled study, showing the impact of their public information campaign on whole, low-fat, and skim milk consumption. Now that was amazing data."

YOU CAN'T SAY the citizens of neighboring Bridgeport and Clarksburg, West Virginia, didn't know what hit them. Over a seven-week period in 1995 CSPI bombarded the local airwaves with bluntly worded ads. "A glass of whole milk has the artery-clogging fat of five strips of bacon," says a trustworthy-looking mom standing in front of a supermarket dairy case. "And 2 percent milk isn't much better. But with 1 percent or skim, you get great taste and all the vitamins, with little or no fat."

The group ran taste tests in markets and poster contests in schools; it even prodded local ministers to preach on the links between health and spirituality. Citizens were invited down to the county courthouse to view a 400-pound block of fat—what they would avoid over a lifetime if only they switched from whole milk to skim.

Though many locals were skeptical at first, the campaign quickly struck a nerve. Sales of whole milk fell 20 percent, while sales of skim and 1 percent milk more than doubled. As for any backlash against the message or the methods, it didn't materialize. A year and a half after the last ad ran, the lowest-fat milks continue to hold their gains in the towns' markets.

"We're very pleased with the campaign," says Jacobson, between bites of his garden burger at TGIFriday's. "Hopefully it will serve as a prototype for other, more widespread public information projects. Of course," he adds, "milk is a very important food to change, but it's also an easy switch to make. Switching from buffalo wings to veggie burgers is much harder."

But do we need to make that switch? Can't we be good most of the time and still eat buffalo wings at happy hour?

Not if you're really trying to keep your fat calories down to 20 or even 30 percent, Hurley says. It's just too difficult to keep track of the fat you're eating. You're more likely to stay under the 30 percent mark when you consistently avoid fatty foods.

"This idea that any food can be part of a healthy diet is absurd," says Hurley. "To make fettuccine alfredo part of a healthy diet, you'd have to eat only fruit and vegetables and rice for two and a half days. The problem is, most people who indulge in this kind of food aren't eating that way the rest of the time."

"We're not fanatics," says Jacobson. "We believe in moderation. But we also know that we've got to be heard. So we have become very good at getting our message—however condensed—out through the media. Our whole mission is making this kind of information public."

It's true that despite what hits the headlines, CSPI's message is not all sour grapes and grim statistics. When the restaurant critiques appear in CSPI's own newsletter, *Nutrition Action*, they're always full of upbeat tips for healthful choices (such as the garden burger and the sirloin steak with baked potato) as well as for improving even the fattiest, saltiest selections (hold the mayo and sour cream).

Besides, the group's boldest moves are made behind the scenes. At the moment it's pressing baby-food makers to stop using starch and sugar as fillers, lobbying against Olestra, and arguing that hydrogenated vegetable oils should be counted with other types of artery-clogging fats on cookie and cracker boxes.

The record speaks loudly. Without CSPI's campaigning, Americans would still be eating cookies laced with cholesterol-raising tropical oils; shoppers would find far fewer low-salt soups and crackers; salad-bar patrons could still be blindsided by greens steeped in sulfites. The words *light* and *lean* would mean whatever food packagers wanted them to mean, and nutrition labels would still be a hodgepodge of meaningless data printed in tiny type.

The new labels, installed with the group's blessing, are bold, consistent, and clear. Consumers can decide to read them or not. The important thing, Jacobson says, is that they now have the chance to make smart choices.

Health-minded restaurant diners will be getting better service, too. In July, following a lawsuit by CSPI and the advocacy group Public Citizen, the government issued rules barring restaurants from displaying little heart symbols or calling menu items "guilt-free" or "heart-smart" if they aren't suitably low in fat and saturated fat.

But those buffalo wings and stuffed potato skins in happy-hour joints probably never will come with nutrition data. So Jacobson, Hurley, and their colleagues have taken it upon themselves to crunch the numbers and spread the news. They have no plan to end their surprise raids.

"Before we started these restaurant studies," Hurley says, "there were very few healthy sections on menus. Now most of the chain restaurants have some kind of health-conscious fare. This shows that we're being heard, that consumers are asking for healthier options, and that the industry is responding in kind."

Minna Morse is an assistant editor at Smithsonian *magazine.*

High price of shelf space

■ **Competition:** *The heavy demand for grocery store shelf space has manufacturers paying retailers "slotting allowances" to guarantee their products are adequately displayed to consumers.*

By SEAN SOMERVILLE

SUN STAFF

Australian conglomerate Burns Philp & Co. wasn't the only loser in a costly war for shelf space against Sparks-based spice giant McCormick & Co. Inc.

Just ask Daniel Martinez, whose family owns Phoenix, Ariz.-based National Spices. He said National Spices lost about $400,000 in annual sales when McCormick gave two grocery chains hundreds of thousands of dollars in 1994 to sack National's line of spices in favor of McCormick's Mojave brand.

"We could never have paid the kind of money that they were paying," said Martinez, 40, who helps his father run the business. "It would have taken six or seven years to recoup. I guess the big dog wins."

McCormick's response is that it pays a slotting allowance determined by the market, and that it never violates an existing contract. "That's the way it's been traditionally done throughout the industry," said Carroll Nordhoff, McCormick executive vice president.

The auction among spice companies is a winner-take-all version of the battle for grocery store shelf space that requires manufacturers to give retailers up-front payments, experts say. The payments, known as slotting allowances, contributed to the financial struggles of Burns Philp, which is selling its spice business. Burns Philp has marketed Durkee, French and Spice Island brands in the United States.

"What you have is a bargaining situation where the retailer has shelf space that's scarce and a lot of manufacturers that want the space and will bid for it," said Greg Shaffer, an Indiana University economist.

Slotting allowances provide part of the answer to an enduring mystery: Why some items are so prominent that they almost grab shoppers and others are so inconspicuous that they seem impossible to find. The practice garnered new attention last month, with the disclosure that the Federal Trade Commission is investigating McCormick's marketing practices.

McCormick said the FTC investigation focuses not on slotting allowances, but on "exclusivity" agreements with a few chains that limit competition. But some analysts say slotting and exclusivity are intertwined because exclusivity agreements would likely translate into higher slotting payments.

Some industry experts say the allowances raise consumer prices and that small manufacturers have been crushed by the practice. But the FTC says it has not challenged slotting allowances because it lacks evidence that they are anti-competitive in a universal sense or harmful to consumers.

Slotting allowances in grocery stores include a broad range of expenditures—"slotting fees" for new products, "pay-to-stay" fees to remain on shelves, "facing allowances" to increase space or improve position and "street money" for aisle displays, Shaffer said.

No one knows precisely how much retailers collect in slotting allowances. But Shaffer estimated it ranges between $6 billion and $18 billion a year.

Marianne M. Jennings, professor of legal and ethical studies at Arizona State University College of Business, called slotting a peculiar part of the grocery store industry. "What you find is this amazing practice that is sort of under the table and sort of not," she said.

Jennings said the fees have helped to drive several smaller manufacturers out of business. "I'm afraid that we're ultimately going to have only Budweiser and Doritos on the shelf because they're the only people who can afford to pay," she said.

Similar practices are growing outside grocery stores. The retail book industry now demands fees from publishers to give books prominent space. Ocean City recently signed a deal to make Coca-Cola products the only beverages sold at city-sponsored events and in municipal vending machines.

Slotting allowances grew so quietly that even their origin is a matter of dispute, Jennings said. As early as the 1930s, A&P supermarkets demanded extra free cases of products as the price of carrying them, Shaffer said.

A key moment came in 1984, when Cincinnati-based Kroger's supermarket chain started demanding cash payments for new products to defray its costs. "What's not in dispute is that the practice of paying for shelf space has grown considerably since" then, Shaffer said.

Some retail chains have a flat fee of $5,000 for new product introductions, Jennings said. Others have a graduated fee schedule tied to location, with eye-level slots costing more than knee- or ground-level spots. Spaces at the end of grocery aisles bring high fees because they guarantee attention.

Grocery stores argue that allowances are necessary to evaluate the 20,000 new products that compete every year to be among the 50,000 items carried by the average grocery store.

"About 90 percent of new products fail or get withdrawn," said Edie Clark, a spokeswoman for the Food Marketing Institute, whose 1,500 members include supermarkets, retailers and wholesalers. "For our industry, the issue has been the cost of a failure."

She said a store's buyer has to decide what product to carry and what product to remove to make room for it—all costs that need to be paid.

Louis Denrich, president of Baltimore-based Valu Food stores, said the chain asks for slotting payments, but does not always receive them. "It's strictly to cover costs," he said. "A lot of companies don't give them. The more desperate a company is to get on the shelves, the more likely they are to pay them."

Giant Food Inc. said it doesn't have a uniform policy when it comes to slotting fees. "If they're available, we take them," said Dave Herriman, senior vice president for grocery, pharmacy and bakery operations. "We ask a manufacturer if he does have one. If he says yes, we say we would like our fair share."

But he said slotting fees do not alone determine whether something gets on the shelves. "Normally our policy is that a product lives or dies by its own merits and not because of size of slotting allowance," Herriman said. "We've taken products with slotting allowances and products without them."

He said slotting fees can hurt business by tying up space for products that don't sell.

The Grocery Manufacturers of America, whose members pay the fees, says it objects to slotting fees when they exceed the cost of doing business—a frequent occurrence, say experts. "Within some retail chains, slotting fees represent net profits," Jennings said.

Manufacturers are generally reluctant to discuss slotting, for fear of alienating retailers and jeopardizing their sales, experts say. Some manufacturers, like Procter & Gamble, don't pay them at all. They rely on advertising that spurs strong demand for their products.

But Jennings said Frito Lay pays $100,000 to chains to carry new products. Truzzolino Pizza Roll was charged $25,000 by one chain to carry its products and Lee's Ice Cream, a Baltimore company, was asked to pay $25,000 for each flavor it wanted stores to carry.

In many cases, the amounts are arbitrary and secret, Jennings said. She believes stores should publish slotting schedules for manufacturers and that the allowances should be uniform and more closely tied to costs.

Scott Garfield, vice president of Lee's Ice Cream, made a run at supermarkets a couple of years ago before giving up. He encountered a particularly hard time because ice cream sections are generally very small.

"You need a certain financial wherewithal to play the game," said Garfield, whose business sells packaged ice cream to stores abroad, but not domestically.

He said stores demand slotting allowances with varying degrees of audacity. "Some are very bold," he said. "They say they're not going to take a product without slotting fees. Another gave me a chance without a fee right off the bat."

Ultimately, the costs of packaging just to get a chance to be on shelves, plus the possibility of continuing fees proved too expensive, he said. Lee's currently sells ice cream domestically only to dipping parlors.

Ann Wilder, whose Towson-based Vanns Spice has operated in McCormick's shadow for 15 years, said her company has lost space to McCormick's deep pockets on a couple of occasions.

Eighteen months ago, Wilder said, she had every reason to believe she was going to get her products into a grocery chain in upstate New York that she would not identify. "The buyer said he would take the product and even told me which distributor to go through," Wilder said. "Then I was told that they had signed an agreement with McCormick."

Because of a scarcity of information about slotting, the effect of the practice on consumers is unclear. Jennings said consumers not only pay higher prices so manufacturers can pay slotting costs, but that the laws of supply and demand are circumvented by the jockeying of manufacturers and retailers.

Shaffer sees it differently. "The consumer is paying higher prices, but on the other hand they also are getting a better selection," he said.

Without slotting allowances, a retailer would have no motive to displace a prod-

uct that is selling. In such instances, he said, slotting costs help manufacturers and retailers share the risk of carrying a new, unproven product.

So far, slotting allowances have attracted scant attention from federal antitrust regulators. "It's a pretty complicated area," said Mike Antalics, the FTC's assistant director for nonmerger litigation. "Even the term slotting allowance is used in different ways by different people. The bottom line is we would be looking at the effect on competition as opposed to the effect on individual competitors. Another way of saying that is the effect on consumers."

Robert A. Skitol, a Washington antitrust lawyer, said the FTC could investigate slotting fees under the Robinson-Patman Act of 1936. One section of the law forbids a seller's favoritism for one buyer over another in regard to price. Another prohibits unreasonable payments from sellers to buyers for services rendered.

"When a manufacturer pays a large allowance to one chain, but doesn't make a comparable payment to every other competing supermarket chain, then there is a substantial question presented of violation of Robinson-Patman," he said.

But Skitol said the FTC has scarce resources and that investigating slotting allowances would be a huge undertaking.

Experts said enforcing reforms would be difficult because slotting payments could be hidden in marketing costs or lower prices for goods. "It's not clear you could stop it even if you wanted to," Shaffer said.

That leaves companies like National Spice with a gnawing feeling that something is amiss. Martinez said the company had supplied the Smitty's chain in Arizona for 27 years, from the time it opened its first store.

One day Smitty's called and told National to take down its displays. McCormick had paid Smitty's $100,000, Martinez said. "The way it was explained to us was that the store was only so big and could carry only one item," he said. "There's no illusion to it. We believe if they hadn't paid slotting fees, we would still be in there."

The Coming Boom(er) Market

In 1996, the first of the 76 million Baby Boomers celebrated their 50th birthday — and changed the meaning of "mature consumer" for decades to come.

Typically, concern about nutrition and health issues increases with age. But the Baby Boomers are not like their parents or any other mature market in history. Considered by demographers to be individualistic, solution-oriented and self-indulgent, the Boomers will reject the symptoms of aging rather than be resigned to them.

"Boomers will grow old, but not gracefully," predicts Cheryl Russell, editor-in-chief of New Strategist Publications and author of *The Master Trend—How the Baby Boom Generation is Remaking America*. "They are already fighting off the signs of aging, buying products and services like relaxed-fit jeans, cosmetics with anti-aging ingredients and elective plastic surgery. In terms of food products, those perceived to 'do more for me' will fly off the shelves," says Russell.

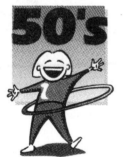

Nutrition and the Mature Market

However "unique" Boomers consider themselves, they will inevitably face the same nutrition and health issues as their parents and grandparents.

"Aging brings some predictable changes in the body — such as decreasing or diminishing senses of taste and smell, along with chewing, swallowing and digestive problems — that affect some older persons' attitudes toward eating," says Nancy Wellman, Ph.D., R.D., F.A.D.A., director of the National Policy and Resource Center on Nutrition and Aging at the Florida International University. "In addition, many older people have illnesses that change the kind and amount of food they can or want to eat."

What and how much older people eat is a complex process, according to Wellman. "Childhood preferences, ideals about how food 'should be,' whether one eats alone or in a social situation, and income level are all important. What is constant, however, are older people's nutritional needs — needs that are not by and large being met."

For example, aging alters the body's need for certain nutrients, such as vitamin D, calcium, the B-complex vitamins and protein—needs that may not be met without conscious changes in the diet. Also, older people may not eat appropriate quantities of food for various reasons. Wellman points out that surveys have found that 18–32 percent of older Americans reported unintended weight loss or gain over a six-month period. In addition, the average person over 65 takes three or more different drugs daily. The side effects can be dramatic, including an altered sense of taste caused by the bitterness of the drugs or a sudden loss of appetite.

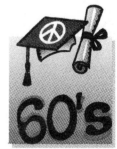

But Wellman believes each of these risk factors represents an opportunity to develop and promote products geared toward solving specific nutrition problems for the aging population. She sees opportunities for food products that are:

- *Convenient.* Foods that need little or no preparation, come in single servings and are easy to open are appealing to the older consumer with limited mobility and smaller appetites.

- *Easy to eat.* Textures need to accommodate chewing and swallowing problems.

- *Flavor and aroma enhanced.* Bacon, cheese or butter flavors, MSG and extracts such as almond and vanilla, can enhance the taste of food and help counter the potentially reduced sense of taste and smell typical in the elderly.

- *Medical foods.* Those that address specific health conditions, such as diabetes, will help a person improve his or her condition.

- *Nutrient dense.* Foods that provide adequate micronutrients with fewer calories help reduce unintended weight loss common among older people.

The (Really) Big Picture

While no one can predict the future, the demographics of the Baby Boomer market are clear, and some data exist on their nutrition attitudes and eating habits. In general, the Boomer market is characterized by:

- *Its sheer size.* Defined as the generation born between 1946 and 1964, the Baby Boomers, 76 million strong, comprise the largest generation in the nation's history. As this huge cohort enters middle age, it is turning the traditional proportions of younger and older generations on its head. In 1970, the country had 70 million people under 18 and 50 million over age 50. However, by 2010, the picture will be upside down, with 96 million people over

50 and only 74 million under 18.

- *The potential for longer lives.* In addition to the size of the market, the life expectancy of Boomers is greater than that of any generation in history. The median age of the Boomers is 40, and most can expect to live almost another 40 years.

By living longer, Boomers also will change traditional lifestyle patterns. "This is the first generation whose life-cycles will change from linear to circular," according to Kathy Hardy, director of the market analysis and assessment department of the American Association of Retired Persons. Instead of following a straight line from college to career and parenthood to retirement, this generation is moving in and out of different roles at various stages of life. "In the more circular life-cycle we're seeing now, mature Americans are going back to school after retirement, going back to work after raising children, starting second or third careers and caring for older parents," said Hardy.

- *Individualistic and anti-authoritarian attitudes.* Better educated than previous generations and taught to think for themselves, the Boomers have a more independent, anti-authoritarian streak, compared to recent generations.

"The Baby Boomer generation is remaking American society because it is the first generation of 'free agents'," Russell observes. Boomers have retreated from the institutions of society like organized religion, marriage and political parties. In Russell's view, the individualistic perspective is not something the Boomers consciously pursue. "It is simply the way they see and relate to the world. Individualism is the master trend of our time."

As a consequence, experts agree that marketing messages must avoid references to "aging," or "the golden years." Instead, Boomers will in all likelihood

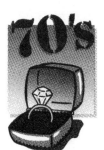

define themselves by events in their life: whether they're a parent, a retiree, an affluent traveler or a new entrepreneur.

Don't Trust Anyone Under 30?

The Boomers' individualistic, anti-authoritarian perspective will also influence where and how they get information on health and nutrition — and whether they trust it.

Boomers traditionally have and will continue to demand more information about the food they eat and be more discerning about that information. As the first generation raised with television and conversant with computers, video, the Internet and other high-tech communication technologies, they have access to many different sources to obtain information about nutrition and foods.

Boomers are eager for more information and will still want to hear about government and university studies focused on the links between nutrition, physical activity and health, according to Jim Hill, Ph.D., of the Center for Human Nutrition at the University of Colorado Health Science Center and chair of the Physical Activity and Nutrition (PAN) Program Scientific Advisory Committee of the International Life Sciences Institute. "Boomers don't just want to know how to live longer, but rather, how to improve the quality of life as they age," he says. "In particular, they want to remain physically active as they age. They also want to know how to avoid obesity and how to guarantee their diets include all the nutrients they need without sacrificing taste."

However, they may not have the type of knee-jerk reaction that consumers have had in the past as every new study comes out, according to Linda Gilbert, a food scientist-turned-president of HealthFocus, Inc., a consumer research firm. Consumers feel more confused today because of the often contradictory messages found in different scientific studies. "Boomers are asking: 'If the experts cannot agree, how can I trust what they say?'" Gilbert says.

The Future is Now

That said, it appears food marketers and communicators need not wait for Boomers to hit middle age to capture that market with health-related messages. According to a 1996 survey conducted by HealthFocus, Inc., 40-year-old Boomers are already making changes in their food-related behavior that reflect a concern with health and nutrition. The survey of more than 2,000 U.S. households assessed the attitudes and behaviors of consumers regarding nutrition and health.

The survey classifies most Boomers as "health investors" — satisfied with their overall well-being and inclined to make choices that will improve and ensure their future health. This group values quality over price and won't sacrifice taste for health benefits.

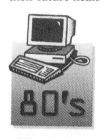

What are Boomers doing? According to the HealthFocus survey, more than three-fourths (78 percent) of those between 40 and 49 report always or usually choosing foods for health reasons. Forty-five (45) percent of the women and 40 percent of the men aged 30-49 report maintaining a heart-healthy diet and 45 percent of women and 39 percent of the men report maintaining a low-fat diet.

Another survey, *Trends in the United States: Consumer Attitudes and the Supermarket*, developed and conducted by the Food Marketing Institute (FMI) for the past 25 years, also found that Boomers are as concerned as other shoppers with the nutritional content of their food (65 percent said 'very concerned'). The survey, a nationwide sample of more than 2,000 supermarket shoppers, found that consumers between the ages of 40 and 49 account for one-fifth (22 percent) of those surveyed. The 1996 survey specifically tracked certain questions related to this group.

Like the HealthFocus survey, "Trends" found Boomers tend to be more concerned about fat content than older shoppers (64 percent) and sodium content than younger shoppers (32 percent). The first wave of Boomers also is more likely than other "Trends" respondents to find the nutrition labels very useful (52 percent vs. 47 percent).

Other market observers foresee the following trends in Boomer food buying behaviors:

- *Emphasis on tasty, flavorful foods.* With a more cultivated palate in general than their elders and a willingness to try new products, Boomers will be seeking out foods that provide new taste sensations.

  Both the HealthFocus and FMI surveys found that taste is the motivating factor in buying a product and often a major influence on the willingness of consumers to try a new product. Boomers may compromise taste for nutrition more often as they get older, but probably not as much as their parents did. Flavorful, ethnic, highly-seasoned (though not necessarily hot and spicy) foods will appeal to those looking for a new food experience. These foods will be more appealing as the sense of smell and taste decline in older years.

- *More demand for "functional" food products.* Boomers are looking for products that may provide benefits beyond basic nutrition, and they will expect to see them in their local supermarket rather than in specialty aisles or stores. For example, the HealthFocus survey found that foods eaten specifically to reduce the risk of disease included broccoli, oranges (or orange juice) and tomatoes (or tomato sauce).

- *Assurance of value.* After taste, Boomers say price and nutritional content are important influences on their willingness to change brands.

- *Convenience.* While Boomers will slow down a bit as they age, they will have a more fast-paced and busy lifestyle than their parents. No-preparation, easy-to-open, single-serving foods will sell well. According to the 1996 "Trends" survey, 38 percent of

Boomers, 45 percent of 50 - 64 year-olds and 46 percent of those over 65 rely on takeout and home delivery meals "fairly often." Convenience will continue to be an important value-added component of a product.

What We Can Expect

When it comes to food, Boomers will, in all likelihood, try to have it all: a practical approach to healthful eating mixed with the occasional, deserved indulgence.

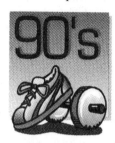

"Boomers are running the other way from the 'quick-fix' approach to health and nutrition. They will look more for practical solutions that they can live with over the long haul," says Gilbert. She expects Boomers to take an "eat more of" approach rather than an "eat less of" approach — emphasizing more whole grains, fruits and vegetables rather than less fat, salt or cholesterol. But it also means enjoying a treat when they want it. Don't expect traditional favorite foods to disappear from their cupboards, pantries, refrigerators and freezers.

The two "seasons" of aging have been characterized by independence and dependence and are loosely defined as under and over age 85. As Wellman says, "Each season of aging has food choice ramifications." In acknowledging the reluctance of Boomers to age, she notes, "Realistically, some of us may eventually need special foods designed to accommodate our dependence. But thanks to a variety of food choices and an active lifestyle, we can look forward to more enjoyable years."

More research needs to be done to track what will change and what will stay the same for Boomers as they make nutrition and health choices through the years. In the meantime, with four million people turning 50 this year and every year until 2015, the Boomers offer food marketers and communicators a sustained — and receptive — audience for messages that link nutrition and food to a healthy, active lifestyle.

Nutrients

One cannot think well, love well, sleep well, if one has not dined well.

—Virginia Woolf

Some basic aspects of nutrition have remained relatively unchanged for many years. The list of nutrients is one of these. Even the specific vitamins and minerals have undergone little revision. Nutrients that provide energy are still identified as carbohydrates, fats, and proteins. Fiber is not a nutrient because it is not essential to life, but it is included in this unit because it clearly performs a significant role in maintaining normal physiological functions.

Significant concepts about each nutrient, however, have changed, often dramatically. With today's available technology, the turnover in data from nutrition studies is so rapid that information may become obsolete even before it is printed and certainly before it is accepted or acted upon. Nor does the availability of voluminous data mean that theories are proven. Studies and experiments must be replicated, subjected to peer review, refined, and tried again. Conflicts in data, a common occurrence, must be resolved before any actionable conclusions can be reached. And, while epidemiological evidence indicates a relationship, this does not prove cause and effect. Years may pass and numerous other studies be concluded before any firm recommendations for either normal or therapeutic diets can be supported. Outside the scientific community this is frequently misunderstood, and sometimes every media report is taken as a new breakthrough.

Compounding the problem of formulating recommendations is the fact that differences among human beings are truly remarkable; an average human being simply

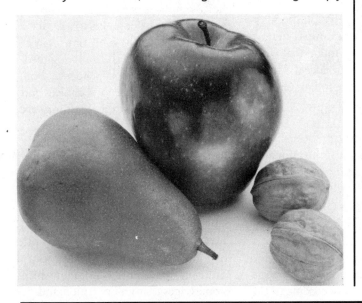

does not exist. Physiological variations preclude accurate predictions of exact nutrient amounts that cause the negative effects of either deficiency or excess. It is the task of the National Academy of Sciences to establish quantity recommendations that more than cover most people's actual requirements but are not high enough to cause harm. The result is the periodically revised Recommended Dietary Allowance (RDA). The current 1989 edition is under review and is certain to undergo changes. Available new evidence regarding nutrient need and performance is being seriously considered. Some of the discussion centers upon evidence that amounts of vitamins higher than RDA allowances may have prophylactic effects that minimize chronic diseases and that exceed the traditional roles of preventing deficiencies. Dr. A. E. Harper, of national renown, rebuts this approach: "The . . . critical question is: Are the effects observed physiologic/nutritional or pharmacologic?"

The articles in this unit were selected because they reflect up-to-date thinking about a variety of nutrients that are currently newsworthy or about which we frequently have questions and/or misconceptions. The first two unit articles on fats are a good example. Current guidelines set one's fat budget at no more than 30 percent of total calories, although the average consumer probably gets closer to 33 percent. Other consumers try to avoid all or most fat, even though some fat is required for a healthy body. Americans may be even less aware that saturated fats, found in animal products and tropical oils, have a major role in promoting disease, while unsaturated fats do not produce the same harmful effects. More confusion results from learning that trans-fatty acids, some of which occur naturally while others form in the process of hydrogenation, have disease effects similar to those of saturated fat. In addition, as the article, "A Type of Fat We May Need More Of" suggests, we might benefit from more dietary emphasis on a particular family of fatty acids called the omega-3s. Even so, exact predictions cannot be made regarding individual reactions and tolerances to fat. Americans remain *very* conscious of fat in food and eagerly look for new products with low-fat and no-fat claims. The food industry, eager to exploit marketing opportunities, has responded with hundreds of new products yearly. However, typical consumers sometimes neglect to note that lower-fat items often have equal or more calories, at the same time, and they remain paradoxically fanatic about super-premium ice creams and other rich desserts high in fat.

Protein, of course, is another matter. Few of us in the United States get too little protein. Even vegetarians, it seems, can easily eat ample amounts that include all of the essential amino acids. Yet many of us grew up with the notion that more protein is always desirable and definitely necessary to increase muscle mass. Experts tell us that this isn't so, that too much protein can even be harmful, and that substituting high carbohydrate foods would often be more beneficial.

Evidence that dietary fiber does, indeed, offer disease protection can be supported by a substantial body of research, although few Americans get the recommended amounts. In "A 'Bran-New' Look at Dietary Fiber," the authors summarize the claims that are both proven and unproven and offer advice about how to get more in one's diet. Eating more fruits and vegetables, legumes, and whole grains is the key.

There follows a series of articles on vitamins, an indication of both the amount of current research and the degree of public interest in them. "Food for Thought about Dietary Supplements" by Paul Thomas is very significant because it addresses the fallacious philosophical mindset that some of us have regarding vitamins. No doubt vitamins seemed to present "miraculous cures" when they were first discovered as the key to terrible diseases such as pellagra, scurvy, and beriberi. But vitamins are workhorses, not magic bullets, that go about their everyday jobs of making the body operate smoothly. In large doses they will have pharmacological effects, some of which may be beneficial, but often they are harmful as well. For many reasons, food sources rather than supplement sources are a better choice.

Vitamin C, ascorbic acid, is a vitamin that has been newsworthy since the days when Linus Pauling first proclaimed that humans should consume more than 3 grams daily rather than the mere 60 mg suggested in the RDA table. Jane Brody's article on vitamin C should be read for its current discussion on this controversial topic. It is certainly not clear that intakes that are greater than currently recommended are desirable and advisable for most people. On the other hand, the issues are much clearer for another water-soluble vitamin, folic acid. Fortification of grain products with folacin has been mandated by the FDA because of a clear connection between a lack of folic acid at the point of conception and neural tube defects in the child.

Vitamins A, D, E, and K, the fat-soluble vitamins, are stored in the body and make significant contributions to health. A plant form of vitamin A, beta-carotene, was originally thought to have beneficial antioxidant effects against cancer and heart disease. However, research trials were stopped due to evidence that high intakes might actually be *causing* death and cancer rates to increase. Vitamin D is vital to bone health because it facilitates calcium absorption. A reduced ability among the elderly to synthesize vitamin D in the skin puts them at still greater risk of osteoporosis and, perhaps, other illnesses as well. In spite of the increasing list of apparent benefits from these and other vitamins, experts have reservations about some of the research and concerns regarding the safety of consuming large amounts. Articles in unit 6 should be read for more information on myths and facts about this subject. Where does the truth lie? Nobody yet knows, but the evidence is generally much stronger for the consumption of foods high in vitamins rather than for supplements. Certainly current knowledge provides strong support for consuming a variety of foods and *at least* the recommended five daily fruit/vegetable servings, something only 10 percent of the U.S. population apparently accomplishes.

In "Fluoridation: A Triumph of Science over Propaganda," Michael Easley describes the fears and misinformation that have interfered with this public health initiative. The evidence that fluoride protects against dental caries is solid, and fluoridation has always been upheld in the court system. And, finally, a discussion of calcium supplements explores the available options. With recommendations for calcium intakes going up and the threats of osteoporosis so ominous, this information may be quite significant.

Much as we would like them, there are few absolutes in the science of nutrition. Perhaps there never will be, for nutrition is an applied rather than a pure science. The present decades are a period of great discovery. For those who marvel at the continued unfolding of the mysteries of human physiology, this is both a confusing and a tremendously exciting era in which to live.

Looking Ahead: Challenge Questions

Are some nutrients more important than others in maintaining health? Support your answer.

What claims are made for vitamins that you know to be false?

Determine the amount of protein you need and the amount you actually get each day. Based on the information in the article on protein, should you make changes? What are they?

How should one decide whether or not to take supplements? Are the issues involving supplements of a single vitamin or mineral any different than for multivitamins?

Should fiber be designated a nutrient? Why or why not?

Determine the percentage of your average daily calories that is contributed by total fat and saturated fat. What did your calculation tell you?

SPECIAL REPORT

A Type of Fat We May Need More Of

Researchers the world over are coming upon more and more evidence that omega-3 fatty acids, found in fish oils, are essential to good health. They appear to play a crucial role not just in staving off heart disease but also in mitigating the symptoms of rheumatoid arthritis, preventing developmental defects in premature babies, and easing depression. Canadian health experts believe omega-3s are important enough that Canada has specific recommendations for how much people should eat every day from fish and other sources. Denmark, too, spells out recommendations to make sure people get enough of these fats, or oils.

Despite the push, the amount of omega-3s that people consume in relation to other fats has never been lower, and it has dropped dramatically in a relatively short time. From the dawn of humankind until the turn of this century, men and women ate a higher proportion of their fat as omega-3s. In the 1900s, other types of fats have edged out these oils in the diet. Thus, it's possible that scientists simply are rediscovering a way of eating for which we were programmed over the course of millions of years.

The evidence for omega-3s and heart disease

Scientists have known for more than a decade that eating fish a couple of times a week is linked to a reduced risk of dying from heart disease. Now the link is getting stronger, particularly for people who already have suffered a heart attack or some other type of coronary problem.

One study showed that men instructed to eat fatty fish after a heart attack (fatty species like herring and mackerel have greater quantities of omega-3s than lean varieties) were 30 percent less likely to die during a 2-year period than heart attack victims not given any recommendations about fish. Similar results occurred in another study of people who had had heart attacks. After about 2

years, there were only 1/5 as many cardiac deaths in the group eating relatively high amounts of omega-3s as in another group. And there were only 1/3 as many non-fatal heart attacks.

Omega-3 fatty acids seem to help by making the blood less likely to coagulate. That, in turn, makes it less likely to form clots that can lead to sudden cardiac death. Omega-3s also appear to stabilize the heart's muscle cells and thereby prevent life-threatening arrhythmias, which are interruptions in heart-pumping rhythm.

One study has even shown that omega-3s can help keep the arteries open after angioplasty. That's a procedure in which a balloon is inserted into a blocked artery and then inflated to compress the clogging "gunk," thereby widening the space through which blood can flow. The problem is that reclogging occurs in up to 45 percent of patients within 6 months. But at Laval University in Quebec, the blood vessels of patients given large, therapeutic doses of omega-3 oils starting 3 weeks before angioplasty and continuing for 6 months of follow-up remained less obstructed than the blood vessels of angioplasty patients not taking omega-3s.

Easing arthritis pain

Many of the 2.5 million people in the U.S. who have rheumatoid arthritis ease the pain in their joints with anti-inflammatory drugs, like aspirin and ibuprofen. But these medications often come with side effects, including stomach discomfort and gastrointestinal bleeding.

Omega-3 supplements may have the potential to replace the drugs, at least to some degree. In more than a dozen studies conducted during the last 10 years, arthritis patients taking omega-3 capsules experienced fewer tender and swollen joints than they had without taking the pills. In addition, morning stiffness lessened. In some instances, patients were able to taper or discontinue their use of anti-inflammatories. It appears that omega-3s suppress a

sequence of events that occurs between the cells of the immune system and those of the joints, a wanted effect because arthritis occurs when the immune system attacks the body's own tissues.

Ongoing investigations will help determine whether omega-3 fatty acids should be used as part of standard arthritis treatment. At present, says Albany Medical College's Joel Kremer, MD, an arthritis researcher who has conducted many of the studies with omega-3s, there remain gaps in knowledge about the bottom-line effectiveness of the fats and about optimal amounts to prescribe. What is known is that omega-3 supplements must generally be taken continuously for at least 12 weeks before patients observe improvements. The improvements appear to increase if treatment lasts at least 18 to 24 weeks.

Unfortunately, it is not possible to get the amounts that appear beneficial from foods alone. A diet with 1 to 2 fish meals every day would be needed to approach the level of omega-3s proven effective in studies, Dr. Kremer says.

For people suffering with arthritis pain who want to try fish oil pills, the senior vice president for medical affairs at the Arthritis Foundation, Doyt Conn, MD, says it's a reasonable idea as long as they discuss it with their physicians. He does point out, however, that the effects generally have been modest. In addition, he says that to portray fish oil as *the* remedy for arthritis would be misleading. "It's fine if it makes someone a little more comfortable," he says. "But it shouldn't be thought of as a replacement for traditional arthritis treatment."

A fish oil regimen also is not something everybody would comply with, Dr. Conn notes. Many capsules contain only about 300 milligrams of omega-3 fatty acids. It would take 8 to 10 horse-pill-sized capsules daily to reach the 2.5 to 3 grams found effective in studies (or 6 ounces of, say, Atlantic salmon every single day).

Note: Do not take large amounts of cod liver oil or any other fish oil preparation

of regular Frosted Flakes has 160 calories. Neither one contains any fat. A cup of either has 4 to 5 teaspoons of sugar.

that has not been stripped of vitamins A and D. Those 2 nutrients can be toxic to the liver in large doses.

Omega-3s for babies?

An omega-3 fatty acid known as docosahexaenoic acid, or DHA, helps make up the membranes surrounding each brain cell, making it one of the most prominent fatty acids in the brain. Researchers believe the availability of DHA to the brain may be particularly important to a developing infant in the last 3 months of pregnancy, when the baby's rate of brain growth is greatest.

Getting enough DHA to the brain is not a problem if the baby is carried for the full 9-month term. A pregnant woman's body releases DHA from stores she has accumulated in her fat tissues throughout her life and delivers it to the fetus through the placenta. But if a baby is born prematurely and then put on formula, it is cut off from the mother's supply of DHA. That could help explain the high risk of damage to the brain and the rest of the central nervous system in children born early. Premature babies may also be at risk of compromised eyesight; the retina has the highest levels of DHA of all tissues in the body.

At issue is whether DHA should be added to American baby formula, not just for the one in 9 babies born prematurely in this country but also for full-term infants who are bottle-fed. Bottle-fed babies miss the DHA supplied by breast milk, which gets into a newborn's still-developing neurologic system.

Formula does contain omega-3 fatty acids that the body is capable of converting to DHA. But it is not known whether newborns, particularly those born prematurely, are able to convert those acids fast enough to meet the needs of the brain and the rest of the nervous system.

Several countries in Europe and Asia already allow DHA in baby formulas. Their decisions were no doubt fueled, at least in part, by studies showing that infants given DHA-containing breast milk have IQs a few points higher than those fed formula.

But the Food and Drug Administration, which oversees the contents of infant formula, is taking a wait-and-see approach. The American Academy of Pediatrics's Committee on Nutrition also believes the data are too sketchy at this point to make a determination.

Consider that the findings thus far have been inconsistent, especially for full-term babies. Some studies have provided evidence that DHA is associated with improved brain and visual function, while others have indicated that babies fed formula without DHA suffer no shortfall in mental or visual development. Still other research shows only a short-term improvement that "washes out" when children get a little older.

One reason it's hard to pin down the effect of DHA in a baby's diet is that so many variables can affect a child's mental abilities. For instance, breast milk contains DHA, but it also contains many other nutrients that could affect such things as IQ measurements. In addition, breast-feeding mothers in the U.S. tend to be relatively well-educated and financially secure, both variables that could positively influence an infant's cognitive, or learning, capacity. It's hard to tease out the effects of those factors, even in well-controlled studies.

A possible treatment for depression

In the last 100 years, the incidence of depression in the U.S. has progressively increased, and it begins at younger ages than it used to. More than 15 million Americans now suffer from the problem.

At the same time that depression rates have gone up, consumption of omega-3 fatty acids in relation to other fats has gone down. Joseph Hibbeln, MD, a psychiatrist at the National Institutes of Health, believes that the shift may not be a coincidence.

To keep mood properly elevated, a chemical in the brain known as serotonin has to fire messages from one brain cell to another. If the fatty membranes surrounding brain cells are relatively fluid like machine oil, the thinking goes, it's easier for the messages to get transmitted properly after serotonin sets things in motion. If the membranes are not so fluid and more like lard, on the other hand, the messages presumably are harder to transmit. That's where omega-3s come in. The brain specifically requires them for an optimal consistency of cell membranes.

It's much too early to suggest that people should eat more fish to stave off or relieve depression, Dr. Hibbeln says. But ongoing experimental work probing a possible connection between depression and an omega-3 shortfall may someday provide a new approach for people suffering from the mood disorder.

Eating More Omega-3s

Two broad categories of fatty acids are found in polyunsaturated fats: omega-3s and omega-6s. Omega-6s, abundant in most cooking oils, currently make up the lion's share of polyunsaturates in the American diet. In fact, the ratio of omega-6s to omega-3s that we eat is about 9 to one. It wasn't always that way.

When humans were still hunter-gatherers who foraged for their food rather than cultivated everything on farms and ranches, and before the advent of technology that enabled the easy manufacture of cooking oil, the ratio of omega-6s to omega-3s was about one to one. Wild game such as deer, rabbits and wild turkeys contain a much higher proportion of omega-3s than ranch-raised animals, and leaves pulled off plants in the jungle and open fields contain more omega-3s than planted crops.

These are not the same omega-3s found in fish, which are the ones scientists generally refer to when they talk about health benefits. But to some degree, the body can convert omega-3s from those sources to the types of omega-3s found in fish—eicosapentaenoic acid (EPA) and docosahexaenoic acid (DHA).

Omega-3s are also available (up to a point) in green leafy vegetables, nuts, canola oil, soybean oil, and tofu. But since we currently get so few omega-3s from non-fish foods to convert to EPA and DHA, the most efficient dietary way to get those 2 substances is simply to eat more fish. The chart shows the amount of EPA and DHA combined in various species of fish. Fatty species have more EPA and DHA than lean fish. Many experts suggest people eat 2 to 3 fish meals a week.

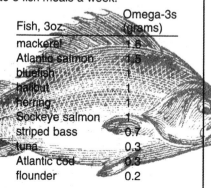

Fish, 3oz.	Omega-3s (grams)
mackerel	1.8
Atlantic salmon	1.5
bluefish	1
halibut	1
herring	1
Sockeye salmon	1
striped bass	0.7
tuna	0.3
Atlantic cod	0.3
flounder	0.2

The facts about fats

Not all fats clog the arteries. Here's how to tell good from bad.

Fat in the diet has a bad reputation, but not all types of fat deserve it. Changes to food labels in recent years have helped consumers tell one type from another—but labels don't tell the whole story. To protect your heart, you need to pay attention not only to how much fat you eat but to which kind of fat—and you need to know how to find out what you're eating.

Saturated or not

The difference between fats that are hazardous to the heart and those that aren't stems from a simple chemical distinction. Fat molecules that have a hydrogen atom at every available binding site, like those in meats, dairy products, and certain tropical oils (such as coconut, palm, and palm-kernel oils), are saturated fats—so called because the binding sites are "saturated" with hydrogen. Fats with a single pair of hydrogen atoms missing, like the main fats in canola and olive oil, are *mono*unsaturated. Fats with two or more pairs of hydrogen atoms missing, like the main fats in corn, soybean, and other vegetable oils as well as in fish oils, are *poly*unsaturated. (All so-called "unsaturated" oils are actually a blend of monounsaturated, polyunsaturated, and even saturated fats.)

Because changing even a single atom in a molecule can profoundly affect its chemical properties, saturated and unsaturated fats have strikingly different effects on health. The clearest difference is that saturated fats increase the risk of coronary heart disease, whereas unsaturated fats do not. Eating saturated fats raises blood levels of cholesterol, which accumulates on the artery walls and can eventually restrict blood flow, especially to the heart. The saturated fat in foods has a far greater effect on blood levels of cholesterol in the body than does the cholesterol in foods. (Contrary to popular belief, cholesterol is not a type of fat.)

In contrast, studies have shown that monounsaturated and polyunsaturated fats can actually *reduce* blood-cholesterol levels, partly by spurring the liver to clear cholesterol from the blood, but particularly when those fats are substituted for saturated fat in the diet. (Over the years, some researchers have proposed that consuming more unsaturated oils would help lower blood-cholesterol levels even if saturated-fat intake was unchanged. But any such effect would be small at best—and would add loads of needless calories.)

Early evidence had suggested that monounsaturated fat might have an edge over polyunsaturated fat: Polyunsaturates appeared to lower the "good" HDL cholesterol along with the "bad" LDL cholesterol, while monounsaturates appeared to cut LDL only. That apparent difference, much ballyhooed several years ago by the olive-oil industry, prompted some health experts to advise people to replace polyunsaturated oils with monounsaturated ones whenever possible. But further research couldn't confirm polyunsaturates' reported negative impact on HDL cholesterol. And some studies even suggested that polyunsaturates were better than monounsaturates at reducing LDL levels. It now appears that, at levels commonly found in the diet, monos and polys have roughly the same effects on blood cholesterol.

Preliminary studies in animals had raised an additional health concern about polyunsaturated fat—that it might increase the risk of certain types of cancer. But no convincing evidence has emerged for such a threat in humans. (However, some evidence suggests an association between intake of *saturated* fat and certain cancers, notably of the colon and prostate.)

Trans fat vs. saturated fat

As awareness grew about the risks of saturated fats, most fast-food chains and food manufacturers switched from beef fat and tropical oils to vegetable oil. To make the vegetable oil firmer and less likely to spoil, food makers bubbled hydrogen through it, producing hydrogenated oil, rich in what's called "trans" fat. Today, trans fat is widely used in deep frying and in prepared foods such as baked goods and snacks. It also gives margarine its butter-like consistency.

For a long time, most researchers assumed trans fat was as safe to eat as the vegetable oil it was derived from. But the molecular changes that make vegetable fat more like animal fat chemically also appear to make it more like animal fat in its health effects. While clinical studies haven't linked trans fats directly to heart attacks, many researchers now believe that, gram for gram, trans fat is nearly as bad for your blood-cholesterol levels as saturated fat is. Recently, Brandeis University scientists went even further. In an extensive analysis of trans-fat research published last summer, they concluded that trans fats may be *worse* than saturated fats because they appear to deliver a double whammy: While both trans fats and saturated fats raise damaging LDL-cholesterol levels, saturated fats also raise protective HDL-cholesterol levels; trans fats, on the other hand, may *lower* HDL.

Many researchers now believe that, gram for gram, trans fat is nearly as bad for your cholesterol levels as saturated fat is.

Those disturbing findings about hydrogenated oils have left people who switched from butter to margarine in a quandary. More than half the readers we recently surveyed thought that neither spread was better for the heart. But butter is still the greater of two evils: It has about 8 grams of saturated fat per tablespoon, more than the combined total of trans and saturated fats in a tablespoon of stick margarine. (Moreover, unlike margarine, butter also contains some cholesterol.) Soft margarine—whether in a tub or in a squeeze container—is better than stick margarine, since it's less hydrogenated. Specially for-mulated "light" margarines, such as *Promise Ultra*, *Smart Beat*, and others, cut fat (and calories) still further by replacing some of the oil with water; a tablespoon of those products contains a gram or less of trans fat and saturated fat combined. They're still just fat, however, not health food. *Promise's* "Get Heart Smart" advertising campaign ran afoul of the U.S. Federal Trade Commission last year for seeming to imply otherwise.

Trans fats aren't listed on food labels, so you have to read between the lines carefully (see box, next page). But keep in mind that while trans fat matters,

Transfats aren't listed on food labels, so you have to read between the lines carefully (see "Finding the hidden trans fat" box). But keep in mind that while trans fat matters, cutting down on saturated fat is still the single most important dietary step you can take to protect your heart, since there's so much more saturated fat than trans fat in the diet.

What you can do

Standard public-health recommendations call for a diet that gets no more than 30 percent of its total calories from fat, and less than 10 percent of calories from saturated fat. The average American now gets about 33 percent of total calories from fat, and just over 11 percent of calories from saturated fat. An additional 3 to 4 percent of daily calories comes from trans fat. While there is no official recommendation for limiting trans-fat consumption, nutrition experts advise counting trans fat as part of your saturated-fat budget.

Here are some ways to reduce your intake of both artery-cloggers:

■ Eat less meat and full-fat dairy foods. Replace those foods with grains, fruits and vegetables, fish, and (skinless) poultry, and choose reduced-fat versions of dairy foods.

■ Beware of so-called tropical oils—coconut oil, palm oil, and palm-kernel oil. They're vegetable oils, but they're highly saturated.

■ To reduce your use of all cooking oils, bake, boil, broil, microwave, poach, or steam foods instead of frying, deep-frying, or sautéing them.

■ If you do sauté, grease a nonstick pan lightly with vegetable oil. Or try a vegetable-oil spray, which allows you to use less oil. You could also sauté foods in broth or wine instead of oil.

■ Replace butter with tub or "squeeze" margarine. (Check the label to see that liquid oil, not partially hydrogenated oil, is listed as the first ingredient.) Or try a reduced-fat "light" margarine.

■ To avoid hidden trans fat, eat less prepared baked goods—pies, doughnuts, ready-made frosting, biscuits, and crackers. And minimize consumption of foods heavy in hydrogenated or partially hydrogenated vegetable oil. (See box next page.)

Summing up

All fats are not equal. Some types clog the arteries, others may even help keep the arteries clear. Here's the overall strategy to follow:

■ Hold down the overall fat content of your diet—and minimize your intake of foods rich in saturated fat in particular.

■ Don't just add "heart-healthy" unsaturated fat to your diet—but do substitute it for saturated fat wherever possible.

■ Choose between monounsaturated oils (such as canola, olive, or peanut oil) and polyunsaturated oils (such as corn, safflower, or soybean oil) based on the desired taste; in terms of health effects, there appears to be no significant difference between the two types of unsaturated oil.

■ Find and minimize the trans fat that's hidden in your diet.

Finding the hidden trans fat

The Nutrition Facts food labels go a long way toward helping consumers know how much total fat, saturated fat, and unsaturated fat they're eating. But the labels say nothing about how much *trans* fat a product contains, even though many researchers now consider it nearly as villainous as saturated fat. These two guides should help.

Reading between the lines

If the ingredients list includes "partially hydrogenated" oils, the product contains trans fat. How much? The label won't tell you directly. But sometimes you can tell indirectly. If the label gives the amount of other fats—saturated, polyunsaturated, and monounsaturated—you can add those figures together and subtract them from the amount of total fat. What remains should be the approximate amount of trans fat the product contains. In this example—*Reduced*

INGREDIENTS: WHOLE WHEAT FLOUR, ENRICHED WHEAT FLOUR (CONTAINS NIACIN, REDUCED IRON, THIAMINE MONONITRATE [VITAMIN B₁], RIBOFLAVIN [VITAMIN B₂]), VEGETABLE SHORTENING (PARTIALLY HYDROGENATED SOYBEAN OIL), SUGAR, SALT, HIGH FRUCTOSE CORN SYRUP, MALTED BARLEY FLOUR, LEAVENING (CALCIUM PHOSPHATE, BAKING SODA), ANNATTO EXTRACT AND TURMERIC OLEORESIN (VEGETABLE COLORS).

	% Daily Value
Total Fat 4g	**6%**
Saturated Fat 0.5g	**3%**
Polyunsaturated Fat 0g	
Monounsaturated Fat 1.5g	

Fat Wheat Thins—adding the amounts of those three fats and subtracting them from the total leaves about 2 grams, or half the fat in the crackers, unaccounted for. It's probably 2 grams of trans fat.

Relying on the USDA

The bar chart below shows data, from the U.S. Department of Agriculture, for several foods that contain particularly high levels of trans fat—in fact, often more trans fat than saturated fat. Each item represents a national brand, which the agency declines to name. In most categories, the trans-fat content of the product we've listed is similar to that of other brands, but not always. To give you the full picture, we've provided the number of grams of total fat, saturated fat, and trans fat per standard serving. Included for comparison purposes are butter, stick margarine, and a "light" tub margarine.

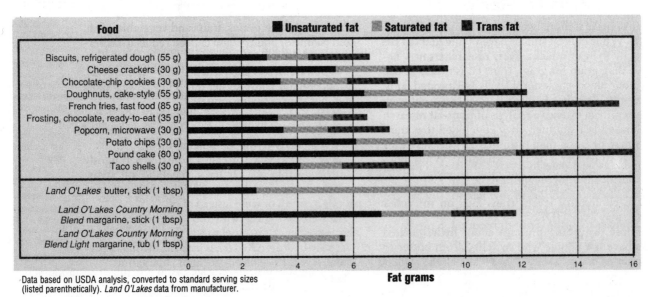

Data based on USDA analysis, converted to standard serving sizes (listed parenthetically). *Land O'Lakes* data from manufacturer.

Should you be eating more protein—or less?

Americans have had a love/hate relationship with protein, and the protein pendulum has been swinging like crazy lately. Many of us grew up thinking only good things about protein. Indeed, we can't live without it. But the trouble may be too much of a good thing. Indeed, some researchers have linked a high intake of animal protein to heart disease and other chronic disorders. On the other hand, high-protein weight-loss diets are the craze once again, as they were in the late sixties and early seventies (see box). If all this increasingly contradictory advice about protein makes your head spin, here's the lowdown.

What's the problem with eating lots of protein?
A diet high in protein—especially animal protein—is associated with an increased risk not only of heart disease and some cancers (such as colon and prostate), but also of osteoporosis and kidney damage. *However, it's hard to prove this link, since we seldom eat pure protein.* People who eat lots of animal protein do have higher rates of heart disease and cancers, but their diets also tend to be high in fat and low in antioxidants and fiber, as well as other potentially beneficial substances. Moreover, those who eat lots of animal protein may also be less health-conscious in general and less physically active than others. It may be such factors, rather than protein intake itself, that account for most of the increased risks.

Is protein from plants more healthful?
In carefully controlled studies, animals fed large amounts of isolated animal protein develop higher levels of blood cholesterol (especially LDL, the "bad" kind) than those fed vegetable protein. This suggests that something about the composition of animal protein boosts cholesterol.

People who get their protein from plants have a lower risk of heart disease and are healthier in general. Last year, for instance, a widely publicized analysis of the benefits of soy protein suggested that it helps lower blood cholesterol and is thus good for the heart (though other compounds in soy may be largely responsible, see *Wellness Letter,* November 1995). Vegetarian sources of protein are also preferable because they're usually low in fat and high in fiber and other potentially beneficial sub-stances. Nevertheless, a few studies have suggested that a very high intake of even plant protein is undesirable, but it's rare for vegetarians to consume such large amounts of protein.

Don't vegetarians have trouble getting enough protein?
Vegetarian diets generally supply more than enough protein. Many grains, legumes, nuts, and seeds are good sources of protein. However, except for soybeans, plant foods contain protein that's incomplete—that is, it has low and sometimes insufficient amounts of one or more of the nine essential amino acids. (Amino acids are protein's building blocks; the essential ones are those the body can't synthesize.) But if vegetarians eat a wide variety of foods each day, they're likely to absorb a full complement of amino acids. They don't need to eat the comple-mentary proteins at the same meal.

What's the link between protein and osteoporosis?
As your protein intake rises, so does the amount of calcium excreted in urine. If you eat lots of protein, this calcium loss may affect the density of your bones and thus may hasten the devel-opment of osteoporosis (bone thinning). This notion is still controversial, but was recently bolstered by a 12-year Harvard study of 86,000 nurses. In it, women who ate lots of animal protein (more than 95 grams a day), especially red meat, had 22% more forearm fractures than those consuming less protein. How-ever, the study didn't actually measure the degree of osteoporosis in the women. In addition, it's likely that a high protein intake endangers your bones only if you consume inadequate amounts of calcium. Thus you should continue to consume milk and other dairy products.

If you exercise a lot, don't you need more protein?
Yes and no. You need adequate protein intake to build and repair muscles, but most active Americans, including vegetarians, get more than enough of it. In the old days, in their quest for added protein, athletes were likely to wolf down T-bone steaks or raw eggs. Today they often turn to high-protein powders, drinks, tablets, capsules, and bars. This is unnecessary. Recent studies do suggest that some endurance athletes or serious weight lifters need more protein than the Recommended Dietary Allowance

(RDA, see below), but because of their greater food intake, they get the extra protein with little trouble. Protein supplements or isolated amino acids won't stimulate muscle growth—only exercise, specifically strength training, does. Excess protein is simply broken down in the body and burned for energy or turned into fat. Strength training, like any exercise, requires extra calories, but the bulk of these should come from complex carbohydrates (starches).

What about the elderly?
This is one group that may have a protein shortfall. Several studies have found that the elderly need a little more protein than the RDA, since the body uses protein less efficiently as it ages. Meanwhile about one-quarter of elderly women actually consume less than the RDA, particularly since they tend to eat less food. This shortfall may compromise their health. If you're over 65, keep an eye on your protein intake.

How much protein do you need?
Proteins are constantly being broken down in our bodies. Most of the amino acids are reused, but we must regularly replace those that are lost.

The daily RDA for protein is the amount the average person needs to stay healthy. It's based on age and weight, and usually works out to about 8% of daily calories—that's fairly little, about as much as is consumed in China. The RDA for adults is 0.8 grams of protein for each kilogram (2.2 pounds) of body weight. That adds up to 64 grams (about 2 ounces) of pure protein for a 175-pound man, and 47 grams for a 130-pound woman. To estimate *your* protein requirement, determine your weight in

---

Do you *really* want to lose weight on a high-protein diet?

High-protein, low-carbohydrate (and usually high-fat) diets are back, and with a vengeance. Newspapers, books, and TV shows are offering testimonials from "carbohydrate dropouts" who swear by them. The fact is, there are basically only a handful of crash diets, and this type pops up every decade or two.

The protein craze has been making headlines because of the growing distrust of "established" nutritional wisdom, and specifically a backlash against high-carbohydrate diets. The protein-diet advocates are now blaming the rise in obesity in this country on excessive carbohydrate intake, which they claim causes insulin resistance and thus weight gain in millions. As we reported in May 1995 in our article on the "pasta scare," this argument doesn't hold water. There's no evidence that carbohydrates, especially complex carbohydrates (starches), stimulate appetite and/or lead to more or easier fat storage and weight gain. And if you do cut down on complex carbohydrates such as grains and vegetables, what are your alternatives? Certainly not more fat: the dangers of a high-fat diet are clear. And not more protein: excessive protein intake carries potential health risks, from kidney damage to osteoporosis, as described above.

Carbo bashers, protein pushers
Among the recent protein-diet books are *Protein Power* by Drs. Michael and Mary Eades, *The Carbohydrate Addict's Diet* by Drs. Rachael and Richard Heller, and *The Zone* by Dr. Barry Sears. The most extreme of these diets is Dr. Robert Atkins's *New Diet Revolution,* a rehash of his 1972 book. It claims that a high-protein, high-fat, low-carbohydrate diet not only promotes weight loss, but also reduces cholesterol and blood pressure and lowers the risk of heart disease and cancer.

On the Atkins diet, you get bacon and eggs for breakfast, but no bread, cereal, or orange juice. Lunch may be a bunless bacon cheeseburger with a small salad. You do without bread, rice, pasta, vegetables, and fruit, eating virtually nothing but protein and fat. Dr. Atkins's plan, like all these diets, is actually a low-calorie diet in disguise. He doesn't specify quantities, but there's not much food in the weight-loss phase of the diet, certainly not enough to supply the vitamins and minerals you need (Atkins recommends pills, preferably the "formulas" he

sells). Cut calories and you lose weight—surprise, surprise.

Your body will indeed begin to burn its own fat on this regimen. Actually, you burn fat all the time, but without carbohydrates your body does not burn the fat completely, and thus substances called ketones are formed and released into your bloodstream. At first, this condition, known as ketosis, may make dieting easier, because it often kills the appetite and even causes nausea. Dr. Atkins and the other protein promoters consider this state "normal" and even "benign." Ketosis is indeed the body's normal way to adapt to this abnormal situation, as it would to fasting. However, ketosis will eventually increase blood levels of uric acid—a risk factor for gout and kidney stones in susceptible people. But before that, if you consume inadequate amounts of carbohydrates, other adverse effects can also occur—weakness, diarrhea, dizziness, headaches, to name just a few. No wonder you lose weight.

What about all the diet doctors' "evidence"?
Their evidence is almost all anecdotal. There are no controlled studies showing that high-protein diets are more effective than any other low-calorie diets. Several of the doctors talk a great deal about eicosanoids, hormone-like substances that control countless physiological functions. They claim that a high carbohydrate intake, by boosting insulin levels, produces a dangerous balance of eicosanoids. However, these compounds are still little understood, and diet (except perhaps for certain fats, such as fish oil) probably has only a minor effect on them.

A diet rich in complex carbohydrates remains the best. Fruits, grains, and vegetables, along with low-fat dairy products and small amounts of meats, provide the vitamins, minerals, and fiber you need. Numerous controlled studies have shown that such a diet helps protect against heart disease, diabetes, and various cancers, as well as aiding in weight control. And it's *not* a crash diet, but a way of eating for the rest of your life.

Words to the wise: In the short term, you could lose weight on these high-protein diets, but they could be dangerous, particularly if followed beyond a few weeks. Like all crash diets, they don't work over the long haul. Quick weight loss is easy—keeping the weight off is the hard part.

kilograms by dividing your weight in pounds by 2.2. Then multiply the result by 0.8. For example, a 150-pound person would require (150 ÷ 2.2) x 0.8 = 55 grams. If you are overweight, you may need less than your result.

Where do those grams of protein come from?
Leading sources of protein are:

- Meat, chicken, and fish: 6 to 8 grams per ounce.
- Dairy products: a cup of milk, 8 grams; yogurt, 10 to 13.
- Eggs: 6 grams each.
- Grains: 1 slice of bread or half cup of pasta, 3 grams.
- Beans: 7 grams per half cup (cooked).
- Nuts: 6 grams per ounce.

Grain products are often overlooked as protein sources—they supply 16 to 20% of the total protein intake in the U.S. Even vegetables contain some protein, albeit smaller amounts (a half cup of broccoli or asparagus has 2 grams).

As you can see, it's hard *not* to get the RDA. For most people, three ounces of lean meat, half a cup of beans, and a cup each of pasta, yogurt, and milk supply more than enough protein for a day. The RDA assumes that you eat a mixed diet of proteins— some from animal sources (high-quality because it offers a complete mix of essential amino acids), some from plant sources (mostly incomplete). Children under 18, along with pregnant or lactating women, need a little more protein per pound of body weight than others.

How much is too much?
Government surveys show that the *average* American man under age 65 consumes 90 to 110 grams of protein per day, and the average woman, 65 to 70 grams—about 50% more than the RDA. There's no evidence that such levels endanger your health, provided the protein isn't accompanied by lots of fat. However, many Americans consume much more than that. A one-pound steak, not unusual fare in restaurants, can supply 100 grams of protein by itself.

The "upper bound" for protein is twice the RDA, according to the National Research Council. Consuming more than that, over the long term, increases the risk of chronic disease and is definitely not recommended. If you eat more than 120 grams of protein a day, cut back. *Most important, try to get more of your protein from plants than from animals.* That way you're likely to get less fat and cholesterol and more of the good things found in grains, beans, and vegetables.

A 'Bran-New' Look at
DIETARY FIBER*

By Kathleen A. Meister and Jack Raso

A couple of generations ago, "bulk" and "roughage" were the prevalent terms for dietary fiber, whose usefulness in the diet was considered limited to preventing constipation. Scientists have since learned that fiber encompasses diverse substances with various potentially important effects on health.

What Is Dietary Fiber?

Dietary fiber consists of plant materials (mostly carbohydrates) that human digestive enzymes cannot break down. Foods of animal origin do not contain any fiber. Whole grains contain substantially more fiber than refined grains, because "refining" entails removal of some of the fiber. Whole grains, legumes, and nuts generally contain more fiber than refined grains, non-leguminous vegetables, and fruits.

There are two types of dietary fiber: *insoluble* and *soluble*. Soluble fibers include gums and some pectins—gluey substances used to make jellies. The distinguishing characteristic of soluble fibers is that, after mixing with water in laboratory studies, particles of purified soluble fibers remain interspersed in the water. The *in*soluble fiber publicized most often is cellulose, the raw material of cellophane and paper.

Table 1 on page 11 indicates the amounts of soluble and insoluble fiber that University of Wisconsin researchers found in various foods. Foods with significant concentrations of soluble fibers include barley, oats, legumes, sweet potatoes, and white potatoes. The insoluble fiber concentration of foods almost always exceeds the soluble fiber concentration. Foods particularly high in insoluble fibers include whole wheat and wheat bran.

Fiber Supplements

Scientific evidence for the healthfulness of a high-fiber diet is much more compelling than that for the healthfulness of fiber itself. Therefore, experts generally recommend increasing dietary fiber intake by increasing consumption of grains, legumes, vegetables, and fruits rather than by taking fiber supplements. There are some exceptions to this rule. Certain kinds of fiber have proved useful against specific health problems—as wheat bran for chronic constipation, or pectins (found in apple peel) for diarrhea.

*Based on *Dietary Fiber*, ACSH Special Report.

Grains, Fruits, and Vegetables

Most of the scientific literature concerning the health effects of consuming plant foods focuses on fruits and vegetables rather than on grains. Some scientific studies associate high grain intakes with good health; others associate high grain intakes with poor health. A partial explanation for this inconsistency is that in many societies high-grain diets are a distinction of the poor, who typically have unmet healthcare needs. It is difficult to tease out information on the health effects of grain consumption from studies of populations in which socioeconomic effects on health are critical. Substantial nutritional differences between whole-grain and refined-grain products may also confound the grain-health connection.

Although information on the health effects of grains is not as plentiful as that on the health effects of fruits and vegetables, daily consumption of grain products as a significant part of the diet is advisable, as grains are low in fat and are a major source of vitamins and minerals as well as fiber.

Fiber and Specific Health Problems

Diverticulosis

Diverticula are small, fingerlike projections or pouches in the colon wall. The term *diverticulosis* refers to the presence of multiple diverticula. Roughly one third of all North Americans over the age of 45—and two thirds of all persons over the age of 85—have diverticula in their colons. Usually, the mere presence of diverticula does not cause any symptoms; between 75 and 90 percent of people with diverticula are asymptomatic.

Diverticulosis usually does not lead to serious problems. In some persons, however, the diverticula become inflamed. This painful acute condition, called *diverticulitis*, may require hospitalization, antibiotic therapy, or surgery.

Many physicians recommend that people with diverticulosis increase their intake of fiber, which may help relieve mild symptoms such as constipation and moderate abdominal discomfort. However, fiber is not used in the treatment of divercul*itis*. (Indeed, the physician may initially order "NPO"—the abbreviation for a Latin phrase that means "nothing by mouth.")

Some studies suggest that a high-fiber diet contributes to the prevention of diverticulosis. One hypothesis is that low-fiber diets promote diverticulosis because they lead to straining at stool, or difficulty

How to Increase Your Fiber Intake

- Eat at least six servings of grain products, at least three servings of vegetables, and at least two servings of fruits daily. Respective examples of servings are: one slice of whole-wheat bread, one-half cup of cooked vegetables, and one orange. Vary your selections within each food group, as foods in the same group may have considerable nutritional differences. For instance, carrots are high in provitamin A but low in vitamin C, while the reverse is true for green peppers.

- Consume whole-grain foods—brown (unpolished) rice, oatmeal, and whole-wheat bread, for example—more often than refined-grain foods, such as white bread and white rice.

- Consume fruits more often than fruit juices.

- Eat legumes (such as kidney beans, lentils, and lima beans) several times a week.

- Increase your fluid intake if you increase your intake of dietary fiber.

in defecating; this increases colon pressure and thus leads to the formation of diverticula.

The findings of a study published in 1994 in the *American Journal of Clinical Nutrition* support the belief that fiber is protective against diverticulosis. This study, which involved more than 40,000 middle-aged to elderly men, showed that higher fiber intakes translated into a lower incidence of symptom-generating diverticulosis. However, this protective effect was attributable largely to fiber from fruits and vegetables, not to fiber from grain products—the source generally recommended to diverticulosis patients.

New Label Claim

A new fiber-related claim will soon appear on the labels of some food products. Last January the Food and Drug Administration announced that the labels of foods with certain levels of *beta-glucan*, a soluble fiber found in whole oats, may include health claims. These claims relate to the finding that, in conjunction with diets low in saturated fat, beta-glucan can decrease blood cholesterol. To bear this claim, a product must provide at least 3/4 gram of soluble fiber per serving. The scientific studies on which the FDA based its decision suggest that, to decrease cholesterol, a daily intake of approximately 3 grams of soluble fiber is necessary. To head off the inference that whole oats or soluble fibers are magic bullets against cholesterol-related heart disease, the FDA-approved claim includes the phrase "diets low in saturated fat and cholesterol."

—*Dr. Ruth Kava*

Colon Cancer

Scientists have long suspected that high intakes of dietary fiber might decrease the risk of colon cancer, one of the most common types of cancer in Western populations. Several plausible mechanisms for a protective effect have been proposed. For example, fiber may protect people against colon cancer by increasing the bulk of intestinal waste, thus diluting carcinogenic substances therein, and/or by accelerating colon contents through the intestinal tract, thus decreasing the exposure of the colon walls to carcinogens. Other, more complex protective mechanisms have been proposed.

However, studies of human populations have not established that high fiber intakes *per se* decrease colon cancer risk. Rather, the data suggest a relationship between diets high in fruits and vegetables—and possibly diets high in whole grains—and a relatively low risk of colon cancer. The apparent protectiveness of fruits, vegetables, and whole-grain products may be attributable, at least in part, to certain plant constituents other than fiber, or to the substitution of fruits, vegetables, and whole-grain foods for less healthful foods. Therefore, taking purified fiber supplements to prevent colon cancer is not advisable.

Blood Cholesterol Levels

The effect of dietary fiber on blood cholesterol levels has been a controversial subject. Many scientific studies have established that (unlike wheat bran and cellulose) the soluble fiber in certain foods and supplements—including guar guam, legumes, oat bran, oatmeal, pectin, and psyllium—can lower serum cholesterol. However, the decrease is modest and requires relatively high daily intakes. For example, consumption of three packets of instant oatmeal daily typically causes a cholesterol decrease of only 2 to 3 percent. Consuming oat bran and other sources of soluble fiber cannot effectively substitute for a low-saturated-fat diet but can augment its cholesterol-lowering effect.

Coronary Heart Disease (CHD)

Several studies of human populations have correlated higher fiber intakes with lower CHD risk and vice versa. Generally, the cholesterol-lowering effect of soluble fiber is too small to account for this correlation. Some researchers have thus theorized that effects unrelated to cholesterol levels—effects on blood clotting, sugar metabolism, and body weight, for example—contribute to fiber's apparent protectiveness against CHD. Other scientists have proposed that fiber is not a protective factor but is primarily a lifestyle marker: People whose diets are, by choice, high in fiber tend to have many healthy habits, and some or all of these habits may decrease their risk of CHD.

Weight Control

Fiber-rich foods are usually low in calories and fat, and they are conducive to *satiety*—a feeling of fullness in the stomach. But whether fiber itself can facilitate weight loss is uncertain. More than 20 scientific studies—none lasting more than three months—have focused on the relationship between fiber intake and the caloric intakes and body weights of volunteers. Wheat-bran fiber, apparently, does not decrease food intake or body weight. Whether other types of fiber can contribute to weight loss remains to be determined. Even more uncertain is whether dietary fiber is useful in long-term weight control.

Fiber Hazards

While moderately high-fiber diets appear safe for healthy adults, fiber supplementation and diets extremely high in fiber may not be.

Many people report gastrointestinal disturbances—gas pains, flatulence, or diarrhea, for example—after increasing their fiber intake. A common assertion is that such effects subside as the body adapts to higher intakes, but evidence of this is scarce. Advice to increase fiber intake gradually to limit gastrointestinal problems arises from clinical experience rather than from controlled scientific studies.

To prevent constipation or an intestinal obstruction, those who take fiber supplements should consume relatively large amounts of fluids. Other side effects are less common: A small percentage of people are severely allergic to psyllium. Guar gum supplements can cause esophageal obstruction but rarely do.

Substances in or accompanying dietary fiber may bind to mineral nutrients and thus impede their absorption. However, such an action is probably inconsequential for most adults on Western-style high-fiber diets, which are also relatively high in minerals. High-fiber diets tend to be higher in minerals than low-fiber diets, because many fiber-rich foods are good sources of minerals. The effect of fiber *supplements* on mineral absorption might be harmful, because (unlike fiber-rich foods) the supplements do not provide minerals.

Fiber in Proper Perspective

Dietary fiber is by no means a universal preventative, and fiber supplements have limited utility. But for most adults high-fiber *diets*—particularly diets high in fruits and vegetables—appear more healthful than low-fiber diets. American adults typically consume fewer servings of vegetables, fruits, and grain products than experts recommend; most would probably benefit from increasing their intakes of these foods.

KATHLEEN MEISTER, M.S., IS A FREELANCE MEDICAL WRITER AND A FORMER ACSH RESEARCH ASSOCIATE. JACK RASO, M.S., R.D., IS ACSH'S DIRECTOR OF PUBLICATIONS.

Food for Thought about Dietary Supplements

The surge of public interest in nutrition supplements has been fired by the recently enacted federal regulations governing health claims, which permits the health food industry to make claims about the function of nutrients not permitted for food products. This article provides healthy skepticism about the common rationales for the use of supplements.

PAUL R. THOMAS, Ed.D., R.D.

Paul Thomas, currently a Fellow at the Georgetown Center for Food and Nutrition Policy, Georgetown University, previously served as a staff scientist for the Food and Nutrition Board, Institute of Medicine, National Academy of Sciences. He is a registered dietitian who received an Ed.D. degree in nutrition education from Columbia University. He is an author and editor of several books on contemporary nutrition issues. Correspondence can be directed to him at the Georgetown Center for Food and Nutrition Policy, 3240 Prospect Street, N.W., Washington, DC 20007.

The dietary supplements industry is very healthy. Sales of vitamins, minerals, and other food concentrates are roughly $4 billion per year. Although at least one quarter of American adults swallow these pills, powders, and potions daily,[1] probably the majority of us take them at least occasionally. What are we getting in return?

I've asked myself this question since the 1960s when, as a teenager, I began taking dozens of supplements after reading about their magical powers in *Prevention* and *Let's Live* magazines, and books by Adelle Davis. Surely they would help cure my adolescent acne; I just needed to find the right combina-tion. But my pizza face only improved when I took tetracycline and topical retinoic acid (the drug, not the vitamin) prescribed by a dermatologist. Growing out of adolescence also helped.

My education about dietary supplements became more comprehensive when I discovered the medical library during my college education as a biology ("pre-med") major. I learned that the hype surrounding them in the popular press was rarely supported by studies in the journals. Dietary supplements have benefited me in that they developed my interest in nutrition to the point where I chose to make a career in this discipline. But over time, and despite the growing popularity of supplements even among nutrition professionals, I have gone from being an enthusiastic vitamin promoter to a skeptic.

Most of us would agree that it's best to meet our nutritional needs with food, which means that everyone should eat a healthy, balanced diet. I believe that, short of that, dietary supplements are at best a poor and inadequate substitute. Supplements are appropriate for some people for specific purposes. But should they be taken every day, by everybody? I don't think so, and I make my case with the following eight points.

POINT 1: NO EXPERT BODY OF NUTRITION EXPERTS RECOMMENDS THE ROUTINE USE OF SUPPLEMENTS

A small number of nutritionists support regular supplement use. But no scientific body of nutrition experts recommends that everyone take supplements on a routine basis as dietary insurance or for optimal health. Expert bodies are by nature conservative and unlikely to recommend a practice until the evidence is convincing and perhaps even overwhelming. That's the point, since dietary guidance for most people should be based on strong evidence.

In 1989, the Food and Nutrition Board of the National Academy of Sciences issued a comprehensive review of the relationships between diet and health.[2] The report stated that dietary supplements should be avoided at levels above the Recommended Dietary Allowances (RDAs). Finally, however, a group of nutrition experts was not warning people to stay away from supplements with pronouncements of dire risks from their use.

The recommendation was not to stay away from supplements, but to take them in no more than RDA amounts. The Food and Nutrition Board acknowledged that the long-term potential risks and benefits of supplements had not been adequately studied and called for more research.

> **The Food and Nutrition Board recommends that those who choose supplements limit the dose to levels of the RDA or less.**

The latest pronouncements on supplements are found in the new (4th) edition of *Dietary Guidelines for Americans*, which was released in January.[3] The report states that "diets that meet RDAs are almost certain to ensure intake of enough essential nutrients by most healthy people," and that people with average requirements are likely to have adequate diets even if they don't meet RDAs.

About supplements, the report states: "Daily vitamin and mineral supplements at or below the Recommended Dietary Allowances are considered safe, but are usually not needed by people who eat the variety of foods depicted in the Food Guide Pyramid." It acknowledged, however, that some people might benefit from supplements. These include older people and others with little exposure to sunlight who may need extra vitamin D. Women of childbearing age might reduce the risk of neural-tube defects in their infants with folate-rich foods or folic acid supplements. Pregnant women usually benefit from iron supplements. And vegans, who avoid animal products, might need some nutrients in pill form. The report urges the public not to rely on supplements.

Surveys show that most supplementers take a one-a-day multiple–vitamin-mineral product. But some take large doses of single nutrients or nutrient combinations as self-prescribed medication for disease

or to try to reach a more optimal state of health, the latter fueled most recently by the enthusiasm for antioxidants. The practices of these aggressive supplementers merit some concern.

POINT 2: NUTRITION IS ONLY ONE FACTOR THAT INFLUENCES HEALTH, WELL-BEING, AND RESISTANCE TO DISEASE

The major chronic diseases that prematurely maim and kill most Americans have multiple causes. However, just as the advent of antibiotics and vaccines led many to think that the cure of diseases awaited specific "magic bullets," some proponents of supplements seem to think that these products are nutritional magic bullets for cancer, heart disease, and other maladies.

Health reporter Jane Brody calls us "a nation hungry for simple nutritional solutions to complex health problems."[4] Edward Golub, in his recent book, *The Limits of Medicine*, warns us against "thinking in penicillin mode."[5] It can be easy to do in nutrition because the first identified nutrient-related diseases (eg, scurvy and beriberi) were

> **Some proponents feel that supplements are "magic bullets" for cancer, heart disease, and other maladies.**

caused by dietary deficiencies. Anyone who doesn't get enough of the proper nutrient will eventually succumb to the relevant deficiency disease. No matter how much you exercise, who your parents are, or whether or not you smoke, you will become scorbutic without sufficient vitamin C.

Unfortunately, there is no such simple cause-effect relationship for diseases such as cardiovascular disease, cancer, stroke, and diabetes. Large doses of vitamin E, for example, may or may not influence the risk of developing heart disease. For some people, it may potentially be important. For most, however, it is at best one factor, and probably not a major one.

A primary contributor to chronic disease risk is our genetic heritage. Nutritionist Elizabeth Hiser writes, "Genes have a powerful influence over body size and disease risk, and though diet helps temper unwanted tendencies, *who* you are is often more important than *what* you eat.... Because of genetics, diet helps some people a lot, some people a little, and a very few people not at all."[6] Genetic endowment accounts in large measure for why some people get heart disease when young, for example, no matter how well they care for themselves, and why others live long lives even when they violate many of the commandments of healthy living.

Chronic disease risk is also affected by whether or not we exercise, refrain from smoking, avoid drinking to excess, limit exposure to unproductive stressors, and have sufficient rest, relaxation, and fun—and, of course, eating a diet that meets dietary guidelines and the RDAs. In our enthusiasm for supplements, however, we run the risk of reducing the importance of these factors.

One example of "thinking in penicillin mode" is linking calcium with the treatment, and especially prevention, of osteoporosis. However, bone health is influenced by many factors, including smoking, alcohol consumption, exercise, and intake of nutrients such as phosphorus, protein, and boron that affect calcium absorption, utilization, and excretion. In fact, osteoporosis is uncommon in several countries with relatively low calcium intakes.

Social commentator H. L. Mencken said, "For every complicated problem there is a simple solution—and it is wrong."[7] Supplements are not the answer to health and disease for the vast majority of people. Who our parents are, how we live our lives, and the food we put into our mouths several times a day affect our health more profoundly.

POINT 3: FOOD IS MORE THAN THE SUM OF ITS NUTRIENTS

Nutritionists used to think that macro- and micronutrients made a food nutritious and good for health. Other food constituents, such as fiber, were seen as nonessential, and therefore unimportant, since death is not directly associated with fiber deficiency. However, we have learned that, while fiber is not essential in the traditional sense, its presence in the diet makes it much easier to defecate and influences blood cholesterol levels and risk of diseases such as diverticulosis and certain cancers.

> **Supplements are not the answer to health and disease for the vast majority of people.**

Many compounds in food that are not classical nutrients can apparently influence health and risk of disease. Several hundred studies show that heavy fruit and vegetable eaters have approximately half the risk of cancer compared with those who don't eat these foods, but the results are not consistently related to one or several nutrients. New biologically active constituents found mostly in plant foods—phytochemicals (or "phytomins" as *Prevention* magazine calls them)—are being discovered regularly. They include flavonoids, monoterpenes, phenolics, indoles, allylic sulfides, and isothiocyanates. Phy-

> **Even, when and if, phytochemicals are reliably found in supplements, it will never be appropriate to take them in that form rather than from foods that contain them.**

tochemicals became a "hot item" in 1994 when they were the subject of a cover story in *Newsweek* that April.[8] The title: "Better than Vitamins: The Search for the Magic Pill." (There's that word too often linked with supplements: magic! So is "miracle.")

Whole natural foods, to quote *Newsweek*, "harbor a whole ratatouille of compounds that have never seen the inside of a vitamin bottle for the simple reason that scientists have not, until very recently, even known they existed, let alone brewed them into pills." Even when phytochemicals can reliably be found in supplements, it will never be appropriate to swallow pills (or consume specially fortified processed foods) instead of eating recommended amounts of the foods that contain them, such as vegetables, fruits, whole grains, and legumes. To do so would be to inappropriately rely on preliminary science, when the future will bring the discovery of new phytochemicals that have always been available from today's natural foods. Determining whether and how isolated food constituents with biologic activity may improve health, treat disease, or extend life is a daunting task that will occupy researchers for decades or longer.

Scientists continue to learn more about the complexity of foods and the myriad of biologically active constituents they contain that can influence health and disease risk. How ironic, then, that the calls this research generates for renewed efforts to persuade people to eat healthier diets—the tried and true—often seems to be drowned out by the acclaim for dietary supplements.

POINT 4: DEVELOPING RDAs AND OPTIMAL NUTRIENT RECOMMENDATIONS IS VERY DIFFICULT

As a staff scientist with the Food and Nutrition Board, I worked with the subcommittee that developed the most recent (10th) edition of the RDAs. I was surprised to learn that the research base for the RDAs is quite limited. There are not as many studies as one would like to determine minimum and average nutrient requirements for each age-sex group, estimate the population variability in need, and to feel more comfortable about the judgments made to derive nutrient allowances. Setting RDAs is tough work!

Now there is substantial discussion about so-called optimal intakes of nutrients, levels of intake

that might allow people to be healthy and fit for a longer time. Some nutrition scientists believe optimal nutrient intakes will typically exceed RDA levels and may require supplements in some cases to achieve. Still, no one doubts that developing optimal nutrient intakes will be orders of magnitude more complex than developing RDAs.

The optimal intake of any nutrient will probably vary substantially among individuals and even throughout one person's life from infancy to old age. It will probably also depend on the parameter of interest. For example, an optimal intake of a nutrient to reduce the risk of heart disease might not be optimal to decrease cancer risk and might actually increase it. Defining, understanding, and assessing optimal nutrition is becoming one of the most exciting challenges for

> **Developing recommendations for optimal nutrient intakes will be many times more complex than developing RDAs.**

investigators in the nutrition and food sciences.

POINT 5: TAKING SUPPLEMENTS OF SINGLE NUTRIENTS IN LARGE DOSES MAY HAVE DETRIMENTAL EFFECTS ON NUTRITIONAL STATUS AND HEALTH

On April 14, 1994, the *New England Journal of Medicine* published the infamous Finnish study.[9] In this clinical trial, 29,000 male smokers in Finland were randomly divided into four groups, receiving either a placebo, 20 mg beta-carotene (approximately four to five times the amount in five servings of fruits and vegetables), 50 IU of vitamin E (about three to four times average dietary intakes, but still a small dose as a supplement), or both the beta-carotene and vitamin E. After 5 to 8 years, the beta-carotene takers had an 18% *higher* incidence of lung cancer, with hints that this carotenoid might also have raised their risk of heart disease. Vitamin E seemed to reduce the risk of prostate cancer but increased the risk of hemorrhagic stroke.

This study is noteworthy, both because of its surprising findings and the fact that it is one of the few large clinical trials on supplements and disease risk. The majority of studies investigating this relationship are epidemiologic in nature. Clinical trials in which subjects are randomly assigned to treatment or control groups help to identify cause-and-effect relationships. Epidemiologic studies, in contrast, can only identify whether the variables under study are related in some way.

The Finnish study showed that antioxidant nutrients might harm rather than help male smokers, so it has been scrutinized intensely. Blumberg, for example, noted that those with the highest plasma concentrations of vitamin E and beta-

> **Clinical studies help identify cause-and-effect relationships, whereas epidemiologic studies can only identify whether variables are related.**

carotene at the start of the study had the lowest risk of developing lung cancer[10]; therefore, these nutrients may have provided some protection to some smokers. But for those who would suggest that the subjects should not have expected any benefits from supplements, given their deadly habit, two points should be made. First, several epidemiologic studies show that fruit and vegetable consumption reduces the risk of lung cancer in smokers—again, foods (containing beta-carotene and many other carotenoids and phytochemicals), not supplements. Second, dietary supplements are often promoted to smokers and those who are not eating or taking care of themselves as well as they should with claims that the products protect health.

The Center for Science in the Public Interest, a consumer advocacy group that had recommended

antioxidants to its readers, changed its position after the Finnish study.[11] "Shelve the beta-carotene," it said, or take no more than about 3 mg per day, the amount found in many multivitamins. It also advised people to "reconsider taking vitamin E." *New York Times* medical writer Nicholas Wade, commenting on the Finnish study, said: "The vitamin supplement industry . . . would like everyone to believe the issue of benefits is settled. . . . For all who assumed the answer was already known, the Finnish trial offers two lessons. One is that science can't be rushed. The other is not to put all your bets on those convenient little bottles: back to broccoli and bicycles."[12]

Time shows the wisdom of Wade's advice. Two large clinical trials were completed in January of this year that further debunk beta-carotene as a magic bullet. After 12 years of taking either 50 mg beta-carotene or a placebo every other day, 22,071 physicians learned that the phytochemical provided no protection against cancer or heart disease. In the second trial, 18,314 men and women at risk for lung cancer due to smoking or exposure to asbestos were given supplements of beta-carotene (30 mg/day), vitamin A (25,000 IU/day), or a placebo. Those receiving the supplements had a *higher* rate of death from lung cancer and heart disease; although the results were not statistically significant, the study was halted. Dr. Richard Klausner, the director of the National Cancer Institute, which financed both trials, concluded, "With clearly no benefit and even a hint of possible harm, I can see no reason that an individual should take beta-carotene."

> **A major concern with supplements is potential toxicity.**

A major concern with supplements is potential toxicity. Fat-soluble vitamins like A and D, which are stored in the body, are obviously harmful in excess, but so are some water-soluble nutrients. Large doses of vitamin B6, for ex-

ample, can produce neuropathy in the arms and legs, leading to partial paralysis. Some people taking tryptophan have developed and died from eosinophilia-myalgia syndrome, a connective tissue disease characterized by high levels of eosinophils, severe muscle pain, and skin and neuromuscular problems. (It is not yet certain whether the syndrome was caused by the tryptophan itself, by a contaminant produced in the manufacturing process, or by the two in combination.) High-dose niacin supplements, especially in the time-released form, have caused liver damage. Large amounts of beta-carotene can be dangerous to alcoholics with liver disorders. And antioxidant nutrients can act as prooxidants under certain conditions, generating cell-damaging free radicals.[13]

Another concern with supplements is the possibility of adverse nutrient interactions. Calcium, for example, affects the absorption of iron and vice versa. Various amino acids compete with each other for absorption from the small intestine and to cross the blood-brain barrier. Large doses of one nutrient or phytochemical can adversely affect

> **Large doses of one nutrient can adversely affect nutritional status in relation to another nutrient.**

nutritional status in relation to another. In one study, for example, very large doses of beta-carotene, 100 mg/day given for 6 days, decreased the concentration of another important carotenoid, lycopene, in the low-density lipoproteins by 12 to 25%.[14] Beta-carotene is not the only carotenoid of benefit to health, or perhaps even the most important one. I am reminded of Walter Mertz, the renowned nutrition and trace mineral expert, who was asked if he took beta-carotene as a supplement. He replied he would be "afraid" to take it, not knowing how extra beta-carotene would affect the balance of all the other carotenoids in his body that he obtained from food.

Little information is available to demonstrate that the long-term and possibly lifetime intake of large doses of nutrients is completely safe. Studies on the consequences of large nutrient intakes in humans rarely have a large sample size and go beyond several months. If high levels of iron in the body, for example, really increase the risk of heart disease, as at least one study suggests,[15] the chances are remote that a physician will think that a patient who died of a heart attack possibly did so because of supplemental iron. In other words, nutrient toxicity may be a cause of more illness and death than suspected, because the problems will not be linked (or even thought to have a possible link) to use of supplements.

POINT 6: DIETARY SUPPLEMENTS VARY SUBSTANTIALLY IN QUALITY

Few federal manufacturing and formulation standards exist for supplements, in part because they fall into a regulatory gray area between foods and drugs.[16] A decade ago, investigators discovered that many calcium supplements did not disintegrate or dissolve in the digestive tract; the calcium was simply excreted. These results prompted the development of disintegration and dissolution standards for some types of supplements by the US Pharmacopoeia, the scientific organization that establishes drug standards. . . .

Garlic supplements provide an example of not necessarily getting what you think you paid for. They have become popular because several studies suggest that garlic may help to lower blood cholesterol and reduce the risk of cancers of the breast, colon, and other organs. Attention has focused on two compounds that may be responsible for these effects: allicin and s-allyl cysteine. The Center for Science in the Public Interest analyzed garlic powder and various garlic pills and found major differences by brand in their content of these two compounds.[17] Plain garlic powder was best and least expensive, whereas the most popular brand of garlic supplement contained no allicin (Table 1). Similarly, Consumers Union recently found that ginseng products varied greatly in their content of ginsenosides, the root's supposed active ingredients.[18]

It is difficult to find a comprehensive, one-a-day type of supplement that supplies nutrients at RDA levels. Most products are not well balanced. They contain, for example, many times the recommended amount of inexpensive B vitamins like thiamin and riboflavin but only small amounts of calcium and magnesium, because recommended amounts of these minerals can add substantially to the size of the pill. Some supplements contain superfluous ingredients such as bee pollen, hesperidin complex, and PABA, which do little more than boost the price (see Refs. 19 and 20 for good advice on choosing a supplement).

POINT 7: SUPPLEMENTS ARE PROMOTED BY COMMERCIAL AND OTHER FORCES ON THE BASIS OF INCOMPLETE OR PRELIMINARY SCIENCE

I stated earlier that the bulk of evidence linking supplements to reduced risks of heart disease, cancer, and other diseases is epidemiologic in nature, or based on *in vitro*, mechanistic, or biochemical studies. They show correlations and indicate the possibility of protective effects, but do not prove cause and effect. So we do not know whether most of these suggestive data are of practical importance to people over the long run as they eat good or bad diets, smoke or refrain from smoking, live in polluted or clean environments, and are either exercisers or couch potatoes.

The scientific community tends to blame journalists for distorted reporting about nutrition. True, there are both good and mediocre reporters on the subject. And too often the reporting is bad, incomplete, prepared from press releases, or focused on one study without placing it in perspective–a poor foundation for people to make intelligent decisions.

A recent study illustrates this point. Houn and colleagues examined popular press coverage of research on the association between alcohol consumption and breast

Table 1
Comparison of Garlic Supplements

Name of Supplement	Cost per Tablet* (cents)	Allicin (µg)†	SAC (µg)‡
McCormick Garlic Powder§	6	5,660	590
KAL Beyond Garlic	18	4,800	270
Garlique	33	3,840	130
Garlicin	18	2,165	145
Nature's Way	8	1,530	140
Kwai	11	815	60
Quintessence	9	535	185
Natural Brand (GNC)	10	300	45
P. Leiner (private label)‖	5	115	45
Kyolic¶	11	0	255

© 1995, CSPI. Adapted from *Nutrition Action Healthletter* (1875 Connecticut Ave., N.W., Suite 300, Washington DC 20009-5728. $24.00 for 10 issues).

* Based on list price when available or average price paid.
† One large clove of fresh garlic supplies about 5,000 µg allicin.
‡ S-allyl cysteine.
§ One third teaspoon.
‖ Product usually carries the name of the drugstore or other chain where it is sold.
¶ The best-selling garlic supplement.

> *Responsibility for distorted reporting of nutrition rests as much with some nutritional scientists as with the media; many major journals reach reporters before medical professionals.*

cancer.[21] Of the 58 published journal papers on this topic over 7 years, only 11 were cited by the press. Three studies published in the *New England Journal of Medicine* and the *Journal of the Medical Association* were featured in more than three quarters of the news stories. And almost two thirds of the stories gave recommendations to women on alcohol consumption based on one study. Reporters ignored the published review articles and editorials that would have provided a better basis for advice. This highlighting of a few studies, which seems to occur in many other nutrition areas, tends to confuse people and lead them to think that a new study will undoubtedly contradict the findings of the previous one. It's the new math of media nutrition coverage: $1+1 = 0$. As syndicated columnist Ellen Goodman puts it, "Fresh research has a sell-by date that is shorter than the one on the cereal box."[22]

Responsibility for distorted reporting of nutrition does not rest with the media alone. Increasingly, it involves nutrition scientists. Although they tend not to make exaggerated claims when reporting their work at scientific meetings, some are more bold when they speak to reporters or the public. Sometimes their institution's press office encourages this boldness. As research funds become harder to secure, scientists and their employers are learning that being in the news raises their visibility, which can help to raise money.

Now, major journals like the *New England Journal of Medicine* and *Journal of the American Medical Association* reach reporters before they reach biomedical professionals. And because a growing

amount of research is financed by industry, a company might seek publicity about a new finding to enhance the value of its stock or draw attention to itself. A good book on the changing nature of reporting scientific advances is *Selling Science*, by sociologist Dorothy Nelkin.[23]

The dietary supplements industry is busy making bold claims for its products on the labels, in advertising, and in product literature using preliminary science. The 1990 Nutrition Labeling and Education Act, which resulted in the new nutrition labels on packaged foods, allows supplement manufacturers to present the same health claims that are allowed on foods—claims supported by "significant scientific agreement" and preapproved by FDA. Two of the authorized health claims are relevant to supplements: the links between calcium and osteoporosis and between folate and neural tube defects.

However, the Dietary Supplement Health and Education Act passed in 1994 allows the industry to make claims pertaining to the structure and function of a nutrient. For example, a supplement could not claim that it helps cure AIDS, but it might be possible to state that the product "boosts the immune system." The legal basis for a claim is that (1) some substantiation exist, (2) FDA be notified of the claim within 30 days of its presence on the label, and (3) two additional sentences be added to such claims: "This statement has not been evaluated by FDA. This product is not intended to diagnose, treat, cure, or prevent any disease." Along with these so-called "structure-function" claims, a retailer may now provide literature on supplements, although it is supposed to be balanced scientifically and not be misleading. Some members of the dietary supplements industry are fighting even these limitations, arguing that their absolute freedom of speech to provide whatever information they think is appropriate is being threatened.

An advertisement in *Time* magazine last October for Bayer Corporation's One-A-Day Brand Vitamins suggests the growing boldness of

claims for even mainstream dietary supplements. The copy states: "It's been all over the news. Findings on folic acid studies were announced recently at a medical conference in Bar Harbor, Maine, suggesting that adequate intake of folic acid may significantly lower elevated homocysteine levels, one of the risk factors for heart attacks and strokes in men. One-A-Day Men's Formula contains 100% of the US RDA of folic acid. Why not start taking your One-A-Day today?"

Public health may benefit from the promotion of supplements by increasing the public's awareness of nutrient, diet, and disease relationships. But I fear the risks outweigh the benefits. The promotional copy typically fails to give information on food-related alternatives to supplements. In addition, the public rarely has the expertise to evaluate the information in the promotion. Furthermore, consumers' expectations of a product's effectiveness may be heightened by the hype and lead to irrational use of the product.

There can be a great difference between *a* truth and *the* truth. A truthful statement may inevitably be misleading. This lesson was made clear in the plethora of ridiculous health claims on foods back in the late 80s and early 90s. Some high-fat products, for example, were truthfully labeled as being cholesterol free, because manufacturers knew many people would think the product was more healthful.

Supplements supplying nutrients at levels beyond what can reasonably be obtained from food should be viewed as nonprescription drugs. High-potency products should not be used without careful thought and perhaps expert help.

POINT 8: FOCUSING ON NUTRIENTS AND SUPPLEMENTS CAN TAKE ATTENTION AND CONVICTION AWAY FROM IMPROVING ONE'S LIFESTYLE

Nationally representative surveys of American adults show that approximately one third are interested in nutrition and think they are on the right track to healthy eating. In contrast, another third couldn't care less about meeting dietary guidelines. Those in the middle third claim they are trying to eat better, but find it difficult.

So, the good news is that two thirds of adult Americans say they care about their nutrition. But the bad news is that perhaps only 5 to 10% of the US population meets dietary recommendations regularly, such as eating five or more servings of fruits and vegetables per day and limiting fat to no more than 30% of calories. Furthermore, obesity is a growing epidemic in this country, now affecting one third of adults and one quarter of children. The irony is that people who eat well are most likely to take supplements, whereas those most likely to benefit from higher nutrient intakes are least likely to take them.

> **Dietary supplements provide a false sense of security.**

My greatest concern about dietary supplements is the false sense of security it provides some people, those who use supplements to an extent as substitutes for a good diet. It is natural for us to want an easier way or, ideally, some magic bullet, to achieve health short of being vigilant or saintly all the time. We're especially likely to cut corners when we are short of time and feeling stressed, such as by choosing foods on the basis of convenience and ease of preparation and by not exercising. Taking a basic supplement as one small part of a health-promoting lifestyle may be reasonable and perhaps even prudent. But taking supplements is a problem for people, probably the majority, who are not making the lifestyle changes they know they should. A recent advertisement by Hoffman-La Roche, Inc. for vitamin E states ... "Many doctors ... believe taking supplements or eating fortified foods containing vitamins and minerals is a sound health measure, particularly for people who don't eat a good diet.... " Unfortunately, some people use supplements as a deliberate or unconscious excuse for not trying to improve their diets and lifestyles.

A reporter called me some time ago to ask how people could use vitamins to stay healthy. I replied that people should pay more attention to their diets. He told me to be realistic and used himself as an example. He said he leads a very busy life, has little time to shop for food and prepare it, and there are few places near work that serve nutritious lunches. So what supplements would help him cope more productively with his situation? Here is an example where supplements may harm more than help, by being used as a surrogate for tackling the hard things that would really improve his nutritional status, such as preparing lunches the night before, convincing nearby restaurants to offer more nutritious fare, and making sure he eats a very nutritious breakfast and dinner. This reporter was looking for what he acknowledged to be a second-best solution, but taking a supplement will make him even less likely to attempt the best but more difficult solution.

CONCLUDING THOUGHTS

... Those who recommend that healthy people supplement their diets with extra vitamins and minerals often call it a form of dietary insurance, as essential to have as car or home insurance. I disagree. When you purchase insurance, the benefits and costs of the policy are detailed and you choose a specific level of protection. The terms of a dietary insurance policy, though,

> **Concentrating anything in the food chain, be it vitamin C, beta-carotene, salt, or fat, increases the likelihood of mistakes.**

can never be known, much less specified. Taking supplements without a clear need is more analogous to playing the lottery. You hope to win some money, and ideally the jackpot, by buying lottery tickets. You won't hurt yourself unless you buy more tickets over time than you can afford, but you are not likely to win anything either, especially the big prize.

Even comprehensive dietary supplements are, at best, poor substitutes for nutrient-rich foods. Foods, about which we know little, are more than the sum of their parts, about which we have some knowledge. Furthermore, it's harder to hurt yourself with foods than with supplements. Concentrating anything in the food chain—be it vitamin C, beta-carotene, salt, or fat—increases the likelihood of mistakes. Nutrients and other nonnutrient substances relevant to health are readily available in familiar and attractive packages called fruits, vegetables, legumes, grains, and animal products. And they come in concentrations and in combinations with which humans have had long cultural familiarity.[29] ...

REFERENCES

1. Slesinski MJ, Subar AF, Kahle LL. Trends in use of vitamin and mineral supplements in the United States: The 1987 and 1992 National Health Interview Surveys. *J Am Diet Assoc* 1995;95:921–3.
2. National Research Council. *Diet and Health: Implications for Reducing Chronic Disease Risk.* Washington, DC: National Academy Press, 1989.
3. US Department of Agriculture, Department of Health and Human Services. *Nutrition and Your Health: Dietary Guidelines for Americans,* 4th ed. Washington, DC: Government Printing Office, 1995.
4. Brody J. Personal health: Sorting out the benefits of taking extra vitamin E. *New York Times,* July 26, 1995:C8.
5. Golub E. *The Limits of Medicine: How Science Shapes Our Hope for the Cure.* New York: Times Books, 1994.
6. Hiser E. Getting into your genes. *Eating Well* 1995;6(1):48–9.
7. Herbert V, Kasdan TS. Misleading nutrition claims and their gurus. *Nutr Today* 29(3):28–35, 1994.
8. Begley S. Beyond vitamins: The search for the magic pill. *Newsweek,* April 25, 1994:45–9.
9. The Alpha-Tocopherol, Beta-Carotene Cancer Prevention Study Group. The effect of vitamin E and beta carotene on the incidence of lung cancer and other cancers in male smokers. *N Engl J Med* 1994;330:1029–35.
10. Blumberg JB. Considerations of the scientific substantiation for antioxidant vitamins and β-carotene in disease prevention. *Am J Clin Nutr* 1995;62:1521S–1526S.
11. Liebman B. Antioxidants: Surprise, surprise. *Nutr Action Healthletter* 1994;21(5):4.
12. Wade N. Method and madness: Believing in vitamins. *New York Times Magazine,* May 22, 1994:20.
13. Herbert V. The antioxidant supplement myth. *Am J Clin Nutr* 1994;60:157–8.
14. Graziano JM, Johnson EJ, Russell RM, Manson

JE, Stampfer MJ, Ridker PM, Frei B, Hennekens CH, Krinsky NI. Discrimination in absorption or transport of β-carotene isomers after oral supplementation with either all-*trans*- or 9-*cis*-β-carotene. *Am J Clin Nutr* 1995;61:1248–52.

15. McCord JM. Free radicals and prooxidants in health and nutrition. *Food Tech* 1994;48(5):106–11.

16. Anon. Buying vitamins: what's worth the price? *Consumer Rep* 1994;59:565–9.

17. Schardt D, Schmidt S. Garlic: Clove at first sight? *Nutr Action Healthletter* 1995;22(6)3–5.

18. Anon. Herbal roulette. *Consumer Rep* 1995;60:698–705.

19. Anon. A 9-point guide to choosing the right supplement. *Tufts Univ Diet & Nutr Letter* 1993;11(7)3–6.

20. Liebman B, Schardt D. Vitamin smarts. *Nutr Action Healthletter* 1995;22(9):1,6–10.

21. Houn F, Bober MA, Huerta EE, Hursting SD, Lemon S, Weed DL. The association between alcohol and breast cancer: Popular press coverage of research. *Am J Publ Health* 1995;85:1082–6.

22. Goodman E. To swallow or not to swallow. *Liberal Opinion Week*, April 24, 1994.

23. Nelkin D. *Selling Science: How the Press Covers Science and Technology*, revised edition. New York: WH Freeman and Company, 1995.

24. Anon. Many shoppers not yet aware of nutrition facts label. *Food Labeling News* 1995;3(32):21–3.

25. Gussow JD. *A Word on Behalf of Food.* Presentation at the Alumni Advances Conference of the dietetic internship program at Oregon Health Sciences University, Portland, OR, May 1995.

26. Shepherd SK. Nutrition and the consumer: Meeting the challenge of nutrition education in the 1990s. *Food & Consumer News* 1990;62(1):1–3.

27. Goodman E. Food literacy. *Liberal Opinion Week*, December 14, 1992.

28. Stacey M. *Consumed: Why Americans Love, Hate, and Fear Food*. New York: Touchstone Books, 1994.

29. Gussow JD, Thomas PR. *The Nutrition Debate: Sorting Out Some Answers*. Palo Alto, CA: Bull Publishing Co., 1986.

The views expressed in this article are those of the author and do not reflect the position of the Center for Food and Nutrition Policy.

Vitamin C: Is Anyone Right On Dose?

JANE E. BRODY

HOW much vitamin C is enough? Is it the 60 milligrams a day—the amount in half a cup of fresh orange juice—that is the current Recommended Dietary Allowance (R.D.A.), the 30 to 40 milligrams that some nutritional biochemists think it should be, the hundreds of milligrams that millions of Americans now take as a daily supplement or the thousands of milligrams that Dr. Linus Pauling believed would protect against serious illnesses, including cancer?

A new study says 200 milligrams a day is optimal.

A detailed new federally sponsored study, by far the most comprehensively done to date, says none of the above. The study, directed by Dr. Mark Levine and published today in The Proceedings of the National Academy of Sciences, found that the "optimal" daily intake of vitamin C was more like 200 milligrams, although only about 10 milligrams are needed to prevent vitamin C deficiency.

More than 1,000 milligrams a day of vitamin C may even be hazardous.

The researchers, at the National Institutes of Health, also concluded that daily doses above 400 milligrams "have no evident value" and that amounts of 1,000 milligrams (1 gram) or more, which many people now take as daily supplements or on occasion to prevent or treat illness, could be hazardous. Beyond a dose of about 400 milligrams, the study

showed, the body's ability to absorb vitamin C sharply declines and excess vitamin is excreted.

Megadoses of vitamin C are said to do nothing in healthy people.

Unlike previous studies used to establish recommended amounts, this one looked beyond the levels needed to prevent scurvy.

"This means Linus Pauling was all wrong, at least with respect to healthy people," Dr. Levine remarked in an interview. "He had the best of intentions, but he did not have the science to support his hypothesis." Dr. Levine said that "in healthy people, megadoses are doing nothing and may do harm, and in sick people, I don't think they will be helpful either."

Industry sources estimate that 30 to 40 percent of Americans now take vitamin C supplements, and that about 1 in 5 supplement users take more than 1,000 milligrams a day.

Although the 200-milligram level is more than three times the currently recommended amount, it is a level that can still be readily obtained from foods, especially if one follows the latest Federal advice to eat five or more servings a day of fruits and vegetables. For example, one would exceed the 200-milligram level by consuming four ounces of orange juice, half a cup of cooked broccoli, one baked potato and one kiwi fruit.

But the most recent national survey indicated that less than a third of Americans consumed five or more servings of fruits and vegetables a day. This suggests that unless significant improvements are made in people's eating habits, it would be necessary to take supplements or fortify commonly eaten foods with vitamin C for most of the population to consume 200 milligrams each day.

Dr. Adrianne Bendich, assistant director of human nutrition research at Hoffman-La Roche, a major manufacturer of bulk vitamin C, said a recent review she had conducted of dozens of well-designed studies of vitamin C showed that even at daily doses of a 1,000 milligrams or more, no adverse effects had been reported in otherwise healthy people. Dr. Bendich said she saw "no problem with raising the current R.D.A." The R.D.A.'s are established by the academy's Food and Nutrition Board as safe and desirable levels of intake by healthy people to prevent nutritional deficiencies.

Martin Hirsch, public policy director for Hoffman-La Roche, said the company "welcomes publication of new data that support a shift from thinking about the R.D.A.'s as a means of preventing nutritional deficiency to viewing them as a way to promote optimal health."

But other nutrition scientists who served on the last R.D.A. committee challenged the study's conclusions that 200 milligrams of vitamin C, also known as ascorbic acid or ascorbate, are necessary or desirable. Dr. Victor Herbert, a nutrition researcher at the Bronx Veterans Affairs Medical Center who generally disputes the need for supplements, called the study's conclusions "fraudulent." He noted that the study had excluded people with health conditions, like a family history of kidney stones or a tendency to accumulate iron, which could be worsened by taking amounts of vitamin C beyond the current R.D.A. He said that even consuming 200 milligrams a day could be harmful to as many as one-third of Americans. For example, he said, 12 percent of Americans have iron overload and could be made worse by this amount of vitamin C.

A study does not suggest dosages for children or ill adults.

Dr. Levine said he had excluded people with various illnesses because he did not want to risk harming anyone with the high doses used in part of the study. He also said that the findings strictly applied "only to young, healthy men," and he noted, "We don't know what will happen to sick people, women, the elderly or children." A similar study is under way in young, healthy women.

Dr. John N. Hathcock, director for nutritional and regulatory science at the Council for Responsible Nutrition, a[n] organization supported by the supplement industry, agreed that "you can't say from this study that 200 milligrams of vitamin C is safe or harmful for people with conditions that were excluded." But, he added, "If a person has such a condition, that person should be under the care of a physician and should take his or her advice regarding vitamin C intake."

Dr. James Allen Olson, a biochemist at Iowa State University in Ames who, like Dr. Herbert, served on the committee that established the current R.D.A.'s, questioned the study's assumption that because the 200-milligram dose was best absorbed and utilized by body tissues, that this would mean that it was the most desirable amount.

But Dr. John Erdman Jr., a nutritional scientist at the University of Illinois who is a member of the academy's Food and Nutrition Board, said the group was already considering a change in the basic concept of the R.D.A. "to consider outcomes that would go beyond just the prevention of deficiency diseases." For vitamin C, for example, such outcomes might include "enhancing the immune response," he said. He added that the new study provided "the kind of data the R.D.A. committee would look at very strongly." He said the committee "would have to decide whether saturation of cells with vitamin C was a necessary and a desirable goal."

The study, sponsored by the National Institute of Diabetes and Digestive and Kidney Diseases in Bethesda, Md., analyzed the biochemical effects of various amounts of vitamin C administered to seven healthy young men who lived in a hospital ward for four to six months. Nutrient requirement studies, which are very costly and time-consuming, are typically done on small numbers of participants. Although most researchers would prefer that the studies be larger, their exacting nature can yield meaningful results, unlike clinical and epidemiological studies that require many participants to achieve statistical significance.

The men's blood levels of vitamin C were first depleted by placing the men on a daily diet that contained less than five milligrams of this essential nutrient. Then, while continuing their vitamin C-deficient diet, the men were given seven different doses of the vitamin to determine which level was best absorbed and would result in peak amounts in the blood and tissues. The doses studied, which were administered sequentially, were 30, 60, 100, 200, 400, 1,000 and 2,500 milligrams a day.

The team of 11 researchers determined which doses were fully absorbed, which produced "saturation levels" in blood plasma, white blood cells and other tissues and which resulted in excretion of vitamin C or its metabolic products in the stool and urine. The white blood cells, a vital component of the immune system, were saturated at a dose of 100 milligrams a day. That is, beyond this dose no more vitamin C was absorbed by the cells. The blood plasma was nearly saturated by a dose of 200 milligrams and fully saturated at 1,000 milligrams, the researchers found.

But beyond 100 milligrams, the volunteers began to excrete some vitamin C in their urine, indicating that the body was not using all that it absorbed. Absorption levels through the gut also declined as dosages were increased beyond 200 milligrams. At 500 milligrams, less than three-fourths of the vitamin C administered to the volunteers was absorbed, and at 1,250 milligrams, less than half was absorbed, Dr. Levine said.

At 1,000 milligrams or more, the urine was found to contain oxalate, a breakdown product of vitamin C that in some people can result in the formation of kidney stones. A second substance, urate, which results from the breakdown of nucleic acids, the building blocks of genes, also accumulated in urine at these high doses, Dr. Levine reported. An endocrinologist by training, Dr. Levine is chief of the molecular and clinical nutrition section at the Federal institute.

"It looks as if the body is very tightly regulated with respect to vitamin C," Dr. Levine said. "It seems to be saying 'enough is enough.' Beyond 200 milligrams, the cells don't fill up any more, plasma fills up very little, absorption goes down and excretion goes up."

Dr. Levine said there was no "absolute proof" that it was best to be saturated with vitamin C. "Our study doesn't prove that 200 milligrams a day will prevent heart disease, cancer or infectious illnesses," he said. But he added that he and his colleagues were impressed by the fact that many pieces of evidence "converge on 200 milligrams as the right dose," including the amount that people get from diets rich in fruits and vegetables, how much is absorbed by the body, the dose that results in saturation of cells and blood, the amount that may be toxic and the amount that is consumed by people who are relatively protected against various serious diseases.

Dr. Levine said: "The current R.D.A. for vitamin C is based on flawed studies and that its very concept—to prevent scurvy—is outmoded. We should be basing our recommendation on what is best for the population, not just to prevent a deficiency disease."

The trials of beta-carotene: Is the verdict in?

It hasn't been glamorous or provocative, and it may have sounded ultra-conservative. But despite the steady stream of news stories and the constant barrage of advertising touting the magic-bullet benefits of vitamins C and E and beta-carotene, we've urged our readers to think twice before popping antioxidant supplements. The best way to get your antioxidants, we've held firmly, is to eat a diet rich in fruits and vegetables.

Of course, it's easy to see why Americans have been spending $40 million annually on beta-carotene supplements alone. After all, vitamin pills, sold over-the-counter, have seemed so harmless.

Yet the National Cancer Institute recently put the brakes on a long-term, $42 million beta-carotene research trial because of findings that the antioxidant might be harming participants. At the same time, another major study concluded that beta-carotene did not improve the health of more than 22,000 men who had been swallowing supplements for a decade.

Did scientists miss the mark? Have the potential benefits of beta-carotene been overblown? Worse still, have people taking beta-carotene supplements been harming themselves?

Circumstantial evidence

Exactly 15 years ago, in March 1981, a group of internationally renowned cancer researchers published a landmark paper that tossed into the scientific arena a theory rife with possibility. They pointed to a number of studies showing that in populations where consumption of fruits and vegetables rich in beta-carotene runs high, the risk of cancer runs low. These findings suggested that beta-carotene may somehow help stall the development of malignant tumors. Evidence of a link between high blood levels of beta-carotene and low cancer rates lent weight to the theory.

Naturally, the idea that beta-carotene might offer protection against cancer was an enticing one. It had been 10 years since Richard Nixon declared the "war on cancer," yet researchers were making little headway in their search for ways to prevent the disease. If an inexpensive, easy-to-swallow, seemingly harmless substance like beta-carotene could solve the problem, it would be a boon to public health.

So scientists embarked on numerous studies, and the results looked promising, especially for lung cancer. Between 1983 and 1993, more than two dozen studies linking beta-carotene to a reduced incidence of lung cancer were published. Overall, the reports consistently indicated anywhere from a 10 to 70 percent drop in the risk of lung cancer in people whose diets were high in beta-carotene.

Deliberations

While the studies were insightful, their conclusions were far from definitive. They mostly showed loose associations: for example, people with high blood levels of beta-carotene tended to have lower rates of cancer than people with lower beta-carotene blood levels. But that doesn't prove that taking beta-carotene pills will reduce cancer risk.

To learn whether the connection is more than a coincidence, a chemoprevention trial is necessary. In this type of study, people are given the substance in question and then followed to see if they are less likely to develop disease than people not given the test substance.

Because cancer can take decades to develop, chemoprevention trials typically last many years. And they often involve thousands of people. The duration and number of participants make for a very high price tag. But given the enormous potential of beta-carotene, the National Cancer Institute began pouring millions of dollars into a number of beta-carotene chemoprevention trials during the mid-1980s.

In 1994, the results came in for one of the first of these studies, the Alpha-Tocopherol, Beta-Carotene Cancer Prevention Trial—the ATBC Trial, for short. The news was disturbing. After more than 29,000 male smokers in Finland took supplements of either vitamin E, beta-carotene, or a "dummy" placebo pill daily for five to eight years, 18 percent more cases of lung cancer and 8 percent more overall deaths occurred in the beta-carotene group than in the other groups. Because these results countered those of earlier studies, however, scientists chalked them up to a possible statistical fluke and punctuated them with a large question mark.

Then in January of this year, an independent watchdog committee monitoring a similar, ongoing study called the Beta Carotene and Retinol Efficacy Trial

(CARET) noticed the same trend. After an average of four years, 28 percent more cases of lung cancer and 17 percent more overall deaths had occurred in the group taking beta-carotene. Because it looked as if beta-carotene wasn't helping and may actually have been *harming* participants, the trial was halted in January.

Simultaneously, yet another eyebrow-raising announcement was made about the Physicians' Health Study, a 12-year look by Harvard researchers at more than 22,000 male physicians. Again, beta-carotene came up short, apparently conferring no protection against cancer or heart disease.

Rush to judgment?

On the face of it, the newly released results suggest that millions of consumers who have been taking beta-carotene pills may have been hurting themselves—or at least wasting their time. But experts maintain that even in light of the negative findings, the beta-carotene case is not closed.

Consider that the ATBC trial involved only male smokers. And CARET included only smokers, former smokers, and workers exposed to asbestos. Scientists suspect that something about long-term exposure to cigarette smoke or asbestos in combination with beta-carotene supplements may promote lung cancer. It might be that some component of cigarette smoke interacts with beta-carotene to generate particularly harmful by-products in the body, according to Norman Krinsky, PhD, a beta-carotene expert at the Tufts University School of Medicine. But at this point, he says, "We know zilch about what these by-products might be," and more research is required to pinpoint them.

Another unanswered question is why study after study has revealed a significant association between diets rich in beta-carotene and a reduced risk of lung cancer, but the major supplement trials have "failed." Again, possibilities abound. Maybe beta-carotene "works" only in the presence of some other substance in fruits and vegetables, like chlorophyll. Or perhaps it's not beta-carotene at all, but some other substance in produce that confers protection against cancer.

Back in the 1980s, when interest in beta-carotene took off, it was the only member of a group of substances called carotenoids that scientists had singled

Beta-carotene and beyond

Time was when nutritionists viewed beta-carotene and other members of the carotenoid family as nothing more than vitamin A precursors, that is, substances that were converted into vitamin A in the body. Today we know of more than 500 different carotenoids, many of which appear to function as much more than just vitamin A precursors.

Scientists have only begun to scratch the surface to learn about how these substances work in the body. Preliminary research suggests that two carotenoids—lutein and zeaxanthin—protect the eyes against age-related macular degeneration, which afflicts one in three people over age 75. Another carotenoid, lycopene, may help stave off prostate cancer.

Despite the potential of carotenoids, food composition tables currently used by nutritionists still lump beta-carotene and its relatives together under vitamin A, making it difficult to identify good sources of particular carotenoids. Fortunately, the U.S. Department of Agriculture and the National Cancer Institute have begun putting together the first carotenoid database, from which the following chart is derived.

Note that there is no recommended dietary allowance for the various carotenoids. The table however, highlights good sources of carotenoids and underscores the benefits of eating a wide variety of produce. It also helps you see what you're missing if you rely on supplements alone rather than eating fruits and vegetables.

	Beta-Carotene (micrograms)*	Lutein & Zeaxanthin (micrograms)	Lycopene (micrograms)
½ cup cooked broccoli	1,014	1,404	0
½ cup Brussels sprouts	374	1,014	0
1 medium raw carrot	5,688	187	0
½ medium pink grapefruit	1,611	0	4,135
½ cup cooked kale	3,055	14,235	0
1 medium peach	86	12	0
1 cup raw spinach	2,296	5,712	0
1 medium tomato	640	123	3,813
¾ cup tomato juice	1,638	0	15,616

*A microgram is a thousandth of a milligram. Amounts are averages taken from a number of samples and should be viewed as estimates rather than hard-and-fast values.

out as a possible disease fighter. And because beta-carotene was available in pill form, it was a convenient substance to test in large-scale trials. During the past few years, however, scientists have come up with more and more research suggesting that beta-carotene is just one of many members of the carotenoid family that may fight disease.

For example, researchers now suspect that the carotenoids called lutein and zeaxanthin, found in spinach, kale, and broccoli, help protect against an eye condition called age-related macular degeneration, which ranks as the leading cause of irreversible blindness among older adults. And in December, Harvard University researchers published a study linking diets rich in another carotenoid named lycopene, found primarily in tomatoes, with a decreased risk of prostate cancer. Because beta-carotene is found along with other carotenoids in fruits and vegetables, it may serve as a marker of fruit and vegetable consumption but not be the ingredient that is staving off disease (see box).

The trials continue

Another reason experts say the jury is still out on beta-carotene concerns the design of the studies that have been concluded or stopped thus far. The Physicians' Health Study was a primary prevention trial aimed at determining if beta-carotene helps prevent cancer or heart disease in a healthy population. The ATBC trial and CARET were both *secondary* prevention trials, which were designed to see whether beta-carotene helps prevent cancer in high-risk groups like smokers or people exposed to asbestos. But if beta-carotene supplements were tested in, say, a secondary prevention study of a large group of men at high risk for a disease other than lung cancer, the outcome might be different. What's more, all three trials involved only men; beta-carotene may behave differently in women.

Because so many questions remain, some of the trials on beta-carotene are continuing despite the latest round of negative findings. One is a secondary prevention trial called the Women's Antioxidant and Cardiovascular Study, designed to evaluate the effect of vitamin E, vitamin C, and beta-carotene in some 8,000 women at high risk for heart disease. Besides acting as an antioxidant, beta-carotene is thought to help relax the artery walls, making them more flexible and less likely to become blocked.

"We haven't seen any evidence of harm from beta-carotene in these women, and there's good reason to believe beta-carotene may benefit them," says JoAnn Manson, MD, a Harvard researcher who is spearheading the trial. "But we're going to be monitoring the interim results very closely."

Too little sun?

Overexposure can cause wrinkles and skin cancer. But underexposure can dangerously lower vitamin-D levels.

Americans have been warned repeatedly to cover up or use sunscreens to avoid the dangers of too much sun. But they're seldom warned about the consequences of too *little* sun. Sunlight stimulates the skin to synthesize vitamin D. Insufficient exposure to sunlight can lead to insufficient levels of the vitamin, since many people don't get enough from diet alone. Indeed, recent evidence suggests that insufficient vitamin-D levels may be far more prevalent than previously believed, particularly in older people. It may be far more harmful as well, weakening the bones, possibly worsening arthritis, and perhaps even increasing the risk of cancer.

The dangers of little D

Here's what research shows about the three most important risks, proven or potential, of getting too little vitamin D.

■ **Weakened bones.** Vitamin D helps the body absorb calcium from food; that, in turn, increases calcium absorption by the bones. Outright deficiency of the vitamin causes a condition known as rickets in children, osteomalacia in adults, in which new bone tissue fails to harden due to lack of calcium. Vitamin-D deficiency also worsens osteoporosis, or porous bones, through direct and indirect effects on existing bone tissue.

But mounting evidence indicates that even moderately low levels of the vitamin, traditionally considered within the normal range, may also weaken the bones. Such "low normal" levels stimulate secretion of a hormone that pulls calcium out of the skeleton; some research suggests that such levels increase the risk of fractures as well. Clinical trials have shown that boosting consumption of vitamin D, with or without extra calcium, can slow bone loss or increase bone density in older women who have low-normal blood levels of the vitamin. And one large clinical trial has proved that boosting consumption of both vitamin D and calcium can actually reduce the risk of fractures in such women.

■ **Arthritis.** Osteoarthritis, the most common kind of arthritis, develops when the cartilage lining the joints breaks down, causing painful friction between the bare ends of the bones. As the disease progresses, the bone itself may start to break down or develop spurs, increasing the pain. In theory, vitamin D might slow that progression, by helping the bones maintain their normal shape and possibly helping the remaining cartilage stay healthy. In the first test of that theory, published last September, Boston researchers studied 75 arthritic knees for up to 10

Getting enough vitamin D may be harder for older people.

years. They found that the risk of the disease worsening was three times greater in people with average or lower blood levels of vitamin D than in those with higher levels. Both bone and cartilage deteriorated faster in those with less of the vitamin.

■ **Cancer.** Vitamin D has inhibited the development and growth of many different cancers in both test-tube and animal studies. In humans, the risk of various cancers—notably breast, colon, and prostate, the three most common kinds in nonsmokers—is substantially lower in sunny regions than in areas with less sunlight, both around the world and within the U.S. One possible reason: The skin produces more vitamin D in sunnier climes. Studies of vitamin-D consumption tentatively support that explanation. Four of five large observational studies have found at least some evidence linking low intake with an increased risk of colorectal cancer. Studies of blood levels, the most accurate measure of vitamin-D status, have yielded mixed results: One study of colon cancer and another study of prostate cancer linked relatively low levels of the vitamin with increased risk, but two other prostate-cancer studies found no such link.

Who's at risk?

Younger people almost always get enough vitamin D, either from sunshine or from diet. But getting enough may be harder for older people, for several reasons. First, they need more than younger people do, to fight bone loss. And the rate of vitamin-D synthesis by the skin is two to four times slower in older than in younger individuals. Many older people, fearing skin cancer and other damaging effects of the sun, wear protective clothing and apply strong sunscreens whenever they go outside. Others simply don't like to bare their arms or legs in public, or seldom go outdoors in the first place. Further, older people are more likely to take certain drugs, notably laxatives and the cholesterol-lowering drug cholestyramine (*Questran*), that interfere with the absorption or action of vitamin D.

Despite those obstacles, healthy older residents of sunny regions, including the American South, generally get adequate amounts of vitamin D from sunshine alone, just by going about their daily affairs—even if they wear sunscreen (apparently because it's rarely applied perfectly and at all times). Only those Southerners who never get outdoors need to be concerned about vitamin D. (Note that sitting by a window doesn't help, since glass absorbs virtually all ultraviolet light, the component of sunshine that stimulates vitamin-D synthesis.) But getting enough sunlight is somewhat harder in the North.

Northern exposure

The best time to expose the skin in the northern U.S. is mid-morning or mid-afternoon during the spring, summer, and fall. That's because the sunlight is too weak to stimulate much vitamin-D production in the early morning or late afternoon—or to stimulate any production during the winter. And the skin is more susceptible to damage or sunburn at midday.

At the optimal hours, a light-skinned older person in Boston or Chicago would need roughly 15 to 20 minutes of exposure—on the face, hands, and lower arms—about three times a week during the warmer months to produce an adequate year-long supply of vitamin D. (The body can store extra vitamin D for the winter.) Briefer, more frequent exposure would work equally well. But a darker-skinned person would need up to 50 percent more exposure. And the requirement is higher in regions north of Boston or Chicago—50 percent higher in Toronto, for example—and lower in regions to the south. In general, you produce enough vitamin D in about one-third the time it takes for your skin to start turning red.

Many older Northerners may not get even that much exposure, and thus may not get enough vitamin D. Studies have found insufficient levels of the vitamin—low enough to increase bone loss—in at least 25 percent of healthy older people in Boston. The numbers are even higher during the dark, winter months. (Indeed, average bone density drops and fracture risk rises in winter, an increase that's only partly due to slips on ice and snow.) And more than half of people who never get outside—due to illness, frailty, or disease—have low levels of vitamin D.

Directions for D

If you're an older person in the North, you may need to change your habits to ensure an adequate supply of the vitamin. One way is to expose your skin to the sun as described above. Such modest exposure is generally safe. If you stay out longer than that, however, be sure to apply sunscreen with an SPF (sun-protection factor) of 15 to 30 after the initial period.

You may be able to get all the vitamin D you need from your diet (see table). People with insufficient sun exposure probably require about 400 IU (International Units) per day during their 50s and 60s, 600 to 800 IU during their 70s and 80s. Fortified milk is supposed to contain 100 IU per cup. A few years ago, studies found that milk often contains significantly less than that. While the fortification process has improved since then, studies have not confirmed that milk is now a fully reliable source of the vitamin. Still, it's wise to drink several cups of low-fat or skim milk per day: The milk generally supplies at least a moderate amount of vitamin D and invariably supplies lots of calcium. People who do consume plenty of milk and often eat fatty fish, the other main source

of vitamin D, are almost surely meeting the 400 IU daily requirement. However, meeting the higher requirement from dietary sources alone may be difficult.

If the guidelines presented in this report suggest that you're not getting enough vitamin D—either the full amount from sunlight or diet, or a partial contribution from both—consider taking a supplement.

That's particularly appropriate during the winter and for people who are at increased risk for osteoporosis. The risk is much higher for older women than older men, especially if their menopause started early or they consumed little calcium before menopause. Other factors increase risk in both sexes: lack of weight-bearing exercise, heavy alcohol consumption, cigarette-smoking for many years, being thin, and being white or Asian. Individuals over age 70 or so who rarely or never gets outdoors generally need a supplement, regardless of where they live or what they eat.

If you do take a vitamin-D pill, be sure it contains no more than the dose that brings you up to roughly the suggested intake (including diet) for your age group. Too much vitamin D can lead to elevated calcium levels in the blood and, in turn, to severe kidney damage and calcium deposits in many parts of the body. However, you can't get a toxic dose of vitamin D from sun exposure, even if you consume lots of the vitamin; that mechanism is self-regulating.

Summing up

Insufficient vitamin-D levels appear to be more common and more hazardous than previously believed. Young people and Southerners generally don't need to worry, unless they never go outside. But older Northerners need to ensure an adequate supply, by taking any of these steps:

■ Regularly expose your skin for a short while; the older you are, the darker your skin, and the farther north you live, the more exposure you need. (But cover up or apply sunscreen before you start to redden.)

■ Consume plenty of milk and fatty fish.

■ Consider taking a supplement if you're not meeting at least one of the preceding requirements fully, or both of them partly—particularly if you are an older postmenopausal woman or have other risk factors for osteoporosis. The pill should contain no more than you need to reach the total suggested intake for someone your age.

Vitamin D in the diet [1]

Food	Serving size	Vitamin D (IU)
DAIRY		
Milk [2]	1 cup	100 [3]
Egg, whole	1	26
FISH AND SHELLFISH		
Oysters	3 oz	544
Cod liver oil	1 tsp	452
Catfish	3 oz	424
Mackerel	3 oz	394
Salmon	3 oz	238
Sardines, canned in oil	3 oz	231
Tuna, bluefin	3 oz	170
Halibut	3 oz	170
Tuna, canned in water	3 oz	136
Shrimp	3 oz	122
Sole/flounder	3 oz	51
Cod	3 oz	48
Bass, freshwater	3 oz	34
Swordfish	3 oz	34
Clams	3 oz	7
MUSHROOMS (fresh)		
Shiitake	2 oz	57
Chanterelle	2 oz	48
Button (common)	2 oz	0

IU = International Units

[1] In addition to milk, other foods that may have added amounts of vitamin D include breads, breakfast cereals, fruit drinks, chocolate beverages, and cocoa powder.

[2] Whole, reduced-fat, low-fat, or nonfat milk.

[3] While each cup of milk is supposed to be fortified with 100 IU of vitamin D, studies have not yet proved the reliability of the fortification process.

Source: USDA and ESHA Research, Salem, Ore.

Fluoridation:

A Triumph of Science over Propaganda

By Dr. Michael W. Easley

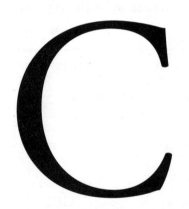

Community water fluoridation (herein called simply "fluoridation") is the precise adjustment of the concentration of the essential trace element fluoride in the public water supply to protect teeth and bones. In 1945 Grand Rapids, Michigan, became the first city in the world to fluoridate its public water supply. Since then, communities throughout the United States have adopted the practice. Fluoridation is similar to food fortification and enrichment, which encompass the addition of iodine to table salt; vitamins to fruit drinks, milk, and various kinds of pasta; and vitamins and minerals to breakfast cereals and bread.

Fluoridation is the perfect public health intervention. Whole towns are protected in a nondiscriminatory manner. The protection is continuous and received without effort. The fluoride in the water is incorporated into the enamel

The overwhelming weight of scientific evidence confirms fluoridation's safety and effectiveness, and hundreds of peer-reviewed studies on fluoride have discredited antifluoridation propaganda.

of developing teeth in children below the age of 16, making their teeth more resistant to decay for a lifetime. It also promotes remineralization of early decay in adults and interferes with the life cycle of decay-causing bacteria present in the mouths of both children and adults.

Fluoridation is remarkably simple to implement and mimics nature: Virtually all sources of drinking water in North America naturally contain fluoride. Fluoride levels in the United States are adjusted to about one part fluoride per million parts of water—a minute concentration.

The Antifluoridationists

While only a minuscule percentage of Americans opposes fluoridation, an extremist minority urges avoidance of fluoridation. These antifluoridationists or fluorophobics falsely allege that fluoridation is unsafe, ineffective, or costly. They assert that exposure to fluoridated water increases the risk of contracting AIDS, cancer, Down's syndrome, heart disease, kidney disease, osteoporosis, and many other health problems. But the overwhelming weight of scientific evidence confirms fluoridation's safety and effectiveness, and hundreds of peer-reviewed studies on fluoride have discredited antifluoridation propaganda.

Almost at the moment Grand Rapids became the first community to adjust the fluoride content of its water supply, small groups of ill-informed people began objecting to water fluoridation. Early opponents included chiropractors, health food advocates, and members of fringe political and religious groups. The convergence of such individuals and groups led to the formation of small but highly active regional societies whose primary mission was to fight fluoridation. Most of these organizations lacked the funds, political expertise, or scientific credibility to have an impact outside their respective communities. Eventually, however, a few better-funded national organizations appeared whose agendas included opposition to fluoridation.

By exploiting scientific illiteracy, common phobias, paranoia concerning communist plots and Big Brotherism, and occasional acceptance of folk medicine, these organizations persuaded a minority of Americans. Their tactics included attracting the media; holding demonstrations at the local-government level; promoting referenda; lobbying public health agencies, state legislatures, and the United States Congress; and litigating at state and federal levels.

The effects of such activities did not have lasting importance, and antifluoridation efforts have diminished significantly in recent years.

No American court of last resort has ever ruled against community water fluoridation.

Today, most fluoridation initiatives are successful; court challenges by antifluoridationists are rare; and effective antifluoridation lobbying at both state and federal levels is virtually nonexistent. A latter-day antifluoridationist highspot was the movement's extensive campaign in 1995 to prevent enactment of mandatory statewide fluoridation in California. The campaign failed.

. . . And Justice for All

Despite the decrease in antifluoridation activities, they remain a factor—albeit a minor one—in the success or failure of profluoridation efforts in most American cities. The tactics of contemporary antifluoridationists tend more to delay fluoridation than to stop it, but in some areas of the United States fluoridation remains in limbo. This lack of implementation translates into tooth decay, pain, infection, and dental-care expense (See "Dollars and Sense," next page). Moreover, antifluoridation efforts cost taxpayers money by compelling defense of fluoridation to legislators, judges, and the media.

But litigation, which antifluoridationists once considered the ultimate solution to the "fluoridation menace," has failed as an antifluoridation tactic. No American court of last resort has ever ruled against community water fluoridation. And court decisions that uphold fluoridation as an acceptable public health measure within the police powers of state and local government have bolstered profluoridation efforts.

Furthermore, with only two exceptions, American courts have never ruled on the scientific merits of fluoridation but have allowed the scientific method—which includes clinical research and peer review—to determine whether community water fluoridation is acceptable. In both of the exceptions, higher courts overruled

Viable options to community water fluoridation as a public health measure do not exist.

lower-court judges and decreed continuance of fluoridation in the communities in question.

"Quackery" versus Science

Fluoride is harmless at the levels necessary for maximum benefits. Thousands of studies on fluorides and fluoridation have been completed in the last 50 years—more than 3,700 since 1970 alone. Over 50 peer-reviewed epidemiological studies have dealt with the claim that fluoridation increases cancer risk. None has substantiated the claim. A number of nationally and internationally recognized scientific organizations, including the National Cancer Institute, have reviewed all the available scientific studies on the health of populations with fluoridated water supplies and the health of fluoride-deficient populations. These reviewers have declared fluoridation safe.

Indeed, no legitimate epidemiological, laboratory, or clinical study has demonstrated that lifelong ingestion of fluoride at optimal levels in water causes disease in any form. We now have over 50 years' experience with water fluoridation. Moreover, many generations of Americans have spent their lives in areas whose water supplies had naturally occurring fluoride levels 800 to 1,300 percent higher than the levels in fluoridated water. There is no evidence that members of communities with fluoridated water supplies, or with naturally high concentrations of fluoride in their water supplies, have had a higher incidence of any disease than have their contemporaries in areas with water supplies low in fluoride. In 1978 *Consumer Reports* magazine summed up the situation well: "The simple truth is that there's no 'scientific controversy' over the safety of fluoridation. The practice is safe, economical, and beneficial. The survival of this fake controversy represents, in our opinion,

Dollars and Sense

The dental benefits—and concomitant cost savings—from fluoridation have been documented for more than half a century. Here are a few facts:

- People who drink fluoridated water for a lifetime will develop up to 70 percent fewer cavities (occurrences of tooth decay) than they would have without fluoridation.
- Because the technology is so simple and the fluoride supplement so inexpensive, fluoridation is extremely cost-effective. Studies indicate that a $100,000 investment in water fluoridation prevents 500,000 cavities.
- Each dollar invested in fluoridation prevents over $80 of dental treatment. Few disease-prevention efforts, and even fewer government-sponsored programs, achieve that level of return on investment.
- The average per capita cost of fluoridating America's public water supplies is 54 cents per year (or $40.50 over a lifetime). The cost of an average single-surface dental restoration is $55. Thus, provision of fluoride in water for a lifetime costs less than one small dental filling.

—M.W.E.

one of the major triumphs of quackery over science in our generation."

Nearly 145 million Americans can avail themselves of water whose fluoride concentration is optimal. Of the 50 largest municipalities in the United States, 43 have fluoridated water supplies, including four of the five largest cities. Eight states, the District of Columbia, and Puerto Rico have mandated fluoridation throughout their respective territories. Three states and the District of Columbia have fluoridated all of their treatable community water supplies.

Viable options to community water fluoridation as a public health measure do not exist. There are other community-based methods of fluoride delivery—school-based programs that involve rinsing the mouth with a fluoride preparation, ingesting fluoride tablets, or submitting to professional dental application of fluoride, for example. But these methods cost considerably more than community water fluoridation, are much more difficult to implement, and are available only to limited numbers of people and only under special circumstances. Such methods are useful to populations without public water systems but are decidedly second-rate.

The Bottom Line

In recent years public resistance to water fluoridation has waned across the United States, partly because of a higher level of education among voters and partly because of consumers' positive experiences with fluoride (as an ingredient in fluoride toothpastes, for example). Healthcare reform movements have made all Americans aware of the importance of disease prevention. Federal, state, and local officials have acted on this awareness, and the pace of efforts to fluoridate America's remaining deficient water supplies has increased markedly.

Fluoridation is the high-water mark of efficient public health intervention.

MICHAEL W. EASLEY, D.D.S., M.P.H., IS AN ASSOCIATE PROFESSOR IN THE DEPARTMENT OF ORAL HEALTH SERVICES AND INFORMATICS, SCHOOL OF DENTAL MEDICINE, STATE UNIVERSITY OF NEW YORK AT BUFFALO.

SPECIAL REPORT

Yes, But *Which* Calcium Supplement?

Guidelines issued by the National Institutes of Health indicate that adults need from 1,000 to 1,500 milligrams of calcium a day, but surveys show that they consume, on average, only 500 to 600 milligrams. Over time, this calcium deficit is a significant risk factor for thinning bones that are prone to fracture.

Experts agree that increasing the intake of calcium-rich foods is the best way to tackle the calcium shortfall. Calcium in food comes packaged with a host of other nutrients essential for a healthful diet. But some people may find it difficult to meet their needs from foods alone. A 70-year-old, for example, would need to drink 5 cups of milk—or the equivalent—to achieve the recommended daily intake of 1,500 milligrams for men and women 65 and older.

Fortunately, the vast majority of people absorb and utilize supplemental calcium as well as the calcium found in food. When it comes to *choosing* a supplement, however, consumers may be met by a dizzying array. When we visited Boston-area drugstores to survey calcium supplements, one store alone boasted 36 different choices.

Ask the following questions while sorting through the options to find a supplement that is right for you.

1. What is the form of calcium in the supplement? Supplemental calcium always comes chemically partnered with another substance. Available forms include calcium carbonate, calcium citrate, calcium phosphate, calcium lactate, and calcium gluconate.

Calcium carbonate is by far the most common form on the market, found in at least 90 percent of calcium pills as well as in antacids such as Rolaids and Tums. It is also a highly concentrated form. Single tablets can contain 600 milligrams of the mineral, providing a distinct advantage to consumers who want to take as few pills as possible to fill their calcium gap.

Common sources of calcium carbonate include ground limestone (specified on labels simply as "calcium carbonate") or ground oyster shell. Unless it is purified, calcium carbonate from oyster shell may contain heavy metal contaminants, such as lead. Thus, we recommend avoiding it.

Note that for 1 out of 5 people over 60 and 2 out of 5 over 80, calcium carbonate taken on an empty stomach will not break down properly for absorption. That's because those people have a condition known as atrophic gastritis, which is a deficiency of stomach acid. Only when they have just eaten and the stomach has secreted acidic juices will enough acid be present to break down a calcium carbonate tablet.

The solution is simple: just take a calcium carbonate pill right after eating. Bess Dawson-Hughes, MD, chief of the Calcium and Bone Metabolism Laboratory at Tufts's USDA Human Nutrition Research Center on Aging, recommends that all people, whether or not they have atrophic gastritis, take their calcium supplements with meals. The presence of food slows the emptying of the stomach, allowing more time for the calcium tablet to be broken down and for the mineral to be absorbed by the body.

Calcium citrate is the best absorbed form of supplemental calcium. And unlike calcium carbonate, it will be properly utilized by anybody who takes it, whether between or with meals.

That might make it sound as though calcium citrate is a better choice than calcium carbonate. But calcium citrate is hard to pack into a pill. As the chart shows, to get at least 500 milligrams of calcium, a consumer would have to swallow 2 or 3 calcium citrate tablets. Even the slight advantage in absorption that calcium citrate has over other forms doesn't justify all that pill popping.

Calcium phosphate, like calcium carbonate, is a highly concentrated form of supplemental calcium. But it is especially difficult for the body to break down and therefore should be avoided, according to Ralph Shangraw, PhD, a Professor Emeritus of the University of Maryland's School of Pharmacy who has studied calcium supplements extensively.

Calcium lactate and calcium gluconate are best skipped, too. As with calcium citrate, too many pills—6 in the case of Osco's calcium lactate—are needed just to reach 500 milligrams. We could not even find a single calcium gluconate preparation at the 3 drug stores, health food store, or K-Mart we visited or at several supermarket chains.

2. How much does the supplement cost? For as little as 5 cents, you can get 500 milligrams of calcium carbonate. Compare that, for instance, to AARP's Formula 687 calcium citrate, at 18 cents for the same amount. Over a year's time, that comes to a difference of $47.

Note that there's no need to pay more for supplements with any of the following claims: "no starch"; "no sugar"; "no preservatives"; "recommended by pharmacists"; "high potency"; "premium quality"; "free of milk"; "free of yeast"; "physician recommended"; "natural"; and "proven release." Most of these claims actually can be made for *any* calcium supplement.

3. How many milligrams of calcium are in each tablet? Consumers looking to supplement their dietary calcium with only a small amount of the mineral can turn to lower-dose preparations, such as Rolaids or Walgreens Chewables. However, those who want to add 500 to 1,000 milligrams should choose a higher-dose pill, like AARP Formula 314 or Sundown Calcium 600, so they can take fewer tablets each day.

Dr. Dawson-Hughes recommends taking no more than 500 to 600 milligrams of calcium at a time. The body may not be able to absorb larger doses all at once. If your supplement is calcium carbonate, splitting the daily dosage over 2 or 3 meals also cuts down on the possibility of constipation, a problem for some calcium carbonate takers.

Note: While some manufacturers clearly list the milligrams of calcium in each tablet, others list the contents of the whole pill—calcium plus carbonate, for example—requiring you to do a bit of math to figure out the actual amount of

year. Argentinians are second, at 114 pounds per person annually. Americans come in third, eating some 98 pounds of beef each.

calcium. For the products in the chart, we have done the arithmetic for you.

4. Does the supplement contain "extras," such as vitamin D, magnesium, or zinc? For the most part, extra vitamins and minerals in calcium supplements are not necessary. The exception in some cases is vitamin D, which is essential for the body's proper utilization of calcium.

Research indicates that older women need from 400 to 800 International Units of vitamin D a day, but people not getting a fair amount of sun or drinking several cups of milk a day (each cup has 100 units) might not be getting that much. In such cases, a calcium/vitamin D preparation like Caltrate 600 + D can be useful.

5. How well does the supplement dis- solve? If a label has the letters "USP," the supplement meets the U.S. Pharmacopeia's strict standard for dissolution. Most calcium pills without the USP designation also dissolve well. But when we tested the products in the chart without the USP mark, we did find 2 clinkers: Schiff Super Calcium '1200' and Twinlab Calcium Citrate Caps.

A Bare-Bones Look at Calcium Supplements

The 27 calcium supplements listed came from Boston-area pharmacies, a health food store, K-Mart, and Safeway and Kroger supermarkets. Others came by mail order from the American Association for Retired Persons (AARP).

Product	Calcium per Tablet in mg	Cost per Tablet	Cost per 500 mg*	Cost per 30 Days†	Form of Calcium	% DV Vit. D**	Comments
AARP Formula 314 Calcium	600	5¢	5¢	$1.50	Carbonate	—	"No starch" claim superfluous
AARP Formula 564 Calcium with Vitamin D	600	5¢	5¢	$1.50	Carbonate	50	"No sugar" claim superfluous; even chewable pills have very little sugar
AARP Formula 687 Calcium Citrate	200	6¢	18¢	$5.40	Citrate	—	Label claim of 950 mg refers to calcium and citrate combined
Caltrate Plus	600	12¢	12¢	$3.60	Carbonate	50	—
Caltrate Plus Chewables	600	12¢	12¢	$3.60	Carbonate	50	Chew well to help dissolution
Caltrate 600 + D	600	12¢	12¢	$3.60	Carbonate	50	"More calcium for your bones than any leading brand" claim not true
Citracal Calcium Citrate Liquitab	500	6¢	6¢	$1.80	Citrate	—	Dissolves in water like Alka-Seltzer
Citracal Calcium Citrate Ultradense Caplets + D	315	13¢	26¢	$7.80	Citrate	50	—
GNC Calcium Citrate	250	7¢	14¢	$4.20	Citrate	—	"No preservatives" claim superfluous
K-Mart/American Fare Vita-Smart Natural Oyster Shell Calcium	500	6¢	6¢	$1.80	Carbonate	—	Best to avoid oyster shell
Nature Made Calcium	500	8¢	8¢	$2.40	Carbonate	—	"Recommended by pharmacists" claim superfluous
Nature Made Calcium and Magnesium with Zinc	333	5¢	10¢	$3.00	Carbonate	—	Magnesium and zinc not proven necessary in calcium pills
One A Day Calcium Plus	500	10¢	10¢	$3.00	Carbonate	25	"High potency" claim superfluous
Os-Cal 500 + D	500	11¢	11¢	$3.30	Carbonate	31	Best to avoid oyster shell
Osco Calcium Lactate	83	3¢	18¢	$5.40	Lactate	—	6 tablets necessary for 500 mg of calcium
Posture-D	600	17¢	17¢	$5.10	Phosphate	63	Calcium from phosphate not well absorbed
Rolaids	220	4¢	12¢	$3.60	Carbonate	—	Sold as antacid
Safeway Select Calcium	600	9¢	9¢	$2.70	Carbonate	—	"Premium quality" claim superfluous
Schiff Calcium Lactate	100	3¢	15¢	$4.50	Lactate	—	"Free of milk" claim superfluous
Schiff Super Calcium '1200'	600	12¢	12¢	$3.60	Carbonate	100	Did not dissolve when tested
Solgar Calci-Chews	500	10¢	10¢	$3.00	Carbonate	—	"Free of yeast" claim superfluous
Sundown Calcium 600	600	6¢	6¢	$1.80	Carbonate	—	—
Tums 500	500	9¢	9¢	$2.70	Carbonate	—	"Physician recommended" claim superfluous
Twinlab Calcium Citrate Caps	300	8¢	16¢	$4.80	Citrate	—	Did not dissolve when tested
Walgreens Calcium Lactate	84	3¢	18¢	$5.40	Lactate	—	6 tablets needed for 500 mg of calcium
Walgreens Finest Natural Chewable Calcium Plus Vitamin D	300	5¢	10¢	$3.00	Carbonate	25	"Natural" claim superfluous
Your Life Calcium + D	600	12¢	12¢	$3.60	Carbonate	31	"Proven release" claim superfluous

* Rounded to the nearest whole pill.   † Cost of 500 milligrams (mg) a day over 30 days.   ** The DV (Daily Value) for vitamin D is 400 International Units.

Through the Life Span: Diet and Disease

Food improperly taken, not only produces diseases, but affords those that are already engendered both matter and sustenance; so that, let the father of disease be what it may, intemperance is its mother.

—Richard E. Burton

When someone says, "You are what you eat," is it literally true? The parents of students who read this book may remember Adelle Davis, sometimes called the high priestess of nutrition. Among other things, she claimed that aging would not occur on the days when one eats right. All of us know that this is not exactly true, but scientists are constantly adding support to the belief that what we eat does affect what we are in both direct and indirect ways. Harry Golden provides an illustration from World War II (*Only in America*, Cleveland, Ohio: The World Publishing Company, 1958, p. 308):

When the Nazis took Denmark they requisitioned everything the Danes produced. The Danes, as you know, are famous dairy farmers and the Nazis took all their butter, animal fats, cheese, and allied products for their own armies. During that period the Danes were forced to lead an austere life and lived mostly on black bread and fish. What they have found out since is that during that austere period the incidence of degenerative diseases went way down—the Danes lived longer—but when the Danes got their butter, cheese, and animal fats back, the health chart went back to "normal" with a tremendous increase in stomach, heart, blood, and vein diseases. It is all a matter of diet, and I should hang my head in shame, being as fat as I am, and with no fewer than eleven thousand stories yet to write.

It is commonly agreed that a good (balanced) diet throughout life will help us all reach our genetic potentials and avoid premature aging, disease, and untimely death. Studies of other populations, as in the quote above, often provide clues to diet/disease connections. Researchers must interpret them cautiously, however, as such studies cannot prove all-inclusive cause-and-effect relationships; sometimes the results even appear contradictory.

Many popular admonitions about what to eat or avoid eating have led to a bad-food/good-food philosophy. High-fat foods are bad for us and will cause unwanted weight gain; carrots and spinach are good for us. A thoughtful person may realize that no food is inherently bad or good, that it is the quantity eaten that is problematic or beneficial. Thus, moderation is a key concept. Add variety in what is eaten, and one is well on the way to a good diet.

The first articles in this unit were selected because they discuss chronic diseases that have a connection to what we eat. During our youth we often feel invulnerable, but then life moves on, slipping eventfully and uneventfully through a few decades. Soon the 50th birthday is celebrated, with the golden years just beyond. Typically, we have gained weight, probably more than is currently considered healthy. And, as we reach the 60s and 70s, more and more of us will be dealing with high blood pressure, coronary disease, cancer, osteoporosis, and other conditions that cause varying degrees of disability. Now major lifestyle changes become inevitable. However, these diseases might have been avoided altogether, or at least delayed, if we had made the appropriate lifestyle choices while we were young.

The diet/cancer connection, the topic of the unit's first two articles, is still controversial. Results of some major studies appear to link high-fat diets to increased risk of some cancers, but not all studies support this connection. A recent study reports that stored trans-fatty acids appear to be at higher levels in women who develop breast cancer. If future studies support this finding and a cause-and-effect relationship is determined, there will be implications for the consumption of margarines and some other fats used in food preparation. Other possible connections to cancer focus on fiber, alcohol consumption, and the availability of antioxidants in the diet. Current research also suggests that antioxidants found in tea, especially in green tea, are particularly powerful in protecting genetic material. Check out the articles on vitamin C and beta-carotene in unit 2 for additional information. It is good news that many substances feared by people as cancer-causing have been ruled out. These include saccharine and aspartame, bioengineered foods, fluoride, food additives, and irradiation. Articles with information on all of these topics can be found in other units of this book.

Some commonly held information about the relationship between diet and both hypertension and heart disease may have been misstated or overstated. While sodium undoubtedly is implicated in raising blood pressure for those who are sensitive to it, far fewer than half of the total population appears to fit into this category. The relationship of other factors is more clear-cut. Weight control is effective in regulating blood pressure and is also helpful in avoiding heart disease. Many people, however, continue to believe that food cholesterol, rather than saturated fat, is the primary dietary culprit in elevated blood cholesterol levels. Other individuals erroneously, and almost fanatically, attempt to eliminate as much fat from the diet as possible. This can have health repercussions as well.

An article on osteoporosis (see "Boning Up on Osteoporosis") deals with one of the significant health threats to the elderly, although some people have it before age 50, and all of us have influenced the health of our bones well before that. It is now clear that elderly men as well as women are frequently subject to thinning bones and the fractures of osteoporosis. Maintaining an active lifestyle and consuming adequate amounts of calcium are key components in preventing this debilitating disease.

Lactose intolerance is a very different health concern. This is not an allergic reaction to milk protein, as some people think. An allergic reaction involves a response of the immune system that may cause extreme physical reactions, even death. A food intolerance, on the other hand, produces unpleasant symptoms primarily of the gastrointestinal tract. In the case of lactose intolerance, there is an insufficiency of the enzyme required to break down milk sugar. However, most people with decreased amounts of the enzyme can consume normal or somewhat smaller amounts of dairy products without difficulty. Alternatively, enzyme supplements or lactose-reduced food products are available.

Babies are the expressions of their parents' hopes and dreams, a fulfillment of themselves. Parents want their children's first experiences with the breast or the bottle to provide the very best start possible. Certainly a bottle-fed baby can be nurtured physically and emotionally, and no mother should be made to feel guilty if that is the method she chooses. At the same time, there is ample evidence that human milk provides the perfect nourishment as well as the ideal environment for bonding. No other method can transfer protection against early childhood diseases or is safe from contamination. The article "Breast-Feeding Best for Babies" identifies the issues that parents should consider very carefully before deciding whether to breast- or bottle-feed.

The article "When Eating Goes Awry: An Update on Eating Disorders" highlights anorexia nervosa, bulimia nervosa, and binge-eating disorder. These are believed to affect 2 million males and females between the ages of 15 and 35. Five percent of college women are bulimic, and 1 percent of teenage females are anorexic. Many will die. These disorders are psychiatric illnesses that bring depression, shame, isolation, and damaged careers and relationships to their victims. In addition, dangerous eating and dieting practices include the use of diet pills, laxatives and diuretics, and extreme fad diets. An additional article on dysfunctional eating in unit 4, "Dysfunctional Eating: A New Concept," is related.

The particular needs of various ethnic, age, and gender groups are addressed in "Nutritional Implications of Ethnic and Cultural Diversity." Children cannot be viewed as little adults, nor does an adult's physiology remain static while aging. Males and females do not necessarily respond in the same way, and variations of significance can also be found among minority groups and between minority groups and whites. We should be reminded that diversity includes other variables as well, including body weight and shape and, perhaps the biggest divider of all, social class. In all cases, knowledge and commitment can help the consumer to avoid the health and dietary pitfalls of either omission or commission.

Finally, an article on alcohol discusses the evidence regarding its benefits in protecting against heart disease and other conditions. As always, this is a case of "some will win and some will lose." Small deviations in the amount of alcohol consumed can spell the difference between benefit and risk.

One should remember that there is still much we do not know about nutrition and that even within age, gender, and ethnic groups, people are physiologically different. Connections between food/nutrition and health can be found in other units in this book. Unit 1 has articles that describe dietary guidelines and useful labeling information. Articles on vitamins and other nutrients are found in unit 2, and unit 6 discusses information leading to harmful dietary practices. The reader might also review articles in previous *Annual Editions: Nutrition* and in reliable periodicals to fully appreciate the extent of the information—and the confusion—surrounding nutrition.

Looking Ahead: Challenge Questions

Pretend that you are planning research projects relative to nutrition and your age group. Rank by order of importance your top three priorities and defend them.

What changes should you make in your lifestyle in order to conform to the best current knowledge about your nutrient needs? Choose one change and brainstorm ways to achieve it.

What products for lactose-intolerant people can you find in your grocery store? Compare their prices to those of similar products.

Find the article on osteoporosis and estrogen replacement mentioned above, and list the issues to be considered. How would you decide?

Compare the content of infant formula to that of human milk and cow's milk. What are the primary differences, and what are the advantages of each?

How do you think eating disorders could be prevented? What can a friend do to help?

Beating the odds: best bets for cancer prevention

New guidelines give the latest word on hedging your bets against cancer

Of the half million cancer deaths in the U.S. each year, a third are related to dietary factors, according to a report recently released by the American Cancer Society. Most people are aware that the lifestyle choices they make today can affect their chances of succumbing to cancer later, but misunderstandings about the culprits behind the disease abound.

For example, many people believe that a high-fat diet is the major risk factor for breast cancer yet think nothing of drinking a couple of glasses of wine or beer daily. In fact, the evidence linking alcohol consumption and breast cancer is much stronger than any suggesting a connection with dietary fat.

Also, cancers often are lumped together when lifestyle factors are considered, even though certain habits have a much stronger relationship to some cancers than to others. Eating lots of fruits and vegetables, for instance, appears to be more protective against colon and rectal cancer than against prostate cancer.

The chart here, based on the latest guidelines issued by the American Cancer Society, shows which habits are most strongly linked to some of the top cancer killers. The questions and answers that follow on page 5 explain the science behind many of the connections and clear up some common points of confusion regarding cancer and nutrition.

Of course, eating lots of fruits and vegetables, not smoking, and the other lifestyle factors in the chart are healthful habits for everyone. But suppose breast cancer runs in your family. It makes sense to limit alcohol intake and exercise regularly, habits that seem to be particularly effective at staving off the disease.

Keep in mind that these habits may prevent cancer over the long run. Once a person is diagnosed and treated for cancer, certain strategies may not apply. Consider that people who are undergoing chemotherapy may need a relatively high fat diet to keep their weight up.

Cancer	Estimated number of deaths in 1996	Smoking†	Fruits & Vegetables	Exercise	Fat	Smokeless Tobacco	Meat	Obesity	Alcohol
Lung	158,700	★★★	★★★						
Colon & Rectum	54,900		★★★	★★	★★		★	★★	
Breast	44,560		★	★★	★			★★	★★
Prostate	41,400		★	★★	★★		★	★★	
Stomach	14,000	★★	★★						
Kidney	12,000	★★★						★★	
Esophagus	11,200	★★★	★★			★★★			★★
Oral Cavity	8,260	★★★	★★			★★★			★★
Endometrium	6,000				★★			★★★	
Larynx	4,250	★★★	★★			★★★			★★

Key: ★★★ A solid body of evidence suggests a link between this habit and cancer.

★★ Numerous studies pointing in the same direction suggest a plausible link.

★ Some research indicates a connection; other studies show no association. The jury is still out.

⬆ Increase to reduce risk.

⬇ Decrease to reduce risk.

† The link between smoking and lung cancer is by far the most significant association on this chart. Cigarette smoking causes more than 80% of lung cancer cases.

7 questions and answers about the diet-cancer connection

Isn't eating a high-fiber diet one of the best ways to cut cancer risks?

A specific type of fiber, insoluble fiber, is believed to reduce the risk of cancer of the colon and rectum, possibly by speeding the movement of potential carcinogens through the lower portion of the intestinal tract. As for other types of cancer, however, fiber has never been shown to be a factor in and of itself.

Fruits and vegetables contain insoluble fiber (as do whole wheat products and bran), which may be why they are strongly linked to a decreased risk of certain cancers. The reason fruits and vegetables appear to be deterrents to so many other cancers as well is that they contain antioxidant nutrients (beta-carotene and vitamins A and C) and dozens of phytochemicals— recently identified compounds that research suggests play a major role in preventing malignant tumors.

The chart indicates a weak connection between eating less fat and reducing the risk for breast cancer. Isn't the link between fat and breast cancer pretty strong?

Scientists have yet to tease out the role fat may play in breast cancer. High-fat diets have long been thought to contribute to the disease, and many studies show an association between fat and breast cancer. But a widely publicized 8-year study of nearly 90,000 women conducted by researchers at Brigham and Women's Hospital in Boston showed no relationship between the amount of fat that women ate and their incidence of breast cancer.

That's not to say that the study ruled out fat as a possible factor. The jury is still out. In an ongoing study at the Ontario Cancer Institute, researchers are finding that a low-fat, high-carbohydrate diet may decrease the density of breast tissue. Highly dense tissue is a known risk factor for breast cancer.

Why is the alcohol-breast cancer link relatively strong?

Numerous studies provide strong evidence that alcohol increases the risk of breast cancer. In fact, the breast cancer risk appears to rise among women who imbibe in just a few drinks a week. Scientists believe that alcohol may change levels of hormones such as estrogen, which play a role in the development of breast cancer. In addition, alcohol may go hand in hand with a high-risk lifestyle. People who drink heavily often fill up on alcohol rather than eat nutrient-rich, cancer-protective fruits and vegetables.

The American Cancer Society suggests that women with a high risk for breast cancer, say, because of their family history, consider abstaining from alcohol completely. Most experts recommend that all women, even those not at high risk for breast cancer, make their daily limit no more than 1 alcoholic beverage— defined as 12 ounces of beer, 5 ounces of wine, or 1.5 ounces of 80-proof liquor.

Why is meat singled out as a possible factor in prostate and colon cancer?

Some studies have linked consumption of high-fat meat, especially beef, pork, and lamb, to cancer of the colon and prostate. Whether the risk is due to the total fat, saturated fat, or some other component in those foods isn't clear. Scientists speculate that a diet high in animal fat raises a man's level of the hormone testosterone, which in turn increases the likelihood that cancerous cells will multiply and form a tumor. Another theory is that the fat in meat may alter cell membranes, making the cells more likely to mutate and become cancerous.

Why is alcohol so harmful to the mouth and esophagus?

Each drink exposes the mouth and esophagus to a direct onslaught of alcohol, which apparently causes alterations in those tissues that set the stage for the growth of cancerous tumors. The risk of those cancers may start to rise substantially with consumption of as few as 2 drinks a day. The more alcohol drunk, the greater the risk.

When tobacco is added to the equation, the chances of getting oral and esophageal cancer soar even higher. The combination of drinking and smoking cigarettes or chewing tobacco is especially lethal because they seem to bolster each other, making the sum of their combined impact greater than their individual effects.

How is exercise involved in cancer prevention?

Physical activity may help ward off cancer by burning calories, which helps people keep their weight down. Obesity is linked to increased risks of cancer of the colon and rectum, prostate, endometrium, breast (among postmenopausal women), and kidney.

When it comes to colon cancer, physical activity may stimulate the movement of food through the colon, decreasing the amount of time that the organ is exposed to potential carcinogens that come from food. As for breast and prostate cancer, exercise may alter levels of hormones that play roles in those diseases.

What does obesity have to do with cancer?

It's not clear why obesity is a factor, but it seems to particularly affect the risk of cancers that are mediated by hormones. For example, many scientists believe that childhood obesity substantially boosts the risk of breast cancer because the numerous fat cells developed in youngsters contain the hormone estrogen, which over time "feeds" breast tumors. Similarly, the strong link between obesity and endometrial cancer is thought to stem from the increase in estrogen levels that occurs among women who are overweight.

MOST FREQUENTLY ASKED QUESTIONS
. . . About Diet and Cancer

AMERICAN CANCER SOCIETY NUTRITION ADVISORY COMMITTEE

Because people are interested in the relationship of specific foods or nutrients to specific cancers, research in this area is often widely publicized. No one study is the last word on any subject, and it is easy to become confused by what may appear to be contradictory and conflicting advice. Each study should be considered in the light of existing knowledge, but in brief news stories, reporters cannot always put new research findings in context. The best advice is to use common sense; it is rarely, if ever, advisable to change your diet based on a single study or news report, especially if the data are reported as "preliminary."

What are antioxidants and what do they have to do with cancer? Certain nutrients in fruits and vegetables appear to protect the body against the oxygen-induced damage to tissues that occurs constantly as a result of normal metabolism. Because such damage is associated with increased cancer risk, antioxidant nutrients are thought to protect against cancer.[12] Antioxidant nutrients include vitamin C, vitamin E, selenium, and carotenoids. Studies suggest that people who eat more fruits and vegetables containing these antioxidants have a lower risk for cancer.[13] Clinical studies of antioxidant supplements, however, have not demonstrated a reduction in cancer risk (see Beta Carotene, Supplements).

Do artificial sweeteners cause cancer? Several years ago, experiments on rats suggested that saccharin might cause cancer. Since then, however, studies of primates and humans have shown no increased risk of cancer from either saccharin or aspartame.

Does beta carotene reduce cancer risk? Because beta carotene, an antioxidant, is found in fruits and vegetables, and because eating fruits and vegetables is clearly associated with a reduced risk of cancer, it seemed possible that taking high doses of beta carotene supplements might reduce cancer risk. In three major experiments, people were given high doses of synthetic beta carotene in an attempt to prevent lung and other cancers. Two of these studies found beta carotene supplements to be associated with a higher risk of lung cancer in cigarette smokers[18,19] and a third found neither benefit nor harm from beta carotene supplements.[44] Thus, research has not reproduced the beneficial effects of fruits and vegetables by giving high-dose supplements of beta carotene. For cigarette smokers, such supplements may be harmful.[18]

What are bioengineered foods, and are they safe? Foods made through techniques of bioengineering or biotechnology have been altered by the addition of genes from plants or other organisms to increase resistance to pests, to retard spoilage, or to improve transportability, flavor, nutrient composition, or other desired qualities. Few such foods have as yet been marketed. At present, there is no reason to believe that these foods will either increase or decrease cancer risk.

Is calcium related to cancer? Some research has suggested that foods high in calcium might help reduce the risk of colorectal cancer, but this relationship is not proven. Whether or not calcium intake affects cancer risk, eating foods containing this mineral is important to reduce the risk of osteoporosis. Low-fat and non-fat dairy products are excellent sources of calcium, as are some leafy vegetables and beans.

What are carotenoids, and do they reduce cancer risk? Carotenoids are a group of pigments in fruits and vegetables that include alpha carotene, beta carotene, lycopene, lutein, and many other compounds. Consumption of foods containing carotenoids is associated with a reduced cancer risk (see Beta Carotene).

Does cholesterol in the diet increase cancer risk? Cholesterol in the diet comes only from foods from animal sources-meat, dairy, eggs, and fats. At present, little evidence is available to determine whether dietary cholesterol itself or the foods containing this substance might be responsible for the increase in cancer risk associated with eating foods from animal sources. Low blood cholesterol has been found to be more common in people with cancer, but is an effect of cancer, not its cause. There is no evidence that lowering blood cholesterol causes an increase in cancer risk.

Does drinking coffee cause cancer? Several years ago, a highly publicized study suggested that coffee might increase risk for cancer of the pancreas. Because caffeine may heighten symptoms of fibrocystic breast lumps in some women, media stories also have focused on concerns about coffee and breast cancer. Many studies in recent years, however, have found no relationship at all between coffee and the risk of pancreatic, breast, or any other type of cancer.

Does cooking affect cancer risk? Adequate cooking is necessary to kill harmful microorganisms in meat. However, some research suggests that frying or charcoal-broiling meats at very high temper-

From *Nutrition Today*, May/June 1997, pp. 125-127. Reprinted by permission of the American Cancer Society from *CA Cancer Journal for Clinicians*, Volume 46, 1996, pp. 333-338. © 1996 by Lippincott-Raven Publishers.

atures creates chemicals that might increase cancer risk. Preserving meats by methods involving smoke also increases their content of potentially carcinogenic chemicals. Although these chemicals cause cancer in animal experiments, it is uncertain whether they actually cause cancer in people. Techniques such as braising, steaming, poaching, stewing, and microwaving meats do not produce these chemicals.

What are cruciferous vegetables and are they important in cancer? Cruciferous vegetables belong to the cabbage family, which includes broccoli, cauliflower, and brussels sprouts. These vegetables contain certain chemicals thought to reduce the risk of colorectal cancer. The best evidence suggests that a wide variety of vegetables, including cruciferous and other vegetables, reduces cancer risk (see Phytochemicals).

What is dietary fiber and can it prevent cancer? Dietary fiber includes a wide variety of plant carbohydrates that are not digested by humans. Specific categories of fiber are "soluble" (like oat bran) and "insoluble" (like wheat bran). Insoluble fiber is thought to help reduce the risk of colorectal cancer, although the mechanism of this action is uncertain. Soluble fiber helps to reduce blood cholesterol and, therefore, to lower the risk of coronary heart disease. Good sources of fiber are beans, vegetables, whole grains, and fruits.

Does eating fish protect against cancer? Like all fats, fish oils are high in calories. Fish fats are rich in omega-3 fatty acids. Studies in animals have found that omega-3 fatty acids suppress cancer formation, but there is no direct evidence for protective effects in humans at this time.

Do fluorides cause cancer? Extensive research has examined the effects of fluorides given as dental treatments or added to toothpaste, public water supplies, or foods. Fluorides do not increase cancer risk.

What is folic acid and can it prevent cancer? Folic acid (sometimes called folate or folacin) is a B vitamin found in many vegetables, beans, fruits, whole grains, and fortified breakfast cereals. Folic acid may reduce the risk of some cancers. Supplements are sometimes recommended for women who are capable of becoming pregnant as a means to reduce the risk of spina bifida and other neural tube defects in their infants. Current evidence suggests that to reduce cancer risk, folic acid is best consumed along with the full array of nutrients found in fruits, vegetables, and other foods.

Do food additives cause cancer? Many substances are added to foods to preserve them and to enhance color, flavor, and texture. Additives are usually present in very small quantities in food, and no convincing evidence exists that any additive at these levels causes human cancers.

Can garlic prevent cancer? The health benefits of the allium compounds contained in garlic and other vegetables in the onion family have been publicized widely. Garlic is currently under study for its ability to reduce cancer risk, but insufficient evidence supports a specific role for this vegetable in cancer prevention.

If our genes determine cancer risk, how can diet help prevent cancer? Genes that increase or decrease cancer risk can be inherited or acquired by mutations throughout life. Nutrients and nutritional factors in the diet can protect DNA from being damaged and can delay or prevent the development of cancer even in people with an increased genetic risk for the disease.

Why are foods irradiated, and do irradiated foods cause cancer? Radiation is increasingly used to kill harmful organisms on foods so as to extend their "shelf life." Radiation does not remain in the foods after treatment, and there is no evidence that consuming irradiated foods increases cancer risk.

Should I avoid nitrite-preserved meats? Most lunch meats, hams, and hot dogs are preserved with nitrites to maintain color and to prevent contamination with bacteria. Nitrites can be converted to carcinogenic nitrosamines in the stomach, which may increase the risk of gastric cancer. Vitamin C and related compounds are often added to foods to inhibit this conversion. Diets high in fruits and vegetables that contain vitamin C and phytochemicals, such as phenols, retard the conversion of nitrites to nitrosamines. Nitrites in foods are not a significant cause of cancer among Americans.

What is olestra and is it related to cancer? Some synthetic fat substitutes are not absorbed by the body. Although several fat substitutes are under development for use in the food supply, only one of this type-olestra (trademarked Olean)-has been approved for marketing. Olestra may reduce fat intake, but it also reduces the absorption of fat-soluble carotenes and other potentially cancer-protective phytochemicals in fruits and vegetables.[45] Although reducing absorption of these substances might also reduce the health benefits of fruits and vegetables, the overall effect of this type of fat substitute on cancer risk is unknown at present.

Does olive oil affect cancer risk? Olive oil, like all fats, is high in calories, but its fat is mostly mono-unsaturated. Consumption of olive oil is not associated with any increase in risk of cancer, and most likely is neutral with respect to cancer risk.[46]

Do pesticides and herbicides on fruits and vegetables cause cancer? Pesticides and herbicides can be toxic when used in high doses. Although fruits and vegetables sometimes contain low levels of these chemicals, overwhelming scientific evidence supports the overall health benefits and cancer-protective effects of eating fruits and vegetables.[47] In contrast, current evidence is insufficient to link pesticides in foods with an increased risk of any cancer.

What are phytochemicals, and do they reduce cancer risk? The term "phytochemicals" refers to a wide variety of compounds produced by plants. Some of these compounds protect plants against insects or have other biologically important functions. Some have either antioxidant or hormone-like actions both in plants and in people who eat them. Because consumption of fruits and vegetables reduces cancer risk, researchers are searching for specific compounds in these foods that might account for the beneficial effects. There is no evidence that taking phytochemical supplements is as beneficial as consuming the fruits, vegetables, beans, and grains from which they are extracted.

Do high levels of salt in the diet increase cancer risk? Some evidence links diets containing large amounts of foods preserved by salting and pickling with an increased risk of cancers of the stomach, nose, and throat. Little evidence suggests that moderate amounts of salt or salt-preserved foods in the diet affect cancer risk.

What is selenium and can it reduce cancer risk? Selenium is a mineral needed by the body as part of antioxidant defense mechanisms. Animal studies suggest that selenium protects against cancer, but human studies are inconclusive. Selenium supplements are not recommended, as there is only a narrow margin between safe and toxic doses. Grain products are good sources of selenium.

Can soybeans reduce cancer risk? Soybeans are an excellent source of protein and a good alternative to meat. Nonfermented soybeans have high levels of phytoestrogens and other phytochemicals that appear to have beneficial effects on hormone-dependent cancers in animal studies.[23] These effects remain to be proven in humans, however.

Can nutritional supplements lower cancer risk? Strong evidence associates a diet rich in fruits, vegetables, and other plant foods with reduced risk of cancer, but there is no evidence at this time that supplements can reduce cancer risk. The few studies in human populations that have attempted to determine whether supplements can reduce cancer risk have yielded disappointing results. Vitamin and mineral supplements have been shown to reduce the risk of stomach cancer in one intervention study in China,[48] but other studies using high doses of single nutrients have shown no benefit and even unexpected evidence for harm (see Beta Carotene). Although supplements do not substitute for healthful diets in reducing cancer risk, it is possible that some people, such as pregnant women, women of childbearing age, and people with restricted dietary intakes, might benefit from taking moderate doses of vitamin and mineral supplements for other reasons.

Can drinking tea reduce cancer risk? Some researchers have proposed that tea, especially green tea, might protect against cancer because of its content of antioxidants (see Antioxidants). In animal studies, some teas have been shown to reduce cancer risk, but beneficial effects of tea on cancer risk in people are not yet proven.

Does vitamin A lower cancer risks? Vitamin A (retinol) is obtained from foods in two ways: as preformed from animal food sources and as derived from beta carotene found in plant foods. Vitamin A is needed to maintain healthy tissues. Vitamin A supplements have not been shown to lower cancer risk, however. If supplements are taken, they should remain within recommended levels, as high doses of preformed vitamin A can be harmful, especially to pregnant women. Because the body does not convert beta carotene to vitamin A when vitamin A levels are within normal ranges, eating fruits and vegetables containing beta carotene cannot lead to vitamin A toxicity.

Does vitamin C lower cancer risk? Vitamin C is found in many fruits and vegetables. Many studies have linked consumption of vitamin C-rich foods with a reduced risk of cancer. The few studies in which vitamin C has been given as a supplement, however, have not shown a reduced risk of cancer.[49,50]

Does vitamin E lower cancer risk? Vitamin E may lower the risk for coronary heart disease. Vitamin E supplements, however, have not been shown to reduce cancer risks.[18,50]

References*

12. Willett WC: Micronutrients and cancer risk. Am J. Clin Nutr 1994;599(suppl 5):1162s–1165s.
13. Steinmetz, KA, Potter JD: Vegetables, fruit, and cancer. I. Epidemiology. Cancer Causes Control 1991;2:325–357.
18. The Alpha-Tocopherol, Beta Carotene Cancer Prevention Study Group: The effect of vitamin E and beta carotene on the incidence of lung cancer and other cancers in male smokers. N Engl J Med 1994;330:1029–1035.
19. Omenn G, Goodman GE, Thornquist MD, et al: Effects of a combination of beta carotene and vitamin A on lung cancer and cardiovascular disease. N Engl J Med 1996;334:1150–1155.
23. Messina M, Erdman JW (eds): First international symposium on the role of soy in preventing and treating chronic disease. J Nutr 1995;125(suppl 3):567s–808s.
44. Hennekens CH, Buring JE, Manson JE, et al: Lack of effect of long-term supplementation with beta carotene on the incidence of malignant neoplasms and cardiovascular disease. N Engl J. Med 1996;334;1145–1149.
45. Westrate JA, van het Hof KH: Sucrose polyester and plasma carotenoid concentrations in healthy subjects. Am J Clin Nutr 1995;62:591–597.
46. Tricopoulou A, Katsouyanni K, Stuver S, et al: Consumption of olive oil and specific food groups in relation to breast cancer risk in Greece. J Natl Cancer Inst 1995;87:110–116.
47. National Research Council: Carcinogens and Anticarcinogens in the Human Diet: A Comparison of Naturally Occurring and Synthetic Substances. Washington, DC, National Academy Press, 1996.
48. Blot WJ, Li JY, Taylor PR, et al: Nutrition intervention trials in Linxian, China: Supplementation with specific vitamin/mineral combinations, cancer incidence, and disease-specific mortality in the general population. J Natl Cancer Inst 1993;85:1483–1492.
49. Block G: Vitamin C and cancer prevention: The epidemiologic evidence. Am J Clin Nutr 1991;53(suppl 1):270s–282s.
50. Byers T, Perry G: Dietary carotenes, vitamin C and vitamin E as protective antioxidants in human cancers. Annu Rev Nutr 1992;12:139–159.
* Missing references do not apply to this article.

DIET AND HYPERTENSION: PROGRESS TOWARDS A BETTER UNDERSTANDING

••• INTRODUCTION

Hypertension (high blood pressure) affects nearly 50 million Americans, or one in four adults (1–3). Uncontrolled high blood pressure increases the risk for coronary heart disease, stroke, cardiac failure, and kidney disease (1,3–5). In 1995, hypertension cost the nation nearly $24 billion in direct medical expenditures, lost wages, and lowered productivity (5). The magnitude of hypertension, its serious health consequences, and its staggering economic burden clearly justify public health efforts to reduce its prevalence. Relatively small reductions in blood pressure can have a major, positive impact on health (6,7).

Blood pressure generally is expressed in two numbers: systolic (i.e., when the heart is contracting) and diastolic (i.e., when the heart is resting) blood pressure (1). A reading of 120/80 (systolic/diastolic) millimeters of mercury (mm Hg) is considered to be normal, whereas hypertension is defined as a blood pressure reading equal to or greater than 140 mm Hg systolic or 90 mm Hg diastolic (1). The risk of hypertension generally increases with advancing age and is higher among African Americans than Hispanic

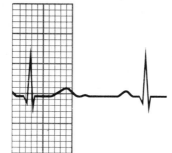

and non-Hispanic whites (3,5,8). At younger ages, men are at greater risk of high blood pressure than women, whereas in later years, the prevalence is higher among women (1,3). Hypertension can also result as a complication of pregnancy (3).

The cause of more than 90% of hypertension is unknown (9). In contrast to this so-called "primary" or "essential" hypertension, a few people develop "secondary" hypertension as a consequence of a disease/condition. Both genetic and environmental factors contribute to the most common or "essential" hypertension. Among environmental factors, lifestyle factors such as diet, alcohol intake, physical activity, stress, and cigarette smoking influence blood pressure (1,10,11). Considerable recent attention has focused on the impact of lifestyle modifications, including diet, on the prevention and management of hypertension (1,3,10,11).

This *Digest* reviews recent research findings related to the role of body weight, sodium (salt or sodium chloride), calcium, potassium, and magnesium in blood pressure regulation. Because the impact of specific nutrients on blood pressure is complicated by the complexity of dietary interactions and because people consume foods, not individual nutrients, researchers have recently assessed the effects of specific dietary patterns on blood pressure (12). Observations from this research, as well as dietary recommendations to reduce the risk of hypertension, also are presented in this *Digest*.

WEIGHT CONTROL AND BLOOD PRESSURE

Evidence related to the role of macro-nutrients (i.e., carbohydrate, fat, protein) on blood pressure regulation is limited and inconclusive (1,10). However, it is generally accepted that excess energy (calorie) intake in association with low levels of physical activity can lead to obesity, a risk factor for high blood pressure (8,13,14). Many hypertensives are overweight and weight reduction lowers blood pressure and may reduce or eliminate the need for antihypertensive medication (13,14).

Body weight or body mass index is a strong, independent predictor of blood pressure (10,14–19). In addition, the location of body fat can influence blood pressure (8,14). Individuals with central or abdominal obesity are at higher risk of hypertension and its complications than those with peripherally located body fat (8,14). Weight control is considered to be the single, most effective lifestyle intervention to reduce blood pressure (14,20).

MICRONUTRIENTS AND BLOOD PRESSURE

Sodium. Historically, dietary sodium has been the nutrient most often linked to blood pressure control (1,11). Worldwide population studies have demonstrated a positive association between sodium intake and blood pressure (8,21–23). In hypertensive patients, severe restriction of dietary salt (sodium chloride) (i.e., <1g/day) often lowers blood pressure, whereas excess dietary salt tends to raise blood pressure (24). However, reducing sodium intake is not uniformly effective for everyone, leading to the concept of salt sensitivity. Indeed, in some individuals, a low sodium intake may adversely impact nutrient intake and increase morbidity and mortality (25,26). Controversy regarding the effect of

New research indicates that blood pressure can be lowered not just by what you take out of your diet, such as sodium, calories, or alcohol, but also by what you add, such as foods rich in calcium, potassium, and magnesium.

sodium on blood pressure is currently being fueled by findings from several investigations (16,17,22,27,28). While a relationship between sodium and blood pressure is generally found when comparing different populations, it is often not observed within a population. Also, the impact of sodium intake on blood pressure appears to be greater for hypertensive than normotensive individuals (28).

Variability in the blood pressure response to dietary salt results from varying degrees of salt sensitivity (24,29–33). In salt sensitive individuals, blood pressure increases with salt loading and decreases with salt restriction, whereas in salt resistant individuals, blood pressure does not change with salt intake (29,31,33).

At present, there is no way to identify salt sensitive from salt resistant individuals (31). However, certain population groups including hypertensive individuals, African Americans, obese persons, patients with kidney disease, individuals with a family history of hypertension, adults aged 65 years and older, and people with low plasma renin levels are more likely to be salt sensitive than others (1,8,29). Genetics may be a major determinant of salt sensitivity and ongoing studies are attempting to identify specific genes, as well as nongenetic factors, that contribute to this trait (29–31,33). Interactions among dietary components such as chloride, calcium, potassium, and magnesium may also contribute to variability in the blood pressure response to dietary sodium (29,34,35).

The estimated minimum requirement for sodium is 500mg/day (36). Because dietary sodium intake in the U.S. typically is about 3,000 to 4,000mg/day (3,37,38), moderation in sodium and salt intake is advised (1,39). About one level teaspoon of salt or a sodium intake of 2,400mg/day (6g salt) is recommended for the general healthy American population (1,39). However, new scientific findings have heightened the debate regarding the appropriateness of universal sodium recommendations (16,25,28).

Nevertheless, reducing dietary sodium may be beneficial for individuals whose blood pressure levels are high, who are salt sensitive, or who are at high risk of low renin hypertension (24). Moderate salt restriction may also enhance the effectiveness of anti-hypertensive medication (24). Another reason to avoid excess salt intake relates to its effect on calcium (39–41). Sodium increases urinary calcium loss and the body's need for calcium (40–44). As discussed below, an adequate intake of calcium may protect against hypertension (32,35).

Researchers have recently considered the possibility that reducing sodium intake may not be risk free. Diets restricted in sodium are potentially low in several essential nutrients which play a beneficial role in blood pressure regulation, including calcium, magnesium, and potassium (32,35,45,46). Also, severely restricting sodium intake may actually increase morbidity and mortality in some individuals (25,35,47). For most people, there is no evidence of long-term adverse effects of sodium intakes between 500 mg to 2,400 mg/day (7).

Calcium. Findings from numerous epidemiological, experimental animal, and clinical intervention studies in humans demonstrate that increasing the intake of calcium or calcium-rich foods such as milk and other dairy foods reduces blood pressure (11,42–44,48–53). The majority of epidemiological studies in this area, especially cross-sectional studies, indicate an inverse relationship between calcium intake and blood pressure levels (18,48,49,54).

In experimental animals, the antihypertensive effect of calcium is fairly consistent (49,50). In both normotensive and hypertensive animals, a high calcium diet lowers blood pressure or attenuates the development of hypertension, whereas calcium deprivation elevates blood pressure (49,50, 55,56). Abnormalities in calcium metabolism in hypertensive animals provide insight into potential mechanisms by which calcium protects against hypertension (55,56).

Clinical intervention trials in humans indicate a beneficial effect of calcium intake on blood pressure levels (49,51–53,57–59). According to a recent meta-analysis of 33 randomized controlled studies involving 2,412 individuals in the general population (51), increasing calcium intake by 1,000 to 2,000 mg/day was associated with a small,

Individuals vary in their blood pressure response to sodium/salt intake and, for some, a low sodium intake may not be risk free.

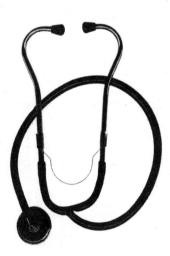

but statistically significant, reduction in systolic blood pressure. However, the modest overall findings may obscure the larger impact of calcium intake on blood pressure in certain subgroups such as calcium deficient and/or hypertensive individuals (51). In support of this concept, the blood pressure-lowering effect of calcium has been demonstrated to be greater in individuals with low rather than high baseline calcium intakes, in hypertensive than normotensive individuals, and in salt sensitive, low renin hypertensives than in salt resistant, high renin hypertensives (44,53,57,58,60). Calcium also lowers blood pressure more when sodium intake is high than when it is low (43).

An adequate intake of calcium during pregnancy is especially effective in reducing risk of pregnancy-induced hypertension and preeclampsia (49,52,61). Consuming the amount of calcium recommended for pregnant women (i.e., 1,200 to 1,500 mg/day) lowered the risk of pregnancy-induced hypertension by 70% and preeclampsia by 62%, according to a recent meta-analysis of 14 randomized controlled trials involving 2,459 pregnant women (52). Pregnancy-induced hypertension occurs in 10% to 20% of all pregnancies, and is characterized by metabolic abnormalities in calcium metabolism (62). Preeclampsia, a life-threatening disorder of late pregnancy that occurs in 2% to 8% of all pregnancies, can endanger the health of both the mother and child (52). Increasing dietary calcium intake to recommended levels during pregnancy is estimated to save several billion dollars a year in health care costs related to hypertensive disorders of pregnancy (63).

Although the mechanism(s) for calcium's hypotensive action is not fully defined, several possibilities have been considered (42–44,56,64). These include a calcium-induced natriuretic (urinary sodium excretion) effect, a decrease in calcium regulating hormones, and a reduction in intracellular free calcium. Because calcium plays an important role in vascular contraction, many of the postulated mechanisms relate to metabolic changes influencing vascular smooth muscle contraction (44,53,58).

A calcium intake of at least the Recommended Dietary Allowance (RDA) (i.e., 800–1,200 mg calcium/day) (36) or the higher levels recommended by a U.S. government consensus panel on optimal calcium intake (i.e., 1,000–1,500 mg) (41) is considered to be a prudent health measure to reduce risk of high blood pressure (49,57,65). Meeting calcium needs with calcium-rich foods such as milk and other dairy foods not only improves the overall nutrient quality of the diet (66), but has also been demonstrated to have no adverse effects on other cardiovascular disease risk factors such as blood lipid levels or body weight (67).

Potassium. Dietary potassium has been demonstrated to protect against hypertension and its associated vascular diseases including stroke, as well as reduce the need for antihypertensive medication (1,8,32,34,68). Epidemiological (10,21), animal (69), and clinical intervention trials (70–72) generally indicate an inverse relationship between potassium intake and blood pressure. However, findings of a hypotensive effect of potassium are not entirely consistent (32). Potassium appears to lower blood pressure more in hypertensive than normotensive individuals and is especially beneficial when potassium intake is low (8,34,70).

The mechanism(s) by which dietary potassium protects against high blood pressure is unknown, but appears to be mediated in part by interactions with other nutrients such as sodium, calcium, and magnesium (32,34,72). Potassium intake may lower blood pressure by increasing sodium excretion. Like calcium, the hypotensive effect of potassium is more pronounced when sodium (salt) intake is high (34,69). Increased potassium intake also reduces urinary losses of calcium and magnesium which have a protective effect on blood pressure (32,69). Ensuring an adequate intake of potassium, preferably from foods such as vegetables, fruits, and dairy foods (milk and yogurt), is recommended to reduce the risk of hypertension (1,39,71).

The blood pressure lowering effect of dietary calcium is particularly beneficial for individuals whose calcium intake is low such as hypertensive persons, African Americans, and mature adults and/or individuals such as pregnant women whose needs for calcium are high.

Magnesium. Magnesium is known to promote vascular smooth muscle relaxation (73). Although epidemiological (10,17,74), animal (75), and clinical intervention trials in humans (76) indicate a protective effect of magnesium on blood pressure, the evidence is more limited and less conclusive than the data for either calcium or potassium (11,32,65, 73). Inconsistent reports regarding magnesium's effects on blood pressure may be explained by its interactions with other nutrients such as calcium and potassium (73). Also, the hypotensive effect of magnesium may be restricted to magnesium-deficient individuals (77). Although many questions remain, consuming an adequate intake of magnesium from foods such as nuts, legumes, unrefined grains, green vegetables, and dairy foods may help prevent hypertension, particularly in susceptible subgroups (65,78).

PUTTING IT ALL TOGETHER: EFFECTS OF DIETARY PATTERNS ON BLOOD PRESSURE

Clearly, the impact of individual nutrients on blood pressure is complicated by the complexity of dietary interactions. To gain increased understanding of the combined effects of nutrients that occur together in foods, the National Institutes of Health sponsored a multicenter feeding trial which examined dietary patterns and blood pressure (12). A diet rich in lowfat dairy foods, fruits, and vegetables significantly and quickly (within two weeks) lowered blood pressure according to the findings from this trial, called the "Dietary Approaches to Stop Hypertension" (DASH). For participants with high blood pressure, this diet reduced blood pressure as effectively as some blood pressure medications (12).

More than 450 adults with systolic blood pressures of less than 160 mm Hg and diastolic pressures of 80 to 95 mm Hg were enrolled in the study (12). About half of the participants were women and nearly 60% were African Americans. For eight weeks, participants were fed one of three diets: a "control diet" similar to what many Americans consume (i.e., low in fruits, vegetables, and dairy foods and containing 36% of calories from fat); a "fruits and vegetables" diet (i.e., higher in fiber, potassium, and magnesium than the control diet, but similar in fat); or a "combination" diet high in lowfat dairy foods, fruits, and vegetables and reduced in total fat (26% of calories), saturated fat, and cholesterol (i.e., higher in fiber, protein, potassium, magnesium, and calcium than the control diet). All three diets were equal in salt content (i.e., 3 g sodium/day) and all participants maintained body weight.

At the end of the eight weeks, the combination diet—the reduced fat diet that added lowfat dairy foods along with fruits and vegetables—produced the largest reductions in blood pressures (12). Overall, this diet reduced systolic blood pressure by 5.5 mm Hg and diastolic blood pressure by 3.0 mm Hg compared to the control diet. For participants with hypertension, the blood pressure lowering effect of the combination diet was even more impressive, with an average reduction of 11.4 mm Hg for systolic and 5.5 mm Hg for diastolic blood pressures (12). The fruits and vegetables diet reduced blood pressure less than the combination diet.

Participants following the combination diet consumed almost three servings of dairy foods a day (i.e., a mean of 1260 mg calcium/day). They also consumed 8 to 10 servings a day of fruits and vegetables. The researchers believe that consuming a diet similar to the combination diet and following other lifestyle recommendations to lower blood pressure could help prevent hypertension and, for some hypertensives, may reduce or eliminate the need for blood pressure medication (12).

Current national guidelines to prevent or treat hypertension include the following:
- Lose weight if overweight
- Limit alcohol intake to no more than one ounce a day
- Increase regular aerobic exercise
- Reduce sodium intake to less than 2.3 g/day (6 g sodium chloride)

Consuming a diet containing 3 servings/day of lowfat dairy foods and 8 to 10 servings/day of fruits and vegetables substantially and quickly (within two weeks) lowers blood pressure, according to a new nationwide U.S. government-sponsored study.

- Consume recommended amounts of dietary potassium, calcium, and magnesium
- Stop smoking
- Monitor blood pressure regularly (1,11).

REFERENCES

1. National High Blood Pressure Education Program. Arch. Intern. Med. *153*: 154, 1993.
2. Burt, V.L., J.A. Cutler, M. Higgins, et. al. Hypertension 26: 60, 1995.
3. Federation of American Societies for Experimental Biology, Life Sciences Research Office. Prepared for the Interagency Board for Nutrition Monitoring and Related Research. *Third Report on Nutrition Monitoring in the United States: Volume 1.* Washington, D.C.: U.S. Government Printing Office, 1995.
4. Kannel, W.B. JAMA 275: 1571, 1996.
5. Dustan, H.P., E.J. Roccella, and H.H. Garrison. Arch. Intern. Med. 156: 1926, 1996.
6. Cook, N.R., J. Cohen, P.R. Hebert, et. al. Arch. Intern. Med. *155*: 701, 1995.
7. Statement from the National High Blood Pressure Education Program Coordinating Committee. Approved March 30, 1995.
8. Adrogue, H.J., and D.E. Wesson. Semin. Nephrol. *16(2)*: 94, 1996.
9. Kaplan, N.M. Arch. Intern. Med. *155*: 563, 1995.
10. Stamler, J., A.W. Caggiula, and G.A. Grandits. Am. J. Clin. Nutr. *65(suppl)*: 338, 1997.
11. National High Blood Pressure Education Program Working Group. Arch. Intern. Med. *153*: 186, 1993.
12. Appel, L.J., T.J. Moore, E. Obarzanek, et. al. N. Engl. J. Med. *336*: 1117, 1997.
13. Preuss, H.G., J.A. Gondal, and S. Lieberman. J. Am. Coll. Nutr. *15(1)*: 21, 1996.
14. McCarron, D.A., and M.E. Reusser. Am. J. Clin. Nutr. *63(suppl)*: 423, 1996.
15. Masaki, K.H., J.D. Curb, D. Chiu, et. al. Hypertension 29: 673, 1997.
16. The Trials of Hypertension Prevention Collaborative Research Group. Arch. Intern. Med. *157*: 657, 1997.
17. Ascherio, A., C. Hennekens, W.C. Willett, et. al. Hypertension 27: 1065, 1996.
18. Dwyer, J.H., L. Li, K.M. Dwyer, et. al. Am. J. Epidemiol. *144*: 828, 1996.
19. Kawamura, M., T. Adachi, J. Nakajima, et. al. Hypertension *27(part 1)*: 408, 1996.
20. Pickering, T.G. Arch. Intern. Med. *157*: 596, 1997.
21. Intersalt Co-Operative Research Group. Br. Med. J. *297*: 319, 1988.
22. Elliott, P., J. Stamler, R. Nichols, et. al. Br. Med. J. *312*: 1249, 1996.
23. Stamler, J. Am. J. Clin. Nutr. *65(suppl)*: 626S, 1997.
24. Haddy, F.J., and M.B. Pamnani. J. Am. Coll. Nutr. *14*: 428, 1995.
25. Alderman, M.H., S. Madhavan, H. Cohen, et. al. Hypertension 25: 1144–1152, 1995.
26. Oparil, S. Am. J. Clin. Nutr. *65(suppl)*: 583S, 1997.
27. Cutler, J.A., D. Follmann, and P.S. Allender. Am. J. Clin. Nutr. *65(suppl)*: 643S, 1997.
28. Midgley, J.P., A.G. Matthew, C.M.T. Greenwood, et. al. JAMA 275: 1590, 1996.
29. Luft, F.C., and M.H. Weinberger. Am. J. Clin. Nutr. *65(suppl)*: 612S, 1997.
30. Ely, D.L. Am. J. Clin. Nutr. *65(suppl)*: 594S, 1997.
31. Cowley, A.W., Jr. Am. J. Clin. Nutr. *65(suppl)*: 587S, 1997.

32. Reusser, M.E., and D.A. McCarron. Nutr. Rev. *52*: 367, 1994.

33. Weinberger, M.H. Hypertension *27(3 Pt.2)*: 481, 1996.

34. Kotchen, T.A., and J.M. Kotchen. Am. J. Clin. Nutr. *65(suppl)*: 708S, 1997.

35. McCarron, D.A. Am. J. Clin. Nutr. *65(suppl)*: 712S, 1997.

36. Food and Nutrition Board, Subcommittee on the Tenth Edition of the RDAs. *Recommended Dietary Allowances, 10th Edition*. Washington, DC: National Academy Press, 1989.

37. Engstrom, A., R.C. Tobelmann, and A.M. Albertson. Am. J. Clin. Nutr. *65(suppl)*: 704S, 1997.

38. Alaimo, K., M.A. McDowell, R.R. Briefel, et. al. Dietary intake of vitamins, minerals, and fiber of persons ages 2 months and over in the United States: Third National Health and Nutrition Examination Survey, Phase 1, 1988–1991. Advance Data from Vital and Health Statistics; No. 258. Hyattsville, MD: National Center for Health Statistics, 1994.

39. U.S. Department of Agriculture, U.S. Department of Health and Human Services. *Nutrition and Your Health: Dietary Guidelines for Americans*. Fourth Edition. December 1995.

40. Itoh, R., and Y. Suyama. Am. J. Clin. Nutr. *63*: 735, 1996.

41. U.S. Department of Health and Human Services, Public Health Service, National Institutes of Health. *Consensus Development Conference Statement. Optimal Calcium Intake*. June 6–8; 12(4): 1–31, 1994.

42. Zemel, M.B., S. Gualdoni, and J.R. Sowers. Am. J. Hypertens. *1*: 70, 1988.

43. Zemel, M.B., S.M. Gualdoni, M.F. Walsh, et. al. J. Hypertens. *4*: S364, 1986.

44. Zemel, M.B. Nutr. Metab. Cardiovasc. Dis. *4*: 224, 1994.

45. Van Buul, B.J.A., E.A.P. Steegers, H.W. Jongsma, et. al. Am. J. Clin. Nutr. *62*: 49, 1995.

46. Morris, C.D. Am. J. Clin. Nutr. *65(suppl)*: 687S, 1997.

47. McCarron, D.A., A.B. Weder, B.M. Egan, et. al. Am. J. Hypertens. *10*: 68, 1997.

48. Morris, C.D., and M.E. Reusser. Semin. Nephrol. *15*: 490, 1995.

49. Hamet, P. J. Nutr. *125(2 Suppl)*: 311, 1995.

50. Hatton, D.C., and D.A. McCarron. Hypertension *23*: 513, 1994.

51. Bucher, H.C., R.J. Cook, G.H. Guyatt, et. al. JAMA *275*: 1016, 1996.

52. Bucher, H.C., G.H. Guyatt, R.J. Cook, et. al. JAMA *275*: 1113, 1996.

53. McCarron, D.A. Keio. J. Med. *44*: 105, 1995.

54. Cappuccio, F.P., P. Elliott, P.S. Allender, et. al. Am. J. Epidemiol. *142*: 935, 1995.

55. Schleiffer, R., and A. Gairard. Semin. Nephrol. *15*: 526, 1995.

56. Porsti, I., and H. Makynen. Semin. Nephrol. *15*: 550, 1995.

57. Allender, P.S., J.A. Cutler, D. Follmann, et. al. Ann. Intern. Med. *124*: 825, 1996.

58. Sanchez, M., A. de la Sierra, A. Coca, et. al. Hypertension *29(part 2)*: 531, 1997.

59. Vaughan, L.A., M.M. Manore, M.E. Russo, et. al. Nutr. Res. *17(2)*: 215, 1997.

60. Zemel, M.B., P.C. Zemel, R. Bryg, et. al. Am. J. Hypertens. *3*: 458, 1990.

61. Hojo, M., and P. August. Semin. Nephrol. *15*: 504, 1995.

62. Zemel, M.B., P.C. Zemel, S. Berry, et. al. N. Engl. J. Med. *323*: 434, 1990.

63. McCarron, D.A., and D. Hatton. JAMA *275*: 1128, 1996.

64. Hatton, D.C., Q. Yue, and D.A. McCarron. Semin. Nephrol. *15*: 593, 1995.

65. Harlan, W.R., and L.C. Harlan. In: *Hypertension: Pathophysiology, Diagnosis, and Management, Second Edition*. J.H. Laragh, and B.M. Brenner (Eds). New York, NY: Raven Press, Ltd., 1995, p. 1143.

66. Duene, A., R.L. Prince, and R. Bell. Am. J. Clin. Nutr. *64*: 731, 1996.

67. Karanja, N., C.D. Morris, P. Rufolo, et. al. Am. J. Clin. Nutr. *59*: 900, 1994.

68. Siani, A., P. Strazzullo, A. Giacco, et. al. Ann. Intern. Med. *115*: 753, 1991.

69. Wu, X., U. Ackermann, and H. Sonnenberg. Clin. Exp. Hypertens. *17(6)*: 989, 1995.

70. Cappuccio, F.P., and G.A. MacGregor. Hypertension *9*: 465, 1991.

71. Brancati, F.L., L.J. Appel, A.J. Seidler, et. al. Arch. Intern. Med. *156*: 61, 1996.

72. Geleijnse, J.M., J.C.M. Witteman, J.H. den Breeijen, et. al. J. Hypertens. *14(6)*: 737, 1996.

73. Paolisso, G., and M. Barbagallo. Am. J. Hypertens. *10*: 346, 1997.

74. Ma, J., A.R. Folsom, S.L. Melnick, et. al. J. Clin. Epidemiol. *48(7)*: 927, 1995.

75. Laurant, P., J.-P. Kantelip, and A. Berthelot. J. Nutr. *125*: 830, 1995.

76. Witteman, J.C.M., D.E. Grobbee, F.H.M. Derkx, et. al. Am. J. Clin. Nutr. *60*: 129, 1994.

77. Zemel, P.C., M.B. Zemel, M. Urberg, et. al. Am. J. Clin. Nutr. *51*: 665, 1990.

78. Resnick, L.M. Am. J. Hypertens. *10*: 368, 1997.

BONING UP ON
OSTEOPOROSIS

Consider an insidious condition that drains away bone—the hardest, most durable substance in the body. It happens slowly, over years, so that often neither doctor nor patient is aware of weakening bones until one snaps unexpectedly. Unfortunately, this isn't science fiction. It's why osteoporosis is called the silent thief.

Carolyn J. Strange

Carolyn J. Strange is a science and medical writer living in Northern California.

There is no cure for osteoporosis, but the onset can be delayed and the severity diminished.

And it steals more than bone. It's the primary cause of hip fracture, which can lead to permanent disability, loss of independence, and sometimes even death. Collapsing spinal vertebrae can produce stooped posture and a "dowager's hump." Lives collapse too. The chronic pain and anxiety that accompany a frail frame make people curtail meaningful activities, because the simplest things can cause broken bones: Stepping off a curb. A sneeze. Bending to pick up something. A hug. "Don't touch Mom, she might break" is the sad joke in many families.

Osteoporosis leads to 1.5 million fractures, or breaks, per year, mostly in the hip, spine and wrist, and costs $10 billion annually, according to the National Osteoporosis Foundation. It threatens 25 million Americans, mostly older women, but older men get it too. One in three women past 50 will suffer a vertebral fracture, according to the foundation. These numbers are predicted to rise as the population ages.

Osteoporosis, which means "porous bones," is a condition of excessive skeletal fragility resulting in bones that break easily. A combination of genetic,

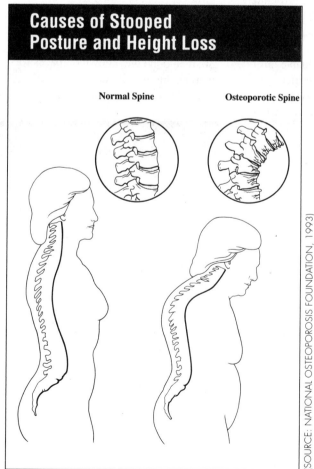

Causes of Stooped Posture and Height Loss

Normal Spine   Osteoporotic Spine

(SOURCE: NATIONAL OSTEOPOROSIS FOUNDATION, 1993)

The spine is made up of a series of small connected bones called vertebrae (left). Healed vertebral fractures become compressed (flattened) or may mend in a wedge shape. Over time, multiple fractures of the spine can result in stooped posture, a loss of height, and continual pain (right).

dietary, hormonal, age-related, and lifestyle factors all contribute to this condition.

Changing attitudes and improving technology are brightening the outlook for people with osteoporosis. Nowadays, many women live 30 years or more—

sponds to the pull of muscles and gravity, repairs itself, and constantly renews itself.

Besides protecting internal organs and allowing us to move about, bone is also involved in the body's handling of minerals. Of the 2 to 4 pounds of cal-

count, but in our skeletal "account" we can deposit bone only during our first three decades. After that, all we can do is try to postpone and minimize the steady withdrawals. Osteoporosis is the bankruptcy that occurs when too little bone is formed during youth, or too

Osteoporosis leads to 1.5 million fractures, or breaks, per year, mostly in the hip, spine and wrist.

perhaps a quarter to a third of their lives—after menopause. Improving the quality of those years has become an important health-care goal. Although some bone loss is expected as people age, osteoporosis is no longer viewed as an inevitable consequence of aging. Diagnosis and treatment need no longer wait until bones break.

There is no cure for osteoporosis, and it can't be prevented outright, but the onset can be delayed, and the severity diminished. Most important, early intervention can prevent devastating fractures. The Food and Drug Administration has revised labeling on foods and supplements to provide valuable information about the level of nutrients that help build and maintain strong bones. FDA has also approved a wide variety of products to help diagnose and treat osteoporosis, including several just last year.

Bone Life

Bone consists of a matrix of fibers of the tough protein collagen, hardened with calcium, phosphorus and other minerals. Two types of architecture give bones strength. Surrounding every bone is a tough, dense rind of cortical bone. Inside is spongy-looking trabecular bone. Its interconnecting structure provides much of the strength of healthy bone, but is especially vulnerable to osteoporosis.

"We tend to think of the skeleton as an inert erector set that holds us up and doesn't do much else. That's not true," says Karl. L. Insogna, M.D., director of the Bone Center at Yale School of Medicine, New Haven, Conn. Every bit as dynamic as other tissues, bone re-

cium in the body, nearly 99 percent is in the teeth and skeleton. The remainder plays a critical role in blood clotting, nerve transmission, muscle contraction (including heartbeat), and other functions. The body keeps the blood level of calcium within a narrow range. When needed, bones release calcium.

A complex interplay of many hormones balances the activity of the two types of cells—osteoclasts and osteoblasts—responsible for the continuous turnover process called remodeling. Osteoclasts break down bone, and osteoblasts build it. In youth, bone building prevails. Bone mass peaks by about age 30, then bone breakdown outpaces formation, and density declines.

The skeleton is like a retirement ac-

much is lost later, or both.

"You've got to get as much bone as you can and not lose it," Insogna says. "The most important risk factor for osteoporosis is a low bone mass."

"The upper limit of bone mass that you can acquire is genetically determined," says Mona S. Calvo, Ph.D., in FDA's Office of Special Nutritionals. "But even though you may be programmed for high bone mass, other factors can influence how much bone you end up with," she says. (See "Reducing Your Risk.") For instance, men tend to build greater bone mass, which is partly why more women face osteoporosis.

But there's another reason. With the decline of the female hormone estrogen at menopause, usually around age 50,

To Learn More

For more information, contact:
• National Osteoporosis Foundation, 1150 17th St., N.W., Suite 500, Washington, DC 20036; (202) 223-2226; World Wide Web: *http://www.nof.org/*. For locations of your nearest bone density testing sites, call (800) 464-6700.
• Osteoporosis and Related Bone Diseases National Resource Center (ORBD-NRC); (800) 624-BONE; TDD: (202) 223-0344.
• Older Women's League (OWL), 666 11th St., N.W., Suite 700, Washington, DC 20001; (202) 783-6686.
• North American Menopause Society, c/o University Hospitals of Cleveland, Department of Obstetrics and Gynecology, 11100 Euclid Ave., Suite 7024, Cleveland, OH 44106; (216) 844-8748; World Wide Web: *http://www.menopause.org/*.
• American Association of Retired Persons (AARP), 601 E St., N.W., Washington, DC 20049; (202) 434-2277; World Wide Web: *http://www.aarp.org/*.

bone breakdown markedly increases. For several years, women lose bone two to four times faster than they did before menopause. The rate usually slows down again, but some women may continue to lose bone rapidly. By age 65, some women have lost half their skeletal mass. Because the changes at menopause increase a woman's risk, many physicians feel it's a good time to measure a woman's bone density, especially if she has other risk factors for osteoporosis.

"The best way to gauge a woman's risk for osteoporotic fracture is to measure her bone mass," says Insogna.

Routine x-rays can't detect osteoporosis until it's quite advanced, but other radiological methods can. FDA has approved several kinds of devices that use various methods to estimate bone density. Most require far less radiation than a chest x-ray. Doctors consider a patient's medical history and risk factors in deciding who should have a bone density test. The method used is often determined by the equipment available locally. Readings are compared to a standard for the patient's age, sex and body size. Different parts of the skeleton may be measured, and low density at any site is worrisome.

Bone density tests are useful for confirming a diagnosis of osteoporosis if a person has already had a suspicious fracture, or for detecting low bone density so that preventative steps can be taken.

"There's a profound relationship between bone mass and risk of fracture," says Robert Recker, M.D., director of the Osteoporosis Research Center at Creighton University, Omaha, Neb.

Readings repeated at intervals of a year or more can determine the rate of bone loss and help monitor treatment effectiveness. However, estimates are not necessarily comparable between machine types because they use different measurement methods, cautions Joseph Arnaudo, in the Center for Devices and Radiological Health. "You always want to go back to the same machine, if you can," he says.

Another new test provides an indicator of bone breakdown. Last year, FDA approved a simple, noninvasive biochemical test that detects in a urine sample a specific component of bone breakdown, called NTx. Clinical labs can get results in about 2 hours. The NTx test, marketed as Osteomark, can help physicians monitor treatment and identify fast losers of bone for more aggressive treatment, but the test may not be used to diagnose osteoporosis.

Expanding Treatment Options

Physicians and patients now have endocrine drug products in FDA's Center for Drug Evaluation and Research.

Before last year, the only choices were the hormones estrogen and calcitonin. While enthusiasm for new weapons against osteoporosis is warranted, one of the old ones is still the top choice.

"Estrogen remains the first thing that women should consider," says Insogna, because the hormone not only helps prevent osteoporosis, but also protects against heart disease.

Last fall, FDA approved the first nonhormonal treatment for osteoporosis.

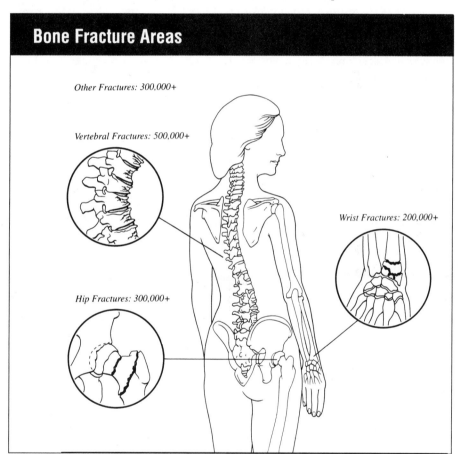

Bone Fracture Areas

Other Fractures: 300,000+

Vertebral Fractures: 500,000+

Wrist Fractures: 200,000+

Hip Fractures: 300,000+

(SOURCE: NATIONAL OSTEOPOROSIS FOUNDATION, 1993)

more treatment options than ever. Under FDA guidelines, drugs to treat osteoporosis must be shown to preserve or increase bone mass and maintain bone quality in order to reduce the risk of fractures. "We want to be sure that the bone is normal or stronger than it was," says Gloria Troendle, M.D., deputy director of the division of metabolism and

Each year, osteoporosis leads to 1.5 million bone fractures, including more than 500,000 vertebral fractures, 300,000 hip fractures, 200,000 wrist fractures, and 300,000 fractures of other bones.

"If you think about what's missing at menopause, it's the hormones," says Paula Stern, Ph.D., a pharmacologist at Northwestern University Medical School, Chicago, Ill.

Estrogen replacement therapy is the best prevention for the drop in bone mass at menopause, and there are more ways to take it than ever. But it's not for everyone. Because estrogen increases the risk of certain cancers and other diseases, taking it may not be appropriate, or it may be given in combination with another female hormone, progesterone, which can also cause undesirable side effects. A woman and her doctor need to carefully weigh the risks and benefits. According to the National Osteoporosis Foundation, a woman's risk of developing a hip fracture is equal to her combined risk of developing breast, uterine and ovarian cancer.

Women who can't or don't want to take hormones—some 30 to 50 percent—have other treatment avenues. Last summer, calcitonin treatment became much easier when FDA approved a nasal spray. Calcitonin, one of the hormones responsible for regulating the level of calcium in the blood, inhibits osteoclasts, the bone dissolvers. The drug, marketed as Miacalcin, is a potent, synthetic version of the hormone, and has been shown to slow and reverse bone loss. The stomach quickly destroys the drug, so before the spray was available, calcitonin had to be injected every day or two.

Last fall, FDA also approved the first nonhormonal treatment for osteoporosis. Alendronate, marketed as Fosamax, falls within a class of drugs called bisphosphonates, which hinder bone breakdown remodeling sites by inhibiting osteoclast activity. In clinical trials lasting three years, alendronate increased the bone mass as much as 8 percent and reduced fractures as much as 30 to 40 percent, depending on skeletal site. Lengthier studies are ongoing.

"Since it's so free of side effects it's a very welcome addition to the armamentarium. But the truth is, we still need a better treatment," says Recker. "We need a drug that will build back bone major league."

"All the drugs approved so far are

Calcium and vitamin D supplements are an integral part of all treatments for osteoporosis.

Calcium (Ac)Counts

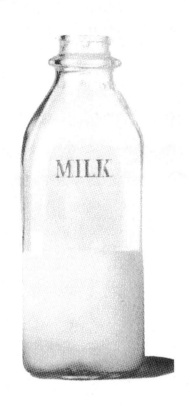

Your skeletal calcium bank has to last through old age. Frequent deposits to this retirement account should begin in youth and be maintained throughout life to help minimize withdrawals. Most women get much less calcium than they need—as little as half.

Nutritionists recommend meeting your calcium needs with foods naturally rich in calcium. Adequate calcium intake in childhood and young adulthood is critical to achieving peak adult bone mass, yet many adolescent girls replace milk with nutrient-poor beverages like soda pop. "Bone health requires a lot of nutrients and you're likely to get most of them in dairy products," says Connie Weaver, Ph.D., who heads the department of food and nutrition at Purdue

University, Indiana. "They're a huge package rather than just a single nutrient." With so many low-fat and nonfat dairy products available, it's easy to make dairy foods part of a healthy diet. People who have trouble digesting milk can look for products treated to reduce lactose. A serving of milk or yogurt contains about 350 milligrams (mg) of calcium. Fortified products have even more.

"People who don't consume dairy foods can meet their calcium needs with foods that are fortified with calcium, such as orange juice, or with calcium supplements," says Mona S. Calvo, Ph.D., in FDA's Office of Special Nutritionals. Other good sources of calcium are broccoli and dark-green leafy vegetables like kale, tofu (if made with calcium), canned fish (eaten with bones), and fortified bread and cereal products.

Nutrition labels can help you identify calcium-rich foods. But keep in mind that the label value is a guideline based on a FDA's Daily Value for calcium, which is 1,000 mg, and your calcium needs may be greater, Calvo says.

What about too much calcium? As much as 2,000 mg per day seems to be safe for most people, but those at risk for kidney stones should discuss calcium with their doctors. Calcium is critical, but even a high intake won't fully protect you against bone loss caused by estrogen deficiency, physical inactivity, alcohol abuse, smoking, or medical disorders and treatments.

—C.J.S.

things that just stop bone turnover. They're not really stimulating more bone production," says Troendle.

Bone mass increases because even though osteoclasts can't start new remodeling sites, osteoblasts continue filling in existing cavities. Increases in bone mass are most pronounced in the first year or two after treatment begins, then taper off. Any gain is helpful, even if it doesn't continue, because increases in bone mass help reduce fracture risk. But experts would like to encourage even greater gains.

Fluoride, known for fighting dental cavities, stimulates bone building, but early studies in osteoporosis patients found that the structure of the new bone was abnormal and weaker than normal bone. Gastrointestinal side effects were also a problem. Investigators are working to find a formulation and dosage regimen that will result in building normal bone.

Drugs Not Enough

Calcium and vitamin D supplements are an integral part of all treatments for osteoporosis. Everyone should make sure they get enough of these two nutrients, but especially those at risk for osteoporosis. Attention to diet and exercise are important not only for treatment, but also for prevention.

"If you go to the doctor and get a prescription, and that's all you do, you're probably not going to be helped very much," Recker says. His prevention clinic is staffed by a physical therapist, a nutritionist, and a nurse, who help people increase their physical activity, improve their diets, and make their homes safer by reducing the risk of falling. "Those three people do more to help the patients than I do with my prescription pad," Recker says.

Calcium intake is critical, and those who need it the most—younger women and girls—don't get enough. (See "Calcium (Ac)Counts.") But calcium alone can't build bone. Without vitamin D, calcium isn't sufficiently absorbed. Most people get enough vitamin D because skin produces it in sunlight. But people confined indoors who have a poor diet—which includes many older

Americans—or who live in northern latitudes in winter may be deficient.

A lifelong habit of weightbearing exercise, such as walking or biking, also helps build and maintain strong bone. The greatest benefit for older people is that physical fitness reduces the risk of fracture, because better balance, muscle strength, and agility make falls less

likely. Exercise also provides many other life-enhancing psychological and cardiovascular benefits. Increased activity can aid nutrition, too, because it boosts appetite, which is often reduced in older people. The biggest reason older people don't get enough calcium, Recker says, is that they simply don't eat much.

"The truth is, you don't have to do

Reducing Your Risk

A host of factors can affect your chances of developing osteoporosis. The good news is that you control some of them. Even though you can't change your genes, you can still lower your risk with attention to certain lifestyle changes. The younger you start, and the longer you keep it up, the better. Here's what you can do for yourself:

• Be sure you get enough calcium and vitamin D.

• Engage in regular physical activity, such as walking.

• Don't smoke.

• If you drink alcohol, do so in moderation.

A sedentary lifestyle, smoking, excessive drinking, and low calcium intake all increase risk. Although coffee has been suspected as a risk factor, studies so far are inconclusive.

Other factors are beyond your control. Being aware of them can provide extra motivation to help yourself in the ways you are able, and aids you and your doctor in health-care decisions. These risk factors are:

• being female: Women have a five times greater risk than men.

• thin, small-boned frame

• broken bones or stooped posture in older family members, especially women, which suggest a family history of osteoporosis

• early estrogen deficiency in women who experience menopause before age 45, either naturally or resulting from surgical removal of the ovaries

• estrogen deficiency due to abnormal absence of menstruation (as may accompany eating disorders)

• ethnic heritage: White and Asian women are at highest risk; African-American and Hispanic women are at lower, but significant, risk.

• advanced age

• prolonged use of some medications, such as excessive thyroid hormone; some antiseizure medications; and glucocorticoids (certain anti-inflammatory medications, such as prednisone, used to treat conditions such as asthma, arthritis and some cancers).

Risk factors may not tell the whole story. You may have none of these factors and still have osteoporosis. Or you may have many of them and not develop the condition. It's best to discuss your specific situation with your doctor.

—*C.J.S.*

very much to get most of the benefits of exercise," Recker says. He suggests 30 minutes of brisk walking five days a week. Add a little weightlifting, and that's even better. It's always smart to ask your doctor before starting a new exercise program, especially if you already have osteoporosis or other health problems.

Brighter Horizons

"A number of new things seem to be in the offing, eventually to come to us, and we're looking forward to getting some additional treatments for osteoporosis," says Troendle.

Uses of existing drugs may be broadened. Early drug trials are often conducted with patients who have severe disease, often after a fracture has occurred or bone loss is quite serious. Some studies under way are testing to see if certain drugs are effective in less severe cases, if they can be started sooner, or used in combination.

The search for bone-building drugs continues. Some naturally occurring bone-specific growth factors have been identified and their use as drugs is being investigated. "The way I visualize the ideal future is that we'll be able to give Drug X that builds up bone to where it's stronger and the risk of fracture is no longer present, then Drug Y maintains it by preventing breakdown," says Stern.

In the realm of devices, researchers are exploring the use of ultrasound to assess bone health. Such tests would eliminate radiation exposure and probably cost less. The study of risk factors also continues. "We consider that to be the research that has the greatest public health significance," says Sherry Sherman, Ph.D., of the National Institute on Aging. Last fall, the institute launched the Study of Women's Health Across the Nation, a large-scale national examination of the health of women in their 40s and 50s. Researchers expect to learn a great deal about the factors affecting women's health during these transitional years and beyond. Studies of genetics, biochemical markers, and life habits are already turning up new insights.

Osteoporosis has been described as an adolescent disease with a geriatric onset, highlighting the importance of beginning to take steps—in exercise and diet—early in life to reduce its disabling impact in later years.

Heart Disease Handbook—Part 2: Deciphering Blood Cholesterol

(Second in a four-part series on heart disease.)

Look around you. Count off every fifth adult you see—nearly 38 million Americans in all—and you have the number of people with high blood cholesterol. All are at risk for atherosclerosis, the type of heart disease that clogs arteries and can eventually stop blood flow to the heart. The sometimes deadly consequences? A heart attack.

Despite the danger of elevated blood cholesterol to an otherwise healthy heart, cholesterol itself is not the enemy. Your body needs cholesterol to build healthy cell membranes and to manufacture hormones and bile acids. The problem is not cholesterol per se, but too much of it. To be accurate, it's too much of the wrong kind that gets you into trouble.

A Little About Lipoproteins. Your risk of heart disease is determined by the transportation system that ferries cholesterol through the body. Just as oil and water do not mix, fat-soluble cholesterol does not mix well with blood. So it relies on carriers called *lipoproteins*, made up of fat (*i.e.* lipid) that's bundled together with protein, enabling it to escort cholesterol through the bloodstream.

Low-density lipoproteins (LDL's) carry cholesterol *to* artery walls, dumping their cholesterol load there, where it congregates to form artery-clogging plaque that can lead to a heart attack or stroke. Such single-minded

evil intent has earned LDL's the nickname "bad cholesterol." About two-thirds of the cholesterol in your blood is transported as LDL's.

High-density lipoproteins (HDL's) carry cholesterol *away* from arteries, scooping it up from artery walls and taking it to the liver for disposal. Such a life-saving role has rightfully earned it the tag "good cholesterol."

To keep the confusing terms straight, remember: You want your *low*-density lipoprotein level to be *low*, and your *high*-density lipoprotein level to be *high*.

Time-Honored Testing for Cholesterol. Adults should get their cholesterol checked every five years, more often if numbers are above the desirable range (see chart) or if there are other risk factors (see Part 1, February 1997).

Besides measuring for total blood cholesterol, it's best to get a separate measure of HDL's. High HDL's temper the risk of a total cholesterol that's above "desirable." Low HDL's, on the other hand, signal heart attack risk even if total cholesterol is well within the desirable range.

If your total cholesterol is high or borderline-high or your HDL's are low, you'll need to check your LDL level. Unlike total cholesterol, LDL's should be measured after a nine- to 12-hour fast. It's still fairly standard practice for labs to indirectly calculate LDL levels from blood levels of triglycerides—the form of fat circulating in your body. But since triglycerides can be affected by a recent meal, you must fast before LDL

testing. It's considered acceptable to measure HDL's without fasting, though a recent government panel of experts recommended fasting even for HDL's.

You can get a complete *lipid profile*—total cholesterol, HDL's, LDL's, and triglycerides—for about $30 to $50. Home cholesterol tests are less costly ($10 to $20), but measure only total cholesterol and are not easy to perform, since you must prick yourself and collect the blood properly.

Connecting the Numbers. To get a better sense of your heart disease risk, you should understand what your blood lipid levels mean and how these numbers relate to one other.

"If LDL's are high, it's a problem, but if, [in addition], HDL's are low, your risk is even higher," says Josef Coresh, M.D., Ph.D., of The Johns Hopkins Medical Institutions in Baltimore.

Also, check your total-cholesterol-to-HDL ratio. Although experts hesitate to pin down an "ideal" ratio, most consider a total-to-HDL ratio of 5:1 (reported as 5) or higher to be risky. (To calculate your ratio, divide total cholesterol by HDL's—e.g. $200 \div 50 = 4$.)

How Bad is Bad? "'Bad' cholesterol is a relative term," explains Coresh. "All LDL's are probably bad, but small, dense LDL's are worse." Worse, that is, than large, buoyant LDL's.

Recent studies suggest that people with a predominance of small, dense LDL's have a greater risk of heart disease than those with larger LDL's.

Reprinted with permission from *Environmental Nutrition*, March 1997, pp. 1, 4. © 1997 by Environmental Nutrition, Inc., and R. L. Polk & Company, 52 Riverside Drive, Suite 15-A, New York, NY 10024.

What Those Numbers Mean

Total Cholesterol

Less than 200	Desirable
200-239	Borderline-High Risk
240 or more	High Risk

HDL ("Good") Cholesterol

60 or more	More Desirable (protective)
35-59	Desirable
Less than 35	High Risk

LDL ("Bad") Cholesterol

Less than 100	Desirable (with heart disease)
Less than 130	Desirable (if no heart disease)
130-159	Borderline-High Risk
160 or more	High Risk

That's the case for about one in three men and one in six postmenopausal women. What's more, small LDL's are linked to other risk factors, like high triglycerides and low HDL's.

Why is small badder than bad? Small LDL's are more easily oxidized than large LDL's. Research has shown that LDL's wreak the most havoc on arteries only after they've been oxidized, that is chemically changed by oxygen, which unleashes destructive molecules called *free radicals*.

The size of LDL's is influenced, in part, by your genes, according to Ronald Krauss, M.D., of Lawrence Berkeley National Laboratory in Berkeley, California. However, LDL size might be increased by weight loss, exercise, a low-fat diet, and to a lesser extent, prescription doses of niacin. LDL size is not something routinely measured. A recent study found it doesn't predict risk any better than a full lipid profile.

A Diet-Drug Partnership. Battling blood cholesterol down to desirable levels is a key step in preventing heart disease or its recurrence. That was demonstrated dramatically in research just published in January. Of more than 1,300 people who had undergone coronary bypass surgery and were following heart-healthy diets, those who were also treated with drugs that aggressively lowered LDL's (to below 100) were able to reduce the progression of atherosclerosis 31% more than those treated with drugs that moderately lowered their LDL's (to 130).

But the first step to keeping blood cholesterol in check is to improve your diet. That means cutting back on fat (especially saturated fats and trans fats), keeping dietary cholesterol within reason, and eating more fruits, vegetables and foods rich in soluble fiber like oats and dried beans. (See Part 4, May 1997.) Losing weight, if necessary, is also part of the equation.

If that's not enough to bring your numbers into desirable range, your doctor may prescribe drugs. There's no question that new cholesterol-lowering drugs called "statins" or the often-overlooked B vitamin niacin can substantially reduce heart disease risk. These drugs are not without possible side effects, however. And taking drugs does not negate the importance of a heart-healthy diet. Without it, medication is not as effective.

Whether you want to prevent heart disease or keep an existing condition from getting worse, you need to take steps *now* to control your blood cholesterol: Eat healthfully, exercise, maintain a healthy weight and don't smoke.

—*Adrienne Forman, M.S., R.D.*

Heart Disease Handbook—Part 3: Triglycerides Turn Troublesome

(Third in a four-part series on heart disease.)

When most people get blood test results, the first thing they want to know is their cholesterol level. Those who are savvy also ask about their HDL's and LDL's (high-density and low-density lipoproteins). But how about triglycerides? If they are high, you probably shrug it off. For that matter, so may your doctor.

That may soon change. For while cholesterol, HDL's and LDL's are now familiar terms in the heart disease lexicon, triglycerides are less well-known, though perhaps equally important for heart disease risk. That's not good news for the 80 to 90 million Americans who may have high levels.

Triglycerides Tamed. Just what are triglycerides? The term is simply a fancy name for fat, or what scientists call lipids. It's what's in the food you eat and in the fat folds on your body.

Triglycerides from food travel through the bloodstream by way of chylomicrons, the largest of the lipid carriers (needed because fat and blood do not mix). Other triglycerides come from the liver, which manufactures them from excess carbohydrates and alcohol as a way to store energy. These triglycerides travel through blood via carriers called very low-density lipoproteins (VLDL's).

Both chylomicrons and VLDL's are broken down by the enzyme, lipoprotein lipase. Some people, however, inherit a lack of this crucial enzyme. Others develop an enzyme defect as a result of conditions like diabetes, alcoholism or kidney disease. The enzyme is present, but ineffective. Either way, triglycerides are elevated; it's the implications that differ.

When Things Are Not What They Seem. It doesn't always follow the higher your triglycerides, the higher your risk of heart disease. In fact, extremely high levels can actually signal less risk than "merely" high levels.

For example, people who lack the lipase enzyme end up with a lot of triglyceride-rich chylomicrons and VLDL's, sending blood triglycerides soaring, often to more than 1,000. Yet, increased risk of heart disease is not a major concern. That's because the triglycerides remain attached to the chylomicrons and VLDL's, which are so large they can't penetrate blood vessel linings and so don't contribute to dangerous build-up of artery-clogging plaque. (Such extremely high triglyceride levels do have serious consequences, however, such as inflammation of the pancreas.)

People with high triglyceride levels between 250 and 700, on the other hand, typically have the lipase enzyme available, but it is ineffective. They *do* risk heart disease. Why? Their triglycerides end up partially broken down. LDL's then take up excess triglycerides floating around and another enzyme breaks them into even smaller particles, called small, dense LDL's. These are the kind most likely to be oxidized and to clog coronary arteries. (See part 2 of series, page 95.)

Triglycerides Now Share Blame. One reason doctors have traditionally paid little attention to triglycerides is that when triglycerides are high, HDL's are invariably low. And low HDL's are a definite warning bell for heart disease risk, so high triglycerides have seemed unimportant in comparison. But scientists are now questioning this.

A recent study of 201 men and women has found that high triglycerides increase heart disease risk independently of HDL's and other factors, and suggests another reason (besides small, dense LDL's) why high levels might be risky. Researchers at the Lipoprotein Research Facility at Rush Medical College in Chicago found that triglyceride levels of 190 or more increase blood viscosity (a measure of blood's ability to flow). And previous studies have shown that people with viscous, or sluggish, blood have increased risk of heart disease, says Robert S. Rosenson, M.D., director of the facility.

"Simply losing weight can lower triglycerides."

Moreover, recent research from the University of Maryland's Center for Preventive Cardiology has found that risk may rise at much lower triglyceride levels than previously thought.

In the study, Michael Miller, M.D., director of the center, showed that of 460 people already at risk for heart disease, those whose triglyceride levels were 100 or more had twice the risk of suffering a heart attack and were twice as likely to die from it as those with levels under 100. While the findings do not necessarily apply to healthy people, Miller suggests the currently accepted triglyceride cut-off of 200—as defined by the National Institutes of Health—needs to be reexamined.

Diminishing the Danger. If high triglycerides are indeed an independent risk factor, then treatment should include ways to control them. Diet is the first choice. Drugs are used only when patients already have heart disease or when triglyceride levels exceed 500.

But designing a diet to reduce triglycerides involves some trial and error. "There's no one diet to recommend across the board for everybody," says Penny Kris-Etherton, Ph.D., R.D., of Pennsylvania State University.

For people who are overweight, simply losing weight can lower triglycerides. For others, Kris-Etherton advises starting with a heart-healthy diet that cuts back on saturated fat. Rosenson echoes her advice, while pointing out that "simple sugars and alcohol are the most offensive dietary substances" for triglyceride levels.

Complex carbohydrates are a better choice than sugars, yet excessive carbs of any type can trigger triglyceride production in some people. As a way to keep carb intake moderate, some research suggests replacing saturated fats with unsaturated fats (instead of more carbs)—in particular, more mono-unsaturated fat, such as that found in olive oil. But will people misconstrue the advice to eat more monounsaturated fats as a license to go overboard?

"My biggest fear is that people will start drizzling olive oil on everything, rationalizing, 'This is good for me'," worries Kris-Etherton. "Well, it's not good if you end up gaining weight, because that will surely cause triglycerides and cholesterol to rise."

Fish oils can also cut triglyceride levels. But, that takes supplements, says Kris-Etherton. Eating fish isn't enough.

EN **Sums It Up.** If your triglycerides are high, adopt a heart-healthy lifestyle that includes the following measures:
- Lose weight if you're overweight.

- Get or stay physically active. Aerobic activity for 30 to 40 minutes, three times a week, can reduce triglycerides 30% to 40%.
- Cut back on saturated fats, like in meat, butter, whole milk and cheese.
- Limit carbohydrates to 55% of calories or less, eaten mostly as complex carbohydrates, like in whole grains, fruits and vegetables. Especially limit simple sugars, like in sweets and soft drinks.
- If the above measures don't work, substitute monounsaturated fats, like olive and canola oils, and peanuts, for the saturated fats in your diet. But be sure total calories don't increase.
- Avoid alcohol; it stimulates triglyceride production in some people.
- Discuss fish oil supplements with your doctor. (Don't take them on your own; they can slow blood clotting, increasing stroke risk.)

—*Marsha Hudnall, M.S., R.D.*

Breast-Feeding Best Bet For Babies

Rebecca D. Williams

Rebecca D. Williams is a writer in Oak Ridge, Tenn.

New parents want to give their babies the very best. When it comes to nutrition, the best first food for babies is breast milk.

More than two decades of research have established that breast milk is perfectly suited to nourish infants and protect them from illness. Breast-fed infants have lower rates of hospital admissions, ear infections, diarrhea, rashes, allergies, and other medical problems than bottle-fed babies.

"There are 4,000 species of mammals, and they all make a different milk. Human milk is made for human infants and it meets all their specific nutrient needs," says Ruth Lawrence, M.D., professor of pediatrics and obstetrics at the University of Rochester School of Medicine in Rochester, N.Y., and spokeswoman for the American Academy of Pediatrics.

The academy recommends that babies be breast-fed for six to 12 months. The only acceptable alternative to breast milk is infant formula. Solid foods can be introduced when the baby is 4 to 6 months old, but a baby should drink breast milk or formula, not cow's milk, for a full year.

"There aren't any rules about when to stop breast-feeding," says Lawrence. "As long as the baby is eating age-appropriate solid foods, a mother may nurse a couple of years if she wishes. A baby needs breast milk for the first year of life, and then as long as desired after that."

In 1993, 55.9 percent of American mothers breast-fed their babies in the hospital. Only 19 percent were still breast-feeding when their babies were 6 months old. Government and private health experts are working to raise those numbers.

The U.S. Food and Drug Administration is conducting a study on infant feeding practices as part of its ongoing goal to improve nutrition in the United States. The study is looking at how long mothers breast-feed and how they introduce formula or other foods.

Health experts say increased breast-feeding rates would save consumers money, spent both on infant formula and in health-care dollars. It could save lives as well.

"We've known for years that the death rates in Third World countries are lower among breast-fed babies," says Lawrence. "Breast-fed babies are healthier and have fewer infections than formula-fed babies."

Human Milk for Human Infants

The primary benefit of breast milk is nutritional. Human milk contains just the right amount of fatty acids, lactose, water, and amino acids for human digestion, brain development, and growth.

Cow's milk contains a different type of protein than breast milk. This is good for calves, but human infants can have difficulty digesting it. Bottle-fed infants tend to be fatter than breast-fed infants, but not necessarily healthier.

Breast-fed babies have fewer illnesses because human milk transfers to the infant a mother's antibodies to disease.

About 80 percent of the cells in breast milk are macrophages, cells that kill bacteria, fungi and viruses. Breast-fed babies are protected, in varying degrees, from a number of illnesses, including pneumonia, botulism, bronchitis, staphylococcal infections, influenza, ear infections, and German measles. Furthermore, mothers produce antibodies to whatever disease is present in their environment, making their milk custom-designed to fight the diseases their babies are exposed to as well.

A breast-fed baby's digestive tract contains large amounts of *Lactobacillus bifidus,* beneficial bacteria that prevent the growth of harmful organisms. Human milk straight from the breast is always sterile, never contaminated by polluted water or dirty bottles, which can also lead to diarrhea in the infant.

Human milk contains at least 100 ingredients not found in formula. No babies are allergic to their mother's milk, although they may have a reaction to something the mother eats. If she eliminates it from her diet, the problem resolves itself.

Sucking at the breast promotes good jaw development as well. It's harder work to get milk out of a breast than a bottle, and the exercise strengthens the jaws and encourages the growth of straight, healthy teeth. The baby at the breast also can control the flow of milk by sucking and stopping. With a bottle, the baby must constantly suck or react to the pressure of the nipple placed in the mouth.

Nursing may have psychological benefits for the infant as well, creating an

The Lactating Breast

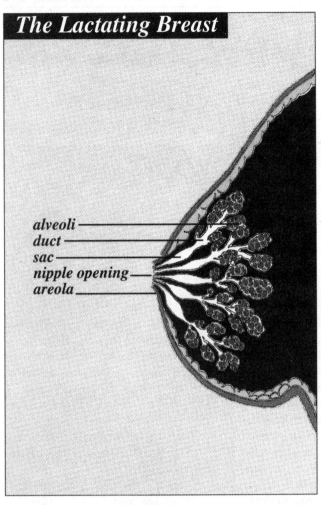

alveoli
duct
sac
nipple opening
areola

When the baby sucks, a hormone called oxytoxin starts the milk flowing from the alveoli, through the ducts (milk canals) into the sacs (milk pools) behind the areola, and finally into the baby's mouth.

early attachment between mother and child. At birth, infants see only 12 to 15 inches, the distance between a nursing baby and its mother's face. Studies have found that infants as young as 1 week prefer the smell of their own mother's milk. When nursing pads soaked with breast milk are placed in their cribs, they turn their faces toward the one that smells familiar.

Many psychologists believe the nursing baby enjoys a sense of security from the warmth and presence of the mother, especially when there's skin-to-skin contact during feeding. Parents of bottle-fed babies may be tempted to prop bottles in the baby's mouth, with no human contact during feeding. But a nursing mother must cuddle her infant closely many times during the day. Nursing becomes more than a way to feed a baby; it's a source of warmth and comfort.

Benefits to Mothers

Breast-feeding is good for new moth-ers as well as for their babies. There are no bottles to sterilize and no formula to buy, measure and mix. It may be easier for a nursing mother to lose the pounds of pregnancy as well, since nursing uses up extra calories. Lactation also stimulates the uterus to contract back to its original size.

A nursing mother is forced to get needed rest. She must sit down, put her feet up, and relax every few hours to nurse. Nursing at night is easy as well. No one has to stumble to the refrigerator for a bottle and warm it while the baby cries. If she's lying down, a mother can doze while she nurses.

Nursing is also nature's contraceptive—although not a very reliable one. Frequent nursing suppresses ovulation, making it less likely for a nursing mother to menstruate, ovulate, or get pregnant. There are no guarantees, however. Mothers who don't want more children right away should use contraception even while nursing. Hormone injections and implants are safe during

nursing, as are all barrier methods of birth control. The labeling on birth control pills says if possible another form of contraception should be used until the baby is weaned.

Breast-feeding is economical also. Even though a nursing mother works up a big appetite and consumes extra calories, the extra food for her is less expensive than buying formula for the baby. Nursing saves money while providing the best nourishment possible.

When Formula's Necessary

There are very few medical reasons why a mother shouldn't breast-feed, according to Lawrence.

Most common illnesses, such as colds, flu, skin infections, or diarrhea, cannot be passed through breast milk. In fact, if a mother has an illness, her breast milk will contain antibodies to it that will help protect her baby from those same illnesses.

A few viruses can pass through breast milk, however. HIV, the virus that causes AIDS, is one of them. Women who are HIV positive should not breast-feed.

A few other illnesses—such as herpes, hepatitis, and beta streptococcus infections—can also be transmitted through breast milk. But that doesn't always mean a mother with those diseases shouldn't breast-feed, Lawrence says.

"Each case must be evaluated on an individual basis with the woman's doctor," she says.

Breast cancer is not passed through breast milk. Women who have had breast cancer can usually breast-feed from the unaffected breast. There is some concern that the hormones produced during pregnancy and lactation may trigger a recurrence of cancer, but so far this has not been proven. Studies have shown, however, that breast-feeding a child reduces a woman's chance of developing breast cancer later.

Silicone breast implants usually do not interfere with a woman's ability to nurse, but if the implants leak, there is some concern that the silicone may harm the baby. Some small studies have suggested a link between breast-feeding with implants and later development of problems with the child's esophagus.

Tips for Breast-Feeding Success

It's helpful for a woman who wants to breast-feed to learn as much about it as possible before delivery, while she is not exhausted from caring for an infant around-the-clock. The following tips can help foster successful nursing:

• *Get an early start:* Nursing should begin within an hour after delivery if possible, when an infant is awake and the sucking instinct is strong. Even though the mother won't be producing milk yet, her breasts contain colostrum, a thin fluid that contains antibodies to disease.

• *Proper positioning:* The baby's mouth should be wide open, with the nipple as far back into his or her mouth as possible. This minimizes soreness for the mother. A nurse, midwife, or other knowledgeable person can help her find a comfortable nursing position.

• *Nurse on demand:* Newborns need to nurse frequently, at least every two hours, and not on any strict schedule. This will stimulate the mother's breasts to produce plenty of milk. Later, the baby can settle into a more predictable routine. But because breast milk is more easily digested than formula, breast-fed babies often eat more frequently than bottle-fed babies.

• *No supplements:* Nursing babies don't need sugar water or formula supplements. These may interfere with their appetite for nursing, which can lead to a diminished milk supply. The more the baby nurses, the more milk the mother will produce.

• *Delay artificial nipples:* It's best to wait a week or two before introducing a pacifier, so that the baby doesn't get confused. Artificial nipples require a different sucking action than real ones.

Sucking at a bottle could also confuse some babies in the early days. They, too, are learning how to breast-feed.

• *Air dry:* In the early postpartum period or until her nipples toughen, the mother should air dry them after each nursing to prevent them from cracking, which can lead to infection. If her nipples do crack, the mother can coat them with breast milk or other natural moisturizers to help them heal. Vitamin E oil and lanolin are commonly used, although some babies may have allergic reactions to them. Proper positioning at the breast can help prevent sore nipples. If the mother's very sore, the baby may not have the nipple far enough back in his or her mouth.

• *Watch for infection:* Symptoms of breast infection include fever and painful lumps and redness in the breast. These require immediate medical attention.

• *Expect engorgement:* A new mother usually produces lots of milk, making her breasts big, hard and painful for a few days. To relieve this engorgement, she should feed the baby frequently and on demand until her body adjusts and produces only what the baby needs. In the meantime, the mother can take over-the-counter pain relievers, apply warm, wet compresses to her breasts, and take warm baths to relieve the pain.

• *Eat right, get rest:* To produce plenty of good milk, the nursing mother needs a balanced diet that includes 500 extra calories a day and six to eight glasses of fluid. She should also rest as much as possible to prevent breast infections, which are aggravated by fatigue.

—R.D.W.

Further studies are needed in this area. But if a woman with implants wants to breast-feed, she should first discuss the potential benefits and risks with her child's doctor.

Possible Problems

For all its health benefits, breast-feeding does have some disadvantages. In the early weeks, it can be painful. A woman's nipples may become sore or cracked. She may experience engorgement more than a bottle-feeding mother, when the breasts become so full of milk they're hard and painful. Some nursing women also develop clogged milk ducts, which can lead to mastitis, a painful infection of the breast. While most nursing problems can be solved with home remedies, mastitis requires prompt medical care.

Another possible disadvantage of nursing is that it affects a woman's entire lifestyle. A nursing mother with baby-in-tow must wear clothes that enable her to nurse anywhere, or she'll have to find a private place to undress. She should eat a balanced diet and she might need to avoid foods that irritate the baby. She also shouldn't smoke, which can cause vomiting, diarrhea and restlessness in the baby, as well as decreased milk production.

Women who plan to go back to work soon after birth will have to plan carefully if they want to breast-feed. If her job allows, a new mother can pump her breast milk several times during the day and refrigerate or freeze it for the baby to take in a bottle later. Or, some women alternate nursing at night and on weekends with daytime bottles of formula.

In either case, a nursing mother is physically tied to her baby more than a bottle-feeding mother. The baby needs her for nourishment, and she needs to nurse regularly to avoid getting uncomfortably full breasts. But instead of feeling it's a chore, nursing mothers often cite this close relationship as one of the greatest joys of nursing. Besides, nursing mothers can get away between feedings if they need a break.

Finally, some women just don't feel comfortable with the idea of nursing. They don't want to handle their breasts, or they want to think of them as sexual, not functional. They may be concerned about modesty and the possibility of having to nurse in public. They may want a break from child care to let someone else feed the baby, especially in the wee hours of the morning.

If a woman is unsure whether she wants to nurse, she can try it for a few weeks and switch if she doesn't

Medicines And Nursing Mothers

Most medications have not been tested in nursing women, so no one knows exactly how a given drug will affect a breast-fed child. Since very few problems have been reported, however, most over-the-counter and prescription drugs, taken in moderation and only when necessary, are considered safe.

Even mothers who must take daily medication for conditions such as epilepsy, diabetes, or high blood pressure can usually breast-feed. They should first check with the child's pediatrician, however. To minimize the baby's exposure, the mother can take the drug just after nursing or before the child sleeps. In the January 1994 issue of *Pediatrics*, the American Academy of Pediatrics included the following in a list of drugs that are usually compatible with breast-feeding:

- acetaminophen
- many antibiotics
- antiepileptics (although one, Primidone, should be given with caution)
- most antihistamines
- alcohol in moderation (large amounts of alcohol can cause drowsiness, weakness, and abnormal weight gain in an infant)
- most antihypertensives
- aspirin (should be used with caution)
- caffeine (moderate amounts in drinks or food)
- codeine
- decongestants
- ibuprofen
- insulin
- quinine
- thyroid medications

Drugs That Are NOT Safe While Nursing

Some drugs can be taken by a nursing mother if she stops breast-feeding for a few days or weeks. She can pump her milk and discard it during this time to keep up her supply, while the baby drinks previously frozen milk or formula.

Radioactive drugs used for some diagnostic tests like Gallium–69, Iodine–125, Iodine–131, or Technetium–99m can be taken if the woman stops nursing temporarily.

Drugs that should never be taken while breast-feeding include:

Bromocriptine (Parlodel): A drug for Parkinson's disease, it also decreases a woman's milk supply.

Most Chemotherapy Drugs for Cancer: Since they kill cells in the mother's body, they may harm the baby as well.

Ergotamine (for migraine headaches): Causes vomiting, diarrhea, convulsions in infants.

Lithium (for manic-depressive illness): Excreted in human milk.

Methotrexate (for arthritis): Can suppress the baby's immune system.

Drugs of Abuse: Some drugs, such as cocaine and PCP, can intoxicate the baby. Others, such as amphetamines, heroin and marijuana, can cause a variety of symptoms, including irritability, poor sleeping patterns, tremors, and vomiting. Babies become addicted to these drugs.

Tobacco Smoke: Nursing mothers should avoid smoking. Nicotine can cause vomiting, diarrhea and restlessness for the baby, as well as decreased milk production for the mother. Maternal smoking or passive smoke may increase the risk of sudden infant death syndrome (SIDS) and may increase respiratory and ear infections.

---

like it. It's very difficult to switch to breast-feeding after bottle-feeding is begun.

If she plans to breast-feed, a new mother should learn as much as possible about it before the baby is born. Obstetricians, pediatricians, childbirth instructors, nurses, and midwives can all offer information about nursing. But perhaps the best ongoing support for a nursing mother is someone who has successfully nursed a baby.

La Leche League, a national support organization for nursing mothers, has chapters in many cities that meet regularly to discuss breast-feeding problems and offer support.

"We encourage mothers to come to La Leche League before their babies are born," says Mary Lofton, a league spokeswoman. "On-the-job training is hard to do. It's so important to learn how to breast-feed beforehand to avoid problems."

Most La Leche League chapters allow women to come to a few meetings without charge. League leaders offer advice by phone as well. To find a convenient La Leche League chapter, call (1-800) LA-LECHE.

Lactose intolerance

You may be able to handle it without treatment

Since he was old enough to remember, Tony always loved ice cream. But as he grew up, he noticed that his stomach got upset after he ate his favorite dessert. Soon, he had diarrhea and cramps nearly every time he had a bowl of ice cream. Eventually, he lost all interest in the once-tempting treat.

Tony isn't alone. As many as 50 million Americans are estimated to have lactose intolerance — an inability to comfortably digest moderate amounts of dairy products like milk and ice cream.

Common worldwide

Worldwide, nearly 70 percent of the adult population is thought to be lactose intolerant. The condition is very common among American Indians and those of Asian, African, Jewish and Hispanic descent.

Northern Europeans, a few African tribes, some Mediterranean peoples and descendants of each of these are the only people who typically do not develop lactose intolerance. No one knows exactly why, but genetics no doubt plays a role.

Incomplete digestion

Lactose intolerance is caused by the incomplete digestion of lactose, the sugar contained in milk. At birth and in early childhood, your body produces large amounts of an enzyme called lactase. Lact*ase* breaks down lact*ose* and allows it to be absorbed.

However, as you grow up, you usually produce less lactase. By the time you're a teenager, you generally produce only about 10 percent of the lactase you did as an infant.

With less lactase available to break down the lactose, your body can no longer comfortably digest the amounts of milk and ice cream that it used to handle easily. If you take in more lactose than you're capable of digesting, the incomplete digestion can lead to gas, stomach cramps, bloating and diarrhea.

Similar symptoms

As obvious as these symptoms may be, lactose intolerance is not easily diagnosed by its symptoms

From *Mayo Clinic Health Letter,* February 1997, p. 7. © 1997 by the Mayo Foundation for Medical Education and Research, Rochester, MN 55905. Reprinted by permission.

Doing a body good

Watching what you eat can be one of the most simple and effective ways to control the symptoms of lactose intolerance.

People who are lactose intolerant generally have fewer symptoms when they drink milk or eat dairy products with a meal. In addition, if you're lactose intolerant, it's a good idea to avoid eating or drinking large helpings of dairy products at one time. Several smaller helpings over the course of a few hours are much easier to digest.

In addition, not all dairy products have the same amount of lactose. Hard cheeses, like Swiss or Cheddar, have small amounts of lactose and generally cause no symptoms.

alone. There are many other conditions, including the stomach flu and irritable bowel syndrome, that can give you similar symptoms.

However, there are ways for your doctor to determine if you're lactose intolerant. One is to measure the hydrogen in your breath after you've taken in a dose of lactose. Large amounts of hydrogen indicate that lactose is not being fully digested and that you're probably intolerant.

Another method involves taking a blood sample after you've received a dose of lactose and testing for signs of lactose breakdown.

Is it normal, or a disorder?

Many doctors are wary of referring to lactose intolerance as a disorder because it's so common all over the world. They suggest that it's a normal development, and since even lactose-intolerant people can often comfortably digest small amounts of dairy products, treatment is usually unnecessary.

However, for people who are lactose intolerant but still want to consume moderate amounts of dairy products, there are options.

The first and perhaps best option is to watch what you eat. A few simple modifications of your eating habits may help control symptoms.

Other options include lactase tablets and drops, such as Lactaid and Dairy Ease. These types of products contain the enzyme that breaks down lactose, reducing the amount your body must digest on its own.

The tablets are taken before you eat dairy foods. They increase the amount of lactase available to your body to increase lactose digestion. The drops are added to milk. They break down the lactose in milk before you drink it.

Simple solutions

With digestive aids, you don't necessarily have to give up your favorite foods just because you're lactose intolerant. However, if you watch what you eat and how much of it you eat, you may find your body can do the job all by itself.

When Eating Goes Awry

An Update on Eating Disorders

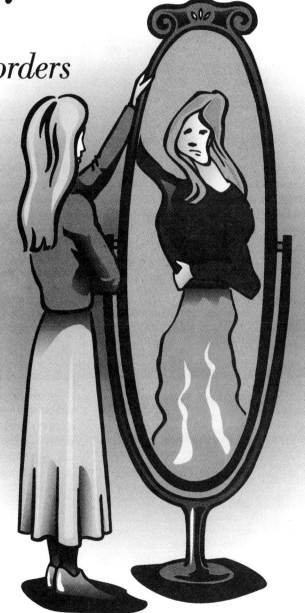

Although eating disorders receive considerable attention and are prevalent in today's society, they are not new in medical history. More than 100 years ago the first case of anorexia nervosa, or self-induced starvation, was documented in England. Yet, it stands to reason that even before the term anorexia was coined, many people struggling with eating disorders were simply diagnosed as having another ailment.

Eating disorders threaten physical health, psychological well-being and sometimes life. Because many people with these problems suffer alone and do not seek professional help, it is difficult to determine the precise number of cases in the United States. However, the American Psychiatric Association (APA) estimates that at any given time, 500,000 people are battling eating disorders. The APA's 1993 Practice Guidelines estimate that between 1 and 4 percent of adolescents and young adults are afflicted. Although the typical patient is a white, middle-to upper-middle-class young woman, some researchers report an increasing number of cases among males and women of other age and ethnic groups.

Types of Eating Disorders

Currently, the APA recognizes two eating disorders: anorexia nervosa and bulimia nervosa. Cases of anorexia nervosa and bulimia nervosa have doubled over the past decade, according to the National Center for Health Statistics (NCHS). Binge-eating, although not yet a recognized eating disorder, is receiving considerable attention as a related disorder.

The major weight loss associated with anorexia nervosa results in a total body weight at least 15 percent below the range of normal weight for age and height. Over time, women suffering from this disorder stop menstruating and may damage vital organs including the heart and brain. Anorexia is believed to affect between 1/2 and 1 percent of women in late adolescence and early adulthood, according to the APA. Its onset is often associated with a stressful life event, such as entering college.

"Anorexia nervosa is most common in white, 15-24 year-old women," says Alexander Lucas, M.D., professor of psychiatry at the Mayo Medical School in Rochester, Minnesota. "It's generally recognized that the disorder is rare among the African-American population for reasons that aren't yet clearly understood. However, there may be both biological and cultural factors that account for the differences in prevalence."

Bulimia nervosa is a serious eating disorder typified by binging (consuming excessive amounts of food in a short time) followed by either self-induced vomiting, use of laxatives, diuretics or enemas, strict dieting or fasting, or vigorous exercise in order to rid the body of the food and prevent weight gain. Although some victims of anorexia nervosa also exhibit symptoms of bulimia nervosa, it is recognized as a distinct disorder. Bulimia nervosa is believed to affect between 1 and 3 percent of adolescent and young women in the United States, although estimates among college-age women reach as high as one out of every five.

Bulimia nervosa victims often are able to hide their problem because they eat normally in public and binge-and-purge in secret. In addition, many are able to maintain a normal body weight while suffering from the disorder. Symptoms of bulimia nervosa, which may be obvious to family and friends, include a chronically inflamed and sore throat that may bleed, decaying tooth enamel (from frequent exposure to stomach acid from vomiting) and swollen salivary glands in the neck and jaw which can make the face appear puffy.

Another type of disorder that is receiving attention is binge-eating. Although less is known about binge-eating disorder, recent estimates suggest that as many as 2 percent of the general population and 30 percent of individuals attending hospital affiliated weight control programs may be afflicted. At a recent American Medical Association (AMA) press conference on compulsive

Eating Disorders Defined

The American Psychiatric Association's Eating Disorders Guidelines are currently being revised. However, to date, the Association lists the following criteria, all of which must be met in order for a case to be recognized as an occurrence of anorexia nervosa or bulimia nervosa

Anorexia nervosa:

- refusal to maintain weight that is above the lowest weight considered normal for age and height
- intense fear of gaining weight or becoming fat, even though underweight
- distorted body image
- in women, three consecutive missed menstrual periods without pregnancy

Bulimia nervosa:

- recurrent episodes of binge eating (minimum average of two binge-eating episodes a week for at least three months)
- a feeling of uncontrollable eating during binges
- regular use of one or more of the following to prevent weight gain: self-induced vomiting, use of laxatives or diuretics, strict dieting or fasting, or vigorous exercise
- persistent over-concern with body shape and weight

mental disorders, Seda Ebrahimi, Ph.D., director of the eating disorders treatment program at McLean Hospital in Belmont, Massachusetts, estimated that one-third of obese patients may be binge-eaters.

Binge-eating, which has been pro-

posed for official recognition as a diagnostic category of eating disorder, is similar to bulimia nervosa in that sufferers may consume extraordinary amounts of food during a single binge. However, they do not compensate for the binge by purging. The morning after a binge, many sufferers experience symptoms similar to a hang-over which may be so extreme that the person is unable to go to school, work or function normally.

"Binge-eating is an avoidance coping mechanism," says Dr. Ebrahimi. "During the binge, the person 'mentally and emotionally checks out' and is unable to stop the out of control eating." Binge-eaters do not purge and tend to minimize the severity of the illness. As a result, doctors may treat binge-eating as an overeating problem rather than a psychiatric disorder, according to Ebrahimi.

Who Develops Eating Disorders and Why?

There are many theories about the causes, but most eating disorder specialists acknowledge that the disorders are very complex and likely involve physical, psychological, societal, cultural and familial aspects.

The development of an eating disorder is not triggered solely by the desire to be thin, according to Amy Tuttle, R.D., M.S.S., a nutrition therapist at The Renfrew Center in Philadelphia, the first residential center for women with eating disorders. "Although much has been said about the the media's role in presenting unrealistic body images to young people, trying to achieve a model-perfect body is not the main reason people develop eating disorders," says Tuttle.

Family dynamics, according to Tuttle, often contribute to the development of an eating disorder. "Some people with eating disorders come from enmeshed families where emotional, relational and physical space boundaries may be blurry. This 'enmeshment' inhibits independence and the development of a separate self," says Tuttle. A prominent theory about eating disorders — that the person with the eating disorder is trying to gain some measure of control in her life — is consistent with this type of family structure. For some people, the act of dieting itself provides an illusion of control.

Depression, feelings of inadequacy, anxiety and loneliness, stress and anger, as well as troubled personal relationships also may contribute to the development of disordered eating patterns. Likewise, major life transitions, the presence of other coping behaviors such as gambling, the presence of another psychiatric disorder such as clinical depression, and alcohol or drug abuse are associated with the onset of eating disorders.

Research also suggests that there may be biochemical imbalances associated with eating disorders. The imbalances — found in certain brain chemicals called neurotransmitters — also are found in people suffering from depression.

Neurotransmitters such as serotonin and norepinephrine control appetite, mood, alertness and sleeping patterns. Low levels of these chemicals may explain the link between eating disorders and depressive illness, as well as why people exhibit abnormal and seemingly illogical eating patterns. However, researchers still are not sure whether neurotransmitter imbalances are the cause of eating disorders or the results of the poor nutrition these disorders bring.

Treatment Offers Hope

Eating disorders are most successfully treated when detected in their early stages. Unfortunately, this is not easy to do. Anorexia nervosa may not be detected until victims become seriously underweight, and bulimia nervosa victims can go for years without anyone knowing about their disease. Fortunately, increasing awareness of the dangers of eating disorders has led more people to seek early help.

According to the APA, simply restoring a person to normal weight or temporarily ending the binge-purge cycle does not address the underlying emotional problems that caused, or are exacerbated by, the abnormal eating behavior.

In addition to addressing any physical complications that result from eating disorders, treatment focuses on correcting the patient's distorted body image, improving self-confidence and self-esteem, treating any underlying depression, establishing normal eating habits and preventing relapse. Many victims can successfully be treated in outpatient programs; however, in critical cases, hospitalization is necessary. Ultimately, success depends on tailoring treatment to the individual's needs.

Generally, a treatment plan will include a combination of physical interventions as well as individual, group or family psychotherapy, cognitive therapy, behavior therapy and medications. To accomplish this level of treatment, a team approach is employed. At The Renfrew Center, the composition of the team depends on the level of care — whether the person is in inpatient or outpatient care — but usually includes a therapist (social worker or psychologist), a dietitian, a psychiatrist, a family therapist, a medical doctor, a nurse and a dentist (for bulimic patients).

The Renfrew philosophy of treatment is two-pronged: therapy for underlying issues, and mealtime support therapy to allow the eating disorder patient to take "food risks." According to Tuttle, "Food risks are behaviors such as eating a certain food which the patient previously considered 'off limits.' Once the patient is able to conquer a food risk, we generally see her display a certain level of self-trust,which often allows her to con-

front underlying issues more directly."

Medications, particularly antidepressants, are commonly prescribed for eating disorder patients. These medications, which regulate the body's level of neurotransmitters, can bring about improved self-esteem and a sense of control, as well as markedly reduce binge-and-purge behavior in bulimics. Currently, the drug Prozac, a serotonin reuptake inhibitor which recently won Food and Drug Administration approval for use in treating bulimia nervosa, is the only drug specifically approved for the eating disorder.

According to John Foreyt, Ph.D., director of the Behavioral Medicine Research Center at Baylor College of Medicine in Houston, Texas, "The use of these medications has shown at least short-term beneficial effects in patients with bulimia nervosa." However, medication is not a stand-alone treatment, cautions Foreyt. "Medications such as Prozac are only adjunct treatments for eating disorders. Therapy to address the multi-factorial nature of the disorders is definitely necessary."

The length of treatment for eating disorders varies, but it can take as long as five years. Success rates for treatment are difficult to estimate because continued treatment does not necessarily mean that the treatment is not working. "Coming back in for day or inpatient treatment is not a sign of failure on the part of either the patient or the treatment process," says Tuttle. "Life brings continual challenges that may need to be addressed with professionals. It's important that people who have or are recovering from an eating disorder stay connected with all of their resources."

Despite the complexities of treating eating disorders, sufferers have an excellent chance for complete recovery, especially if the illness is recognized early.

NUTRITIONAL IMPLICATIONS OF ETHNIC AND CULTURAL DIVERSITY

ETHNIC AND CULTURAL DIVERSITY OF THE U.S. POPULATION

Ethnic minorities comprise nearly 25% of the United States population (1). The four major ethnic minorities include African Americans (12.1%), Hispanic (Latino) Americans (9%), Asian and Pacific Islander Americans (2.9%), and Native Americans and Alaskan Natives (0.8%) (1). These populations differ in many respects, not only from each other, but also from the non-Hispanic white population in the U.S. (1–5). Many major chronic diseases are more common among U.S. ethnic minority populations than among whites (2,3,6–10).

Because eating patterns relate to health risks and are culturally-influenced, diet and nutritional factors may contribute to health status differences between ethnic minorities and whites (3,6). Many aspects of daily living including food preferences and beliefs about the relationship of food to health are influenced by culture (11–13). Culture influences not only what, but also when, where, and how much food is eaten, and how it is obtained, prepared, distributed, and consumed (11,14). Individuals' health perceptions, for example, those related to body weight, are affected by culture (8–10,15).

Because the U.S. population is becoming more ethnically and culturally diverse, individuals in ethnic minority populations may have distinct blends of cultural perspectives and food habits (11,12,14). Acculturation, or the process of adopting or borrowing traits from another culture, may either improve or worsen some dietary practices (11,12).

Percent Distribution of Racial/Ethnic Groups in the United States

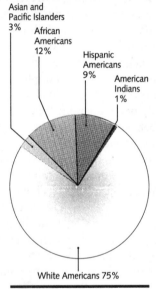

Asian and Pacific Islanders 3%

African Americans 12%

Hispanic Americans 9%

American Indians 1%

White Americans 75%

Source: U.S. Census Bureau

Ethnic minority groups in the U.S. suffer disproportionately from major chronic diseases.

As a result of the growth of ethnic and cultural diversity in the U.S., it is critical that health professionals be aware of how culture influences food behaviors and attitudes, especially those related to health status (16). This *Digest* reviews recent findings regarding dietary patterns and diet-related health problems of ethnic minority populations, with emphasis on the impact of culture. Implications for nutrition intervention and education are also discussed.

NUTRITIONAL IMPLICATIONS OF ETHNIC AND CULTURAL DIVERSITY

African Americans (blacks). The African American (black) population currently constitutes the nation's largest ethnic minority group (1,17). This population is heterogenous and includes several groups with different cultural backgrounds (1,5,13). Although genetics and socioeconomic factors (e.g., high rates of poverty and unemployment) affect the black population's health status, cultural patterns also contribute to blacks' morbidity and mortality from several diet-related diseases (6,17).

Compared to white Americans, blacks are at increased risk of obesity, hypertension, Type II diabetes, cardiovascular disease, and certain cancers (1,6,10,17,18). Differences in risk factor profiles, some of which are culturally-mediated, explain differences in health status between blacks and whites.

Obesity is a serious health problem for blacks, particularly black women (10,15). Data from the most recent National Health and Nutrition Examination Survey (NHANES) III, Phase I (1988–1991) indicate that black women have the highest prevalence of obesity (49.2%) among ethnic and gender subgroups (19). The prevalence of obesity is nearly twice as high for black as for white women (10,16). In addition to their higher rate of obesity, black women are also more likely to have abdominal or upper body obesity which is associated with increased risk of Type II diabetes mellitus, hypertension, and plasma lipid abnormalities (1,16,20).

A combination of genetic, developmental, and environmental factors may contribute to the high prevalence of obesity in black women (8). Preliminary findings from NHANES III indicate that black females consume a slightly higher percentage of energy from fat (35.5%) than do white (33.8%) or Mexican-American (33.7%) females (21). Black women also exhibit lower motivation to manage their weight than white women (8,10,15). Cultural acceptance is thought to be at the core of black women's less intense weight control efforts (7–10,15,22). Black women appear to be more satisfied with their weight than white women (7–10,15, 16,20,22,23).

Hypertension or high blood pressure is also a major health problem for blacks (1,17,24–26). African Americans have a higher prevalence of hypertension (32.4%) than either whites (23.3%) or Mexican Americans (22.6%) (24). Mechanisms that predispose blacks to hypertension may be operative early in life (26,27). Blacks also appear to suffer more from the health consequences of hypertension (e.g., renal damage) than whites (26).

Both genetic and environmental factors contribute to the higher prevalence of hypertension among black individuals (25,26). Among environmental factors, obesity, particularly abdominal or upper body obesity, in black women may contribute to their increased risk for hypertension compared to white women (6,18,26).

Both normotensive and hypertensive black individuals display higher sodium sensitivity and lower plasma renin levels than whites (25,26,28,29). Although blacks do not necessarily consume more sodium than whites,

To improve the effectiveness of weight control programs for African American women, interventions need to be culturally appropriate.

sodium intake for both blacks and whites exceeds recommended intakes (30). Because many blacks are sodium sensitive, they tend to experience a greater increase in blood pressure in response to a given amount of sodium intake than do whites, many of whom are sodium resistant. Cultural preferences for salt and salt-cured foods (6) also may contribute to the higher incidence of elevated blood pressure among African Americans.

A low potassium intake is another dietary factor which may contribute to the increased prevalence of high blood pressure among blacks (26,31,32). Blacks usually consume and excrete less potassium and their blood pressure tends to be higher than whites (30,32). Increasing blacks' intake of potassium (e.g., as found in fruits, vegetables, dairy foods) has been demonstrated to increase plasma renin levels and lower blood pressure (31,32).

The lower calcium intake of blacks (584 mg/day) compared to whites (742 mg/day) (30) may predispose salt sensitive blacks to hypertension (26). Studies have demonstrated that increasing calcium intake reduces blood pressure in salt sensitive hypertensives with low plasma renin activity and ionized calcium levels (29,32,33). Black-white differences in calcium and potassium intake may reflect socioeconomic and cultural differences (25). For blacks who are at risk of hypertension, increasing intake of foods rich in calcium, potassium, and other minerals (e.g., dairy foods), moderately reducing salt intake, and maintaining a healthy weight are recommended (26).

Hypertension and, importantly, overall and upper body obesity contribute to increased coronary heart disease morbidity and mortality in blacks (9,34–36). Psychosocial (e.g., stress, poverty) and cultural factors may also contribute to blacks' higher risk of heart disease (36).

Type II diabetes is an independent cardiovascular disease risk factor that is substantially more prevalent in black than in white individuals (36). Moreover, complications from diabetes generally are more severe for blacks and other ethnic minority populations than for whites (9). Obesity is strongly associated with Type II diabetes. Many cultural factors that influence obesity therefore also affect diabetes.

Compared to whites, blacks are at lower risk for osteoporosis (9,37,38). Nevertheless, a substantial number of black women develop this disease (37,38) and osteoporosis-related disabilities and mortality are higher for black than for white women (38).

Black-white differences in osteoporotic disease and fracture rates may be explained in part by differences in peak bone mineral mass (38–40). Blacks' greater peak bone mass may help protect them from osteoporotic fractures (9,38–40). Genetic differences in calcium metabolism (including vitamin D) and the higher incidence of obesity in blacks than in whites may explain why blacks are at reduced risk of osteoporosis than whites (9,38,41,42).

Milk and milk products are the major dietary source of calcium and vitamin D in U.S. diets (33). Data indicate that black individuals in the U.S. consume fewer servings of milk a week than whites and Hispanics (43). However, whether this lower consumption is due to perceived or actual lactose intolerance and/or cultural factors is unknown. For individuals who have difficulty digesting lactose or milk's sugar, consuming smaller quantities of milk more frequently can maximize milk intake and minimize symptoms (33). Also, other dairy foods such as cheese, yogurt with active cultures, and lactose reduced or lactose free dairy foods are well tolerated by lactose intolerant individuals (33).

The incidence of osteoporosis in blacks is anticipated to rise with the aging of the population (44). In addition, recent findings indicate that some older blacks are at risk of vitamin D deficiency (45). For these reasons, it is important that blacks consume the recommended number of daily servings of milk and other dairy foods, along with other calcium-containing foods that may be traditionally consumed (e.g., dark, leafy green vegetables).

The dietary intake and health status of Hispanic Americans vary widely and are influenced by socioeconomic status, the indigenous culture, and the degree of acculturation.

Hispanic (Latino) Americans.

The Hispanic American population is the second largest ethnic minority in the U.S. and is projected to outnumber the black population by the early 21st century (1,5,17,46–48). Hispanic Americans are a heterogenous mixture of cultures and ethnicity. The majority of these individuals are Mexican Americans (62.3%), with Puerto Ricans (11.1%), Cuban Americans (4.9%), South and Central Americans (13.8%), and others (7.6%) comprising the remainder (1).

Cultural attitudes influence the dietary intake and health status of Hispanic Americans (48). Many Hispanic Americans believe that life events (e.g., disease) are beyond one's control (48). This cultural attitude may jeopardize their willingness to make lifestyle changes to improve health (48). The "hot-cold" theory of disease and its treatment is another common theme. According to this philosophy, foods, herbs, illnesses, and bodily states are symbolically characterized as either "hot" or "cold." A "hot" illness is treated with a "cold" food/medication, and vice versa (48). Believers in this philosophy may unnecessarily restrict certain foods from their diets. Length of U.S. residence also influences dietary patterns and food intake of Hispanic Americans (49–52). With acculturation, dietary intake and health status worsen for many Hispanic Americans (49,50,52).

There are some similarities as well as notable differences in the types and frequency of foods consumed among different groups of Hispanic Americans (48,52–54). For example, tortillas, corn, dried beans, chili peppers, and tomatoes are staple foods of a traditional Mexican American diet, whereas rice and legumes are staples of a traditional Puerto Rican diet (48,53). Dairy products, in particular whole milk and cheese, are an important source of dietary calcium for Hispanic Americans (42,54).

With respect to diet-related health risks, a significant proportion of Hispanic American adults are obese, with the highest percentage occurring in Mexican American females (42.3%) and the lowest (38.2%) occurring in Cuban

American females (1,3,8,10,19,48). Obesity not only is high among Hispanic Americans, but its prevalence appears to be increasing (3). Moreover, Hispanic Americans have a predominance of upper body or centralized adiposity which increases their risk of diabetes mellitus, cardiovascular disease, and gallbladder disease (8,48). Genetics and several environmental factors (e.g., high calorie intake, low physical activity) as well as cultural factors contribute to obesity in Hispanic Americans.

Type II diabetes is approximately three times more common in Hispanic Americans than in non-Hispanic whites (3,10, 46,48,52). Mexican Americans have the highest prevalance of this disease, followed by Puerto Ricans, and to a lesser extent Cuban Americans (52). Rates of diabetes in Hispanic Americans have increased dramatically in recent years (3). Researchers project that obesity and a sedentary lifestyle contribute to the rising incidence of this disease (3,10,48).

Hispanic Americans exhibit a lower risk for hypertension and osteoporosis than whites (1,37,42,44,46). Hispanic Americans' relatively higher protection against these diseases may be due to a variety of genetic, biological, and cultural factors (44).

Calcium intake is similar for Hispanic Americans and non-Hispanic whites and is lower for females than for males (30). Although milk and milk products are the main dietary source of calcium for Hispanics, calcium sources vary among Hispanic ethnic groups (42). Cultural factors and regional availability influence milk intake (55).

Asian and Pacific Islanders.
The Asian/Pacific American population is the nation's third largest ethnic minority and the fastest growing (1,17). Asian/Pacific Americans are characterized by their diversity (1,5,13,17). This population includes Chinese, Japanese, Korean, Filipino, and numerous Southeast Asian (e.g., Vietnamese, Cambodians) Americans and represents a variety of cultures, languages, socioeconomic levels, and educational backgrounds (1).

The ethnic and cultural diversity of the U.S. population presents a major challenge for nutrition and other health professionals.

The dietary intake and health status of Asian Pacific populations are varied and influenced by the cultural heritage of the specific subgroup (14,56). In many Asian cultures, just as in the Hispanic culture, the search for equilibrium or balance is important to health (14,56). Acculturation is another determinant of the dietary intake and health status of Asian/Pacific Americans (57,58). Some traditional Asian foods are good sources of calcium. However, because most Asians are unfamiliar with or unaccustomed to the taste of dairy foods, their overall intake of calcium tends to be low, especially for older adults (57,58).

Information regarding the health status or risk of nutrition-related diseases among Asian/Pacific Americans is limited (59). Nevertheless, some recent findings indicate that the Asian/Pacific American population is at increased risk for several chronic diseases, in part due to acculturation (59). An example is the increase in obesity among native Hawaiians with length of exposure to Western culture (59).

Native Americans.
Although Native Americans represent less than 1% of the total U.S. population, they are an extremely diverse population which includes American Indians and Alaska Natives (Eskimos, Aleuts) (1,5,13,17).

Little is known regarding the food habits and dietary intakes of American Indians as a result of the exclusion of Native Americans living on reservations from national surveys, including the most recent NHANES III (60). Nevertheless, studies of small groups have identified nutritional excesses and shortcomings (60).

Obesity and diabetes are major health problems for Native Americans (1,3,10, 17,60,61). Not only is the prevalence of obesity high and rising, but this disease is an important risk factor for Type II diabetes, hypertension, cardiovascular disease, and gallbladder disease which are prevalent among Native Americans (10,62). The Pima Indians in particular have high rates of obesity and diabetes (6,63,64).

A variety of factors, genetic and environmental (e.g., diet, sedentary lifestyle), are implicated in the development of obesity in Native Americans. Cultural, social, and economic circumstances have decreased Native Americans' use of indigenous foods (e.g., vegetables, grains) and increased their intake of convenience foods, many of which are high in energy and low in essential nutrients (10,60). Although it has been speculated that a cultural acceptance of overweight may contribute to the high prevalence of obesity in Native Americans, findings of a recent study fail to support this assumption (65).

IMPLICATIONS FOR NUTRITION EDUCATION

It is clear that dietary patterns and risk of specific diseases are tied to an individual's ethnic and cultural background (13,48,52,66). Nutrition interventions, including nutrition education programs and materials, must be culturally sensitive to different groups. Cross-cultural counseling skills are also essential for health professionals working with individuals whose traditions, values, and beliefs differ from their own (66). Several resources are available to help dietitians and health professionals meet the challenge of serving the increasing number of clients with different ethnic and cultural backgrounds (12,14,67–69).

REFERENCES

1. National Heart, Lung, and Blood Institute, National Institutes of Health. Fact sheets on Black Americans, Hispanic Americans, Asian/Pacific Islanders, and American Indians. May 1992.

2. National Center for Health Statistics. *Health, United States, 1993.* Hyattsville, MD: Public Health Service, 1994.

3. McGinnis, J.M., and P.R. Lee. JAMA *273*: 1123, 1995.

4. Kumanyika, S. J. Nutr. Educ. *22*: 89, 1990.

5. Newman, J.M. *Melting Pot. An Annotated Bibliography and Guide to Food and Nutrition Information for Ethnic Groups in America.* 2nd ed. New York: Garland Publ. Inc., 1993.

6. Kumanyika, S.K. Ann. Epidemiol. *3*: 154, 1993.

7. Kumanyika, S. Ann. N.Y. Acad. Sci. *699*: 81, 1993.

8. Kumanyika, S.K. Obesity Res. *2(2)*: 166, 1994.

9. Kumanyika, S. J. Am. Diet. Assoc. *95*: 299, 1995.

10. Ernst, N.D., and W.R. Harlan. Am. J. Clin. Nutr. *53(6)*: 1507S, 1991.

11. Terry, R.D. J. Am. Diet. Assoc. *94(5)*: 501, 1994.

12. Gonzalez, V.M., J.T. Gonzalez, V. Freeman, et. al. *Health Promotion In Diverse Cultural Communities.* Palo Alto, CA: Health Promotion Resource Center, Stanford Center for Research in Disease Prevention, 1991.

13. Kittler, P.G., and K. Sucher. *Food and Culture in America. A Nutrition Handbook.* New York: Van Nostrand Reinhold, 1989.

14. Eliades, D.C., and C.W. Suitor. *Celebrating Diversity: Approaching Families Through Their Food.* Arlington, VA: National Center for Education in Maternal and Child Health, 1994.

15. Kumanyika, S.K., C. Morssink, and T. Agurs. Ethn. Dis. *2*: 166, 1992.

16. Melnyk, M.G., and E. Weinstein. J. Am. Diet. Assoc. *94*: 536, 1994.

17. U.S. Department of Health and Human Services, Public Health Service. *Healthy People 2000. National Health Promotion and Disease Prevention Objectives.* DHHS Publ. No. (PHS) 91-50213. Washington, DC: U.S. Government Printing Office, 1991, pp. 31–43.

18. Lenfant, C. Circulation *90(4)*: 1613, 1994.

19. Kuczmarski, R.J., K.M. Flegal, S.M. Campbell, et. al. JAMA *272*: 205, 1994.

20. Allison, D.B., B.S. Kanders, G.D. Osage, et. al. J. Nutr. Educ. *27*: 18, 1995.

21. McDowell, M.A., R.R. Briefel, K. Alaimo, et. al. Energy and macronutrient intakes of persons ages 2 months and over in the United States: Third National Health and Nutrition Examination Survey, Phase 1, 1988–91. Advance data from Vital and Health Statistics; No. 255. Hyattsville, Maryland: National Center for Health Statistics, 1994.

22. Kumanyika, S., J.F. Wilson, and M. Guilford-Davenport. J. Am. Diet. Assoc. *93*: 416, 1993.

23. Food Marketing Institute and PREVENTION Magazine. *Shopping For Health, 1993. A Food Marketing Institute PREVENTION Magazine Report on Diet, Nutrition and Ethnic Foods.* Washington, DC: Food Marketing Institute, 1993.

24. Burt, V.L., P. Whelton, E.J. Roccella, et. al. Hypertension *25*: 305, 1995.

25. Grim, C.E., J.P. Henry, and H. Myers. In: *Hypertension: Pathophysiology, Diagnosis, and Management.* Second Edition. J.H. Laragh and B.M. Brenner (Eds). New York: Raven Press, Ltd., 1995, pp. 171–207.

26. Kaplan, N.M. The Lancet *344*: 450, 1994.

27. Manatunga, A.K., J.J. Jones, and J.H. Pratt. Hypertension *22*: 84, 1993.

28. Sowers, J.R., M.B. Zemel, P. Zemel, et. al. Hypertension *12*: 485, 1988.

29. Zemel, P., S. Gualdoni, and J.R. Sowers. Am. J. Hypertens. *1*: 146S, 1988.

30. Alaimo, K., M.A. McDowell, R.R. Briefel, et. al. Dietary intake of vitamins, minerals, and fiber of persons ages 2 months and over in the United States: Third National Health and Nutrition Examination Survey, Phase 1, 1988–91. Advance Data from Vital and Health Statistics; No. 258. Hyattsville, Maryland: National Center for Health Statistics, 1994.

31. Matlou, S., G. Isles, A. Higgs, et. al. J. Hypertens. *4*: 61, 1986.

32. Langford, H.G., W.C. Cushman, and H. Hsu. Am. J. Hypertens. *4*: 399, 1991.

33. Miller, G.D., J.K. Jarvis, and L.D. McBean. *Handbook of Dairy Foods and Nutrition.* Boca Raton, FL: CRC Press, Inc., 1995.

34. Morrison, J.A., G. Payne, B.A. Barton, et. al. Am. J. Public Health *84*: 1761, 1994.

35. Burke, G.L., P.J. Savage, T.A. Manolio, et. al. Am. J. Public Health *82*: 1621, 1992.

36. Kumanyika, S., and L.L. Adams-Campbell. In: *Cardiovascular Diseases in Blacks.* E. Saunders and A. Brest (Eds). Philadelphia: F.A. Davis Co. Cardiovascular Clin. *21(3)*: 47–73, 1991.

37. Looker, A.C., C.C. Johnston, Jr., H.W. Wahner, et. al. J. Bone Min. Res. *10(5)*: 796, 1995.

38. Grisso, J.A., J.L. Kelsey, B.L. Strom, et. al. N. Engl. J. Med. *330*: 1555, 1994.

39. Gasperino, J.A., J. Wang, R.N. Pierson, Jr., et. al. Metabolism *44(1)*: 30, 1995.

40. Nelson, D.A., G. Jacobsen, D.A. Barondess, et. al. J. Bone Miner. Res. *10(5)*: 782, 1995.

41. Abrams, S.A., K.O. O'Brien, L.K. Liang, et. al. J. Bone Miner. Res. *10(5)*: 829, 1995.

42. Looker, A.C., C.M. Loria, M.D. Carroll, et. al. J. Am. Diet. Assoc. *93*: 1274, 1993.

43. Patterson, B.H., L.C. Harlan, G. Block, et. al. Nutr. Cancer *23*: 105, 1995.

44. Villa, M.L. J. Bone Miner. Res. *9(9)*: 1329, 1994.

45. Perry, H.M., D.K. Miller, J.E. Morley, et. al. J. Am. Geriatr. Soc. *41*: 612, 1993.

46. Stern, M.P. Ethn. Dis. *3(1)*: 7, 1993.

47. Policy and Research, National Coalition of Hispanic Health and Human Services Organizations (COSSMHO). Am. J. Health Promot. *9(4)*: 300, 1995.

48. Sanjur, D. *Hispanic Foodways, Nutrition, and Health.* Needham Heights, MA: Simon & Schuster Co., 1995.

49. American Medical Association, Council on Scientific Affairs. JAMA *265*: 248, 1991.

50. Chavez, N., L. Sha, V. Persky, et. al. J. Nutr. Educ. *26*: 79, 1994.

51. Guendelman, S., and B. Abrams. Am. J. Public Health *85*: 20, 1995.

52. Romero-Gwynn, E., D. Gwynn, L. Grivetti, et. al. Nutr. Today *28(4)*: 6, 1993.

53. Kuczmarski, M.F., R.J. Kuczmarski, and M. Najjar. Nutr. Today *30(1)*: 30, 1995.

54. Block, G., J.C. Norris, R.M. Mandel, et. al. J. Am. Diet. Assoc. *95*: 195, 1995.

55. Rosado, J.L., C. Gonzalez, M.E. Valencia, et. al. J. Nutr. *124*: 1052, 1994.

56. Frye, B.A. Am. J. Health Promot. *9(4)*: 269, 1995.

57. Kim, K.K., E.S. Yu, W.T. Liu, et. al. J. Am. Diet. Assoc. *93*: 1416, 1993.

58. Schultz, J.D., A.A. Spindler, and R.V. Josephson. J. Nutr. Educ. *26*: 266, 1994.

59. Chen, M.S., Jr., and B.L. Hawks. Am. J. Health Promot. *9(4)*: 261, 1995.

60. Brown, A.C., and B. Brenton. J. Am. Diet. Assoc. *94*: 517, 1994.

61. Jackson, M.Y. J. Am. Diet. Assoc. *93*: 1136, 1993.

62. Alpert, J.S., R. Goldberg, I.S. Ockene, et. al. Cardiology *78*: 3, 1991.

63. Warne, D.K., D.R. McCance, M.A. Charles, et. al. Diabetes Care *18(4)*: 435, 1995.

64. Hanson, R.L., D.R. McCance, L.T.H. Jacobsson, et. al. J. Clin. Epidemiol. *48(7)*: 903, 1995.

65. Story, M., F.R. Hauck, B.A. Broussard, et. al. Arch. Pediatr. Adoles. Med. *148*: 567, 1994.

66. Sucher, K.P., and P.G. Kittler. J. Am. Diet. Assoc. *91*: 297, 1991.

67. Diabetes Care and Education, Dietetic Practice Group of The American Dietetic Association. *Ethnic And Regional Food Practices. A Series.* Chicago, IL: The American Dietetic Association, 1989–1994.

68. National Dairy Council. *Guía Para La Buena Alimentación* (Spanish version of the "Guide to Good Eating"). Rosemont, IL: National Dairy Council, 1993.

69. U.S. Department of Agriculture, U.S. Department of Health and Human Services. *Cross-Cultural Counseling. A Guide for Nutrition and Health Counselors.* Washington, DC: U.S. Government Printing Office, May 1990.

Alcohol: weighing the benefits and risks for you

■ Alcohol is associated with about 100,000 deaths from diseases and injuries in this country each year.

■ Alcohol may *prevent* 80,000 deaths from coronary artery disease (CAD) each year, according to a recent American Heart Association report.

These are only rough estimates. It's hard to say exactly how many Americans die as a result of alcohol consumption. And it's even harder to figure out how many deaths from heart disease are prevented by "moderate" drinking. (The 80,000 figure cited above is merely the mean point of a wide range of estimates—anywhere from 12,000 to 136,000—based on data from a dozen studies.) Moreover, such a weighing of the beneficial and adverse effects of alcohol doesn't take into consideration the big differences between the two groups involved. While most alcohol-related deaths occur in relatively young people, the deaths prevented by alcohol are generally in older age groups—those with high rates of cardiovascular disease.

Every month, it seems, there's another study showing that "moderate" amounts of alcohol help protect against heart attacks. And yet the studies often disagree about what type of beverage is beneficial, what the best amount is, and who will benefit. Last year the U.S. government, in its official Dietary Guidelines, as well as the American Heart Association, confirmed the coronary benefits of "moderate" drinking. Encour-

aged by these guidelines, the Wine Institute and several other groups proposed voluntary labeling for alcoholic beverages describing the health benefits of moderate drinking, to balance the current mandatory warning labels.

But wait a minute: the American Cancer Society, in *its* new guidelines, recommends limiting alcohol consumption or abstaining, since even a moderate intake may increase the risk of cancer in some people.

So what is the real bottom line on alcohol? Should you start drinking—or cut down or even quit? Here are some answers to these and other questions.

Which beverages are protective?

Studies have consistently found that a regular consumption of moderate amounts of alcohol helps prevent heart attacks in middle-aged or older men and women by 30 to 50%. Red wine has gotten the most publicity, but some studies have found that white wine also helps, and other studies have found that wine, beer, and liquor are all equally effective. Though wine and various other beverages (even grape juice) contain antioxidant phytochemicals that may help protect against heart disease and cancer, the crucial element is the alcohol itself. Wine may *seem* healthier than other drinks because wine drinkers tend to be better educated and more well-to-do than other drinkers, which may account for other traits (such as a better diet or

Reprinted with permission from *University of California at Berkeley Wellness Letter,* August 1997, pp. 4-5. © 1997 by Health Letter Associates. To order a one-year subscription, call (800) 829-9170.

better health care) that help keep them healthy. People also tend to drink wine with meals, which may be preferable.

Why is it better to drink alcohol with meals?

"Alcoholic beverages have been used to enhance the enjoyment of meals by many societies throughout human history," in the words of the Dietary Guidelines. Food slows the absorption of alcohol, prolonging the potentially beneficial effects on the blood (especially important after a fatty meal) and moderating blood alcohol levels. In addition, people who drink only with meals tend to do so in moderation. Those who drink excessively tend to drink mostly outside of meals.

How does alcohol protect the heart?

Scientists estimate that about half of the protective effect comes from alcohol's ability to boost HDL cholesterol, the "good" kind that removes cholesterol from arterial walls. Thus alcohol reduces atherosclerosis, the hardening and narrowing of the coronary arteries that can cause a blockage and heart attack. Alcohol also reduces the stickiness of the blood and interferes with the formation of clots.

Can alcohol be compared to aspirin as a preventive against heart disease?

Yes and no. Both can reduce the risk of heart disease, and both are not for everybody, since both have serious side effects. With both aspirin and alcohol, the benefits come from low doses, and no one knows yet what the optimal amount is. But unlike aspirin, alcohol is intoxicating and potentially addictive, and its abuse leads to tens of thousands of deaths in this country each year, and wrecks the lives of millions.

What is moderation?

This is the tricky part. Most experts say that moderation means *no more than* one drink per day for women and two drinks for men. A standard drink is 12 ounces of beer, 4 to 5 ounces of wine, or 1.5 ounces of 80-proof liquor, which all supply about the same amount of pure alcohol. In most studies, people who drink that much have the lowest overall mortality rates, especially from heart disease—lower than teetotalers, occasional drinkers, and heavier drinkers.

However, not all studies have agreed with those numbers. A few studies have found that higher intakes can also be beneficial overall. Other studies suggest that "light" drinking is better than a "moderate" intake. For example, the most recent study, from Harvard, followed 22,000 male physicians for 11 years and found that those who drank two to six drinks *a week* (not even one drink a day) had the lowest overall death rates. The men who averaged two drinks or more a day had the highest death rate, because of an increase in deaths from cancer, primarily lung cancer. But this was an unusual study, in that the men (in part because they were doctors) were quite healthy and relatively few died from heart disease. Moreover, only 3% of them fell into the "two or more drinks a day" category. Since the study lumped together moderate and excessive drinkers in this highest, open-ended category, it couldn't determine the risks faced by men who consumed only two drinks a day, nor could it define where the real danger begins. And the results can't be generalized to women.

In general, there are problems with how drinking levels and patterns are categorized in virtually all the studies. For example,

the studies rarely measure when and how alcohol is consumed: ten drinks a week could mean a beer or two with every dinner or two five-beer binges, which would have *very* different effects in the body. And for various reasons, people may not report their alcohol intake accurately.

Why should women drink less than men?

Alcohol affects men and women differently. A woman will get more intoxicated than a man from the same amount of alcohol. Women tend to be smaller than men, and their bodies have proportionately more fatty tissue and less water than men's. Since alcohol is distributed through body water and is more soluble in water than in fat, the blood alcohol concentration from a given intake will be less for a man. Moreover, the stomach enzyme that breaks down alcohol before it reaches the bloodstream is less active in women than in men. Thus excessive drinking tends to have more serious long-term consequences for women. They develop cirrhosis (liver disease) at lower levels of alcohol intake than men, for instance. And women who drink are also at increased risk for osteoporosis.

What about breast cancer?

Several widely publicized studies have suggested that alcohol increases the risk of breast cancer. But other studies have found no increased risk—or only in those who consumed more than two drinks a day, or only in premenopausal women, or only in postmenopausal women. One 1993 study did show that when premenopausal women drink they have higher levels of estrogen in their blood, which, over the course of years of drinking, might increase the risk of breast cancer. On the other hand, one recent study suggested that a compound found in wine may counteract the effect of estrogen in the body.

This has resulted in confusion for women: drink moderately to protect against heart disease, or abstain because of alcohol's potential effect on breast cancer risk? Remember, however, that heart disease kills three times as many women under age 75 as breast cancer (and 20 times as many women over age 75)—and that questions still remain about the link between alcohol and breast cancer. If you're a woman who has a drink a day, there's no health reason to quit, unless you are pregnant or nursing—or possibly if you're at high risk for breast cancer or are on HRT (see box).

What about other cancers?

Alcohol has been linked to several kinds of cancer. The recent Harvard study found an increased risk of lung, esophageal, gastric, pancreatic, urinary tract, and a few other cancers. But studies have yielded inconsistent results about just which cancers are affected. One thing is certain: smoking and drinking act together to increase the risk of several cancers.

What are the other risks?

Long-term, heavy drinking (three or more drinks a day) increases the risk of liver disease, damage to the brain and pancreas, high blood pressure, and hemorrhagic stroke. It can also *cause* heart disease by damaging the heart muscle itself. Even moderate drinking during pregnancy increases the risk of fetal alcohol syndrome, which can result in mental retarda-

Alcohol and hormone therapy: triple dose?

Alcohol consumption may pose an additional quandary for postmenopausal women on hormone replacement therapy (HRT, a combination of estrogen and progestin) or estrogen replacement therapy (ERT, estrogen only). Hormone therapy itself may boost the risk of breast cancer, though as with alcohol, the link is still uncertain. A study last December showed that consuming a large dose of alcohol (equal to about four drinks within 15 minutes) tripled blood levels of estrogen for a prolonged period in 12 women on ERT. And, as we've said, lifetime exposure to estrogen appears to affect the risk of breast cancer. But this was just one small study, using only one type of hormone preparation. Presumably, more moderate amounts of alcohol would have much less of an effect on homone levels in the blood. If you are on ERT or HRT, that may be still another reason to stay within the one-drink-a-day limit. And if you have a strong family history of breast cancer, you may want to avoid both hormone therapy and alcohol. (For more about the risks and benefits of HRT, see *Wellness Letter,* October 1995.)

tion and birth defects. It also increases the risk of osteoporosis, car crashes (often involving impaired pedestrians), workplace injuries, and cycling and firearms injuries, as well as homicides and suicides. Moreover, alcohol abuse alters judgment and creates unhealthy family dynamics, contributing to domestic violence and child abuse.

Who should avoid alcohol?

Do not drink

■ if you are pregnant, are trying to conceive, or are nursing.

■ if you can't restrict your drinking to moderate levels (a special concern for recovering alcoholics and those with a family history of alcohol abuse).

■ if within the next few hours you plan to drive or take part in an activity that requires attention or skill.

■ if you are taking certain medications.

■ if you have very high blood levels of triglycerides, uncontrolled hypertension, liver disease, abnormal heart rhythms, peptic ulcers, sleep apnea, or certain other disorders. (The *Wellness Letter* will discuss triglycerides in an upcoming issue.)

If you don't fall into one of those categories and don't drink, should you start?

Few, if any, medical experts advise nondrinkers to *start* drinking for health reasons. As the two statistics at the start of this article show, alcohol probably kills more people than it saves—and those killed tend to be younger.

First of all, you shouldn't feel pressured to drink if you abstain for religious or personal reasons, or simply don't like the taste or effects of alcohol.

That said, if you don't drink (and don't fall into one of the groups listed above) and are considering starting—or if you do drink and are worried that you shouldn't, **weigh the risks and benefits** *for you,* **considering your age, sex, risk factors for various diseases, and family history.** Your doctor may be able to advise you. In general, men over 45 and women over 55 have a much greater chance of developing heart disease than cancer, so they might consider moderate drinking (no more than two drinks a day for a man, one drink a day for a woman) to improve their odds of staying healthy. Of course, there are even better ways for you to improve your odds: lose weight if you are overweight, stop smoking, have a healthy, low-fat diet, and start exercising if you are sedentary.

Fat and Weight Control

If you wish to grow thinner, diminish your dinner, And take to light claret instead of pale ale; Look down with an utter contempt upon butter, And never touch bread till it's toasted—or stale.

—H. S. Leigh, *A Day for Wishing*

There have been times and places in history when being fat was considered beautiful. Harry Golden, writing in *Only in America* (Cleveland, Ohio: The World Publishing Company, 1958), tells how it was on the Lower East Side of New York when he was a boy. For two cents and accompanied by lots of fanfare, the salesman would guess a person's weight and weigh him or her in public. It was a big social event on Saturday night in a society where women bragged about gaining five pounds and practiced ways to simulate double chins. Harry and his mother, however, had differing views:

When I weigh myself I do not look at the results. I just listen to the gears grind and, when everything quiets down, I simply step off the scales and walk away. By this system I have won the battle, leaving the machine frustrated, if not useless. I was always a fat kid and once when I complained about it my mother said, "Nothing at all to worry about; in America the fat man is always the boss and the skinny man is always the bookkeeper."

Most of today's society, however, does not view fat pounds with pride. Thin is in. It is the willowy person who is seen as beautiful, socially acceptable, and appealing to the opposite sex. Those of us with bulges and bumps will knead and pound, use saunas, and starve ourselves—anything to lose a pound. Surveys indicate that as many as half of adult women and a quarter of adult men are dieting at any given time. Even more telling is the high number of grade school and adolescent girls who have reported weight loss attempts, often at the behest of their mothers.

Despite these attitudes and values, and regardless of national goals to the contrary, America has gained weight. Following a steady trend that began in the 1980s, about one-third of the adult population continues to add pounds. For the first time in this country, there are more overweight people than those of normal size. Although people in their 50s have gained the most, weight increases cut across all ethnic, age, and gender groups. These newest findings are reported in the article "Three Major U.S. Studies Describe Trends" and come from the Third National Health and Nutrition Examination Survey (NHANES III), but they are not unique to the United States. Most of the industrialized world has seen a similar phenomenon since World War I. And, in what seems paradoxical, Weight Watchers now has a growing market among Zimbabwe's black population and expects to move into other developing countries because obesity is increasing. Still, the United States exceeds other countries in prevalence of overweight. This is not good news for the Healthy People 2000 goal, which calls for reducing overweight to no more than 20 percent of adults.

Through the years many methods have been used to lose weight, as the next article on the history of dieting indicates. One school of thought holds that, especially in the presence of other health risks, dieting must be attempted and can produce desired results. Others claim that it is far wiser to focus on lifestyle changes rather than on weight loss and on health rather than on total weight. This philosophy espouses empowerment to increase self-awareness and to effect gradual change, which is more likely to be permanent. If it works, it is a powerful argument, since most dieters regain their lost pounds within a few years.

Although many experts are concerned about negative consequences and the failure to maintain weight loss, some dieters and professionals favor the use of drugs to help lose weight. The highly medicalized state of our culture and the desire for quick fixes has led many women to seek a pill that will provide a quick-fix weight loss. "Diet Pills: Are Millions of Women Playing Russian Roulette with Their Health?" examines the newest generation of pills designed to promote weight loss. While many people see these drugs as a panacea, the *Women's Health Advocate Newsletter* points out that they can have serious consequences and that all of the side effects are not yet known. They are joined in this view by the FDA, which, in late 1997, removed several diet pills from the market.

Finding simple answers to why people gain weight would be a cause for celebration, but many questions about weight are still unanswered. Why do some of us gain too much with extraordinary ease when others try to gain and fail? How much *should* we weigh? Experts simply do not agree. We know a lot more than we did but still not enough to reach absolute conclusions. Yes, an obesity gene has been discovered (see "Obesity: No Miracle Cure Yet"), as have natural body chemicals that participate in the control of appetite. Any practical applications appear to be years away, however, although various news items indicate that companies will try to capitalize on this early information and public interest.

Many experts see prevention of obesity as the most effective strategy for those still at healthy weights, and it is logical that childhood should be targeted as a time when future eating behaviors are established. It is trou-

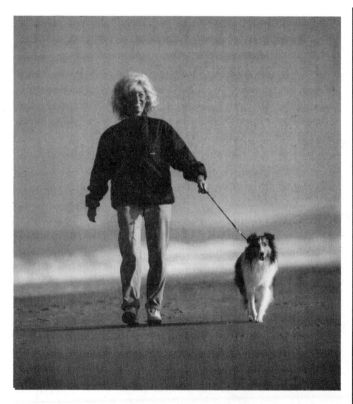

sumption by about 3 percent of total calories. Perhaps there is a lesson to remember, one we would like to forget and one that marketers of the hundreds of low- and no-fat foods would like us to ignore. Calories still count! Recipes can be changed to lower fat content, to be sure, but the fat is often replaced with high amounts of sugar. These facts are discussed in "Reduced-Fat Foods: Dieter's Dream or Marketer's Ploy?" Some studies also suggest that we simply compensate for the reduced-fat foods at a later time. In addition, alcohol accounts for 6 percent of our caloric intake.

If one does decide that losing weight is appropriate, doing so can become a major challenge. Health should be the focus, not societal pressure or fitting into a bathing suit. Most diets will work if adhered to, but weight loss alone is not cause for celebration. The trick is to keep it off, for only then is it effective. Just as important is losing it safely. Put together, this means loss that is slow and gradual, a permanent lifestyle change that includes exercising and maintaining a diet that provides adequate nutrients and calories. This is not exciting, not dramatic, and not easy; in fact, it is just plain hard work. Even then, many Americans are not successful.

Given the intense interest among both health professionals and the public, other ways of controlling weight will no doubt be found in the future. Most people hope that any innovations or new strategies will permit appetite satisfaction and an occasional strawberry shortcake.

Looking Ahead: Challenge Questions

How does concern about your weight affect your life and that of your friends? Analyze your attitudes and behavior and describe what, if any, changes in these are appropriate.

What are the issues of benefit and risk that one should consider before deciding to go on a diet?

Find a description of a new trendy diet and evaluate it for effectiveness and safety.

Which of the many products with fat and sugar substitutes do you like? What is your purpose in using them? Do you reduce total calories by using these products?

In the library, find a review of the Minnesota Experiment or Colin Turnbull's description of starvation among the Ik, which are mentioned in the article on dysfunctional eating. What do you learn about the effects of starvation from these sources?

Do you think weight reduction should be a national goal? Why or why not? What population groups would you target and what strategies would you use?

bling, then, that more than 10 percent of children and teenagers are already overweight. The article "Diet and Exercise: What Kids Need Today" identifies a trend toward more sedentary activity rather than increased energy intake as the cause of this energy imbalance. Using this knowledge to encourage healthy lifestyles now becomes a major challenge, especially since nearly 30 percent of all students nationwide believe that they are overweight, even when many of them are not. Over half of high school girls and a quarter of high school boys report trying to lose weight. Boys tend to diet, while girls often use high-risk methods such as laxatives, vomiting, diet pills, and smoking. These anorexic and bulimic behaviors are at least as unhealthy as excess pounds and require solutions as well. One commonality among students of all weights, especially females, is low self-esteem. A quarter of our high school students, especially girls and Hispanics, reported considering suicide in the previous year. Dysfunctional eating, an umbrella term that includes anorexia, bulimia, and other disorders is discussed in Frances Berg's "Dysfunctional Eating: A New Concept."

It is ironic that weight gain has occurred during the very time period when we have actually reduced fat con-

Three major U.S. studies describe trends

by Frances M. Berg, MS

Obesity and its effects and associations are documented in three nation-wide U.S. studies: the Third National Health and Nutrition Examination Survey (NHANES III), the Youth Risk Behavior survey, and the Third Report on Nutrition Monitoring, also used in the NHANES study. What these reports show is a continuing increase in obesity, mostly at the heavier end, and a tremendous concern about body image and weight loss for young people, especially girls.

NHANES III

According to the latest information, about 14 percent of American children, 12 percent of adolescents, and 35 percent of adults are overweight.

What alarms public health officials is that rates of overweight were fairly stable during the 1960s and 1970s, but during the 1980s and early 1990s both children and adults gained weight. During this time the number of overweight children and adolescents has increased from 5 percent (Fig. 1), and the number of overweight adults has increased from about 25 percent, using somewhat different definitions for the age groups.

The landmark study revealing this striking new evidence is NHANES III, conducted in two 3-year phases from 1988 to 1994 by researchers at the National Center for Health Statistics, Centers for Disease Control and Prevention (CDC), Hyattsville, Maryland. Weight and height were measured as part of a physical exam in a mobile examination center. The stratified, multistage, probability cluster sample is representative of the U.S. civilian, noninstitutionalized population.[1]

Children and teens

For children (6 to 11 yr), the survey finds more black and Hispanic children overweight than white children at all ages. For black children, 15 percent of boys and 18 percent of girls are overweight; for Mexican-American, 19 percent of boys and 16 percent of girls; and for white, 13 percent of boys and 12 percent of girls (Table 1).

Adolescents (12 to 17 yr) reveal a similar pattern. For black adolescents, 13 percent of boys and 16 percent of girls are overweight; for Mexican-American, 15 percent of boys and 14 percent of girls; and for white, 12 percent of boys and 10 percent of girls. Numbers for other racial and ethnic groups were too small for meaningful analysis.

Adults

Approximately 36 percent of women and 33 percent of men are overweight, with more variation between racial and ethnic groups for women than men. White women have about the same rates as white men (33.5 vs 33.7 percent), but black and Hispanic women have rates of overweight that are far higher than men in these populations. Among blacks, 52.3 percent of women and 33.3 percent of men are overweight. Among Hispanics, 50.1 percent of women and 36.4 percent of men are overweight (Table 2).

Trend is up

The prevalence of overweight in the United States apparently increased even as the 6-year study progressed. While

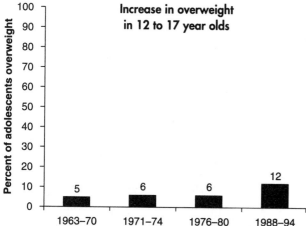

Figure 1. Increase in overweight in 12 to 17 year olds. Note: The prevalence of overweight has increased from 5 to 12 percent during the last three decades for boys and girls aged 12–17 at the 95th percentile. Most of this increase has come during the last decade. From NHANES III, 1988–1994.

Table 1 Overweight among children and adolescent		
	Children No. (%)	*Adolescents* No. (%)
Male		
White, non-Hispanic	446 (13.2)	281 (11.6)
Black, non-Hispanic	584 (14.7)	412 (12.5)
Mexican-American	565 (18.8)	406 (15.0)
Total	1673 (14.7)	1154 (12.3)
Female		
White, non-Hispanic	428 (11.9)	342 (9.6)
Black, non-Hispanic	538 (17.9)	447 (16.3)
Mexican-American	581 (15.8)	412 (14.0)
Total	1606 (12.5)	1274 (10.7)
Total	3279 (13.7)	2428 (11.5)

Percent of children (ages 6–11 yr) and adolescents (ages 12–17 yr) who were overweight in NHANES III, 1988–1994. Overweight is defined as body mass index at or above the 95th percentile. Pregnant females are excluded. Totals include racial/ethnic groups not shown. From NHANES III, 1988–1994.

6 percent between phase 1 (1988–1991) and phase 2 (1991–1994). For adults, it increased 9 percent.

Among adults, overweight prevalence increased by 3.3 percentage points for men and 3.6 percentage points for women between phases 1 and 2. This is consistent with other findings, such as CDC's Behavioral Risk Factor Surveillance System, which indicate that the age-adjusted prevalence of overweight based on self-report increased by nearly 1 percent each year for adults during 1987–1993.

However, analysis of the data shows that the weight increase is not consistent through all ages and ethnic groups. The greatest increase occurs at the upper end of the distribution, especially for children and teens. In other words, the heaviest youth are now heavier than in earlier studies, and more of them have moved above the cutoff point that defines overweight. The weights for leaner children, however, are similar to those found by previous NHANES studies dating back to 1963.

Definitions

Researchers used the 95th percentile of body mass index (BMI), as set in the 1960s, to define the cutoff point for children and adolescents. Using this definition, 5 percent of youth were overweight in the 1960s. It is a more conservative definition than using the 85th percentile, and is believed preferable since it is less likely to include and stigmatize youth who do not belong in the overweight category because of growth and puberty fat changes.

However, NHANES III, phase 1, used the 85th percentile for adolescents, and identified about 22 percent as being overweight at this level. This is the definition used in Healthy People 2000 to set the objective that no more than 15 percent of adolescents would be overweight by the year 2000, an objective now regarded as impossible, with trends moving in the opposite direction.

Adults are defined as overweight at BMI levels of 27.8 for men and 27.3 for women. This was set in the 1960s at the 85th percentile for adults age 20 to 29 years old. Thus, 15 percent of young adults initially were defined as overweight.

Data for 18- and 19-year-olds are not included in the current analysis, to keep the categories comparable with earlier NHANES surveys.

What's happening?

The federal researchers suggest that current weight increases come from a shift in which energy intake from food exceeds energy spent in activity. NHANES III shows that the average calorie intake has increased somewhat for both children and adults since NHANES II (1976–1980) and that recreational activity is low for many Americans.

The methodology on food intake was somewhat different between the two studies, but there was also an increase

estimates are subject to sampling variability, the number of children and adolescents who were overweight increased

in calories for most population subgroups between phases 1 and 2 of NHANES III. This observation has led researchers to conclude that this is a real increase, according to Cynthia Ogden, PhD, MRP, of the nutrition monitoring staff at the National Center for Health Statistics.[2]

Phase 1 also documented a high prevalence of inactivity in the United States and found that rates of inactivity are greater for women than men and for nonHispanic blacks and Mexican-Americans than whites. Leisure-time physical activity among adults appears to be quite stable as shown by the National Health Interview Survey (NHIS) and the BRFSS from the mid-1980s through the early 1990s. Decreasing activity levels may have resulted from changes in work, transportation, and time spent in inactivity, (e.g., watching television and playing electronic games) the NCHS researchers report.

Data for physical activity among children and adolescents have not been collected with comparable methods across surveys through the 1980s and 1990s.

Prevention

Researchers warn that obesity prevention is extremely important, because most methods for achieving weight loss are unsuccessful over time. Reversing the trend in overweight will require changes in individual behavior and the elimination of societal barriers to healthy choices.

"This report tells us again that Americans need to do better in choosing a healthy diet and a sensible plan of physical activity," said Health and Human Service (HHS) Secretary Donna E. Shalala. Just last year, the Surgeon General called attention to the need for regular moderate physical activity in our lives, and for a balanced diet. It's good advice, and we all need to act on it, for the sake of our own good health.

Last July, the first-ever Surgeon General's Report on Physical Activity and Health recommended 30 minutes of moderate physical activity per day. Regular moderate physical activity can substantially reduce the risk of heart disease, diabetes, colon cancer, and high blood pressure, the report said.

The Surgeon General's Report is available from CDC's Nutrition and Physical Activity information line (toll-free): 1-888-CDC-4NRG, or on the World Wide Web at http://www.cdc.gov. The new HHS and Department of Agriculture Dietary Guidelines for Americans are available for 50 cents through the Consumer Information Center, Department 378-C, Pueblo, CO, 81009; or from the World Wide Web at http://odphp.osophs.dhhs.gov. The Morbidity and Mortality Weekly Report can be obtained by mail: CDC, 1600 Clifton Road, Atlanta, GA 30333 or on the World Wide Webb at http://www.cdc.gov. HHS press releases are available on the World Wide Web at http://www.dhhs.gov.

Table 2 Overweight among adults

	Men No. (%)	Women No. (%)
White, non-Hispanic	3285 (33.7)	3755 (33.5)
Black, non-Hispanic	2112 (33.3)	2490 (52.3)
Mexican-American	2250 (36.4)	2128 (50.1)
Total	7933 (33.3)	8748 (36.4)
Total adults	16,681 (34.9)	

Percentage of adults (age 20 and over) who were overweight in NHANES III, 1988–1994. Overweight is defined as body mass index of 27.8 or more for men and 27.3 or more for women (85th percentile from NHANES II for ages 20–29). From NHANES III, 1988–1994.

Table 3 Weight control behaviors of high school students—percent of students

Category	Were attempting weight loss Female	Male	Total	Took laxatives or vomited to lose weight or control weight gain Female	Male	Total	Took diet pills to lose weight or to control weight gain Female	Male	Total	Dieted to lose weight or to control weight gain Female	Male	Total	Exercised to lose weight or to control weight gain Female	Male	Total
Race/ethnicity															
White	64.9	24.1	43.1	8.2	1.2	4.5	10.2	1.1	5.3	52.5	15.6	32.8	69.6	39.9	53.7
Black	44.5	18.9	33.2	4.1	4.3	4.2	4.0	3.6	3.8	31.8	11.7	22.7	49.1	34.6	42.4
Hispanic	58.3	32.1	45.4	10.9	4.1	7.6	8.6	2.8	5.7	48.2	23.4	36.0	61.3	42.5	52.0
Grade															
9th	63.8	25.2	42.6	9.3	1.5	5.0	9.2	1.9	5.2	52.7	16.6	32.7	72.2	42.8	55.9
10th	58.3	23.8	40.5	9.4	2.2	5.7	7.2	1.8	4.4	49.0	15.0	31.5	65.6	39.6	52.2
11th	58.1	25.3	41.2	7.6	3.0	5.2	12.0	2.1	6.9	44.8	17.0	30.4	59.1	37.7	48.0
12th	60.3	23.1	41.6	3.9	2.2	3.1	6.8	1.7	4.2	45.8	15.4	30.6	59.8	37.6	48.8
Total	59.8	24.3	41.4	7.6	2.2	4.8	8.7	1.9	5.2	47.8	16.0	31.2	63.8	39.3	51.0

Percent of high school students who engaged in behaviors with weight control, during the 30 days preceding the survey, by sex, race/ethnicity and grade. From Youth Risk Behavior Survey 1995.

Youth Risk Behavior survey

The Youth Risk Behavior Surveillance System monitors health-risk behaviors among young people, through self-reported questionnaires. The surveys are conducted in alternate years by the Centers for Disease Control and Prevention, Division of Adolescent and School Health. Data from state and local surveys are also used. Several of the behaviors surveyed relate to weight, physical activity, and body image as reported in the 1995 YRBS report on United States high school students.[3]

Perceived overweight

According to this survey, 28 percent of all students nationwide believe they are overweight. This is higher for girls than boys (34 vs 22 percent). Overall, Hispanic and white students are more likely than black students to say they are overweight (32, 29, and 21 percent, respectively).

Attempting weight loss

Sixty percent of high school girls and 24 percent of boys report they are trying to lose weight. This is more common for white and Hispanic students of both sexes than for black students (Table 3).

Many of the students attempt to lose weight using high risk methods. During the 30 days before the survey, 53 percent of white high school girls dieted to lose weight, along with 48 percent of Hispanic and 32 percent of black girls. During those 30 days, 8 percent of white, 11 percent of Hispanic, and 4 percent of black girls had taken laxatives or vomited to lose weight. Nine percent of girls had taken diet pills.

For boys, 23 percent of Hispanic, 16 percent of white, and 12 percent of black students had dieted to lose weight.

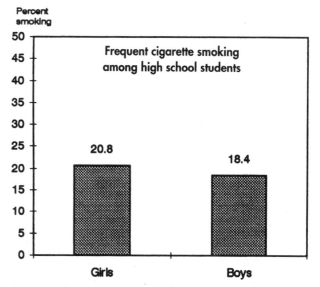

Figure 2. Frequent cigarette smoking among high school students. Note: Cigarette smoking on 20 or more of the preceding 30 days. From Youth Risk Behavior Survey 1995; *Afraid to Eat,* 2nd Edition 1997.

Smoking

Smoking is a common method of weight loss and weight control being used by youth today, especially white girls. Their smoking rates now surpass the rates of boys, for the first time ever. There is one compelling reason: to control their weight (Fig. 2).

One in three high school students smokes occasionally (at least one cigarette a month). This is highest for white students at 38 percent, with 34 percent for Hispanic, and 19 percent for black students. White girls have even higher rates at 40 percent, compared with 37 percent for white boys, and 12 percent for black girls.

Table 4 Physical activity of U.S. high school students—percent of students												
	Participated in vigorous physical activity			Participated in moderate physical activity			Participated in stretching exercises			Participated in strengthening exercises		
Category	Female	Male	Total	Female	Male	Total	Female	Male	Total	Female	Male	Total
Race/ethnicity												
White	56.7	76.0	67.0	16.8	19.7	18.3	53.9	56.1	55.1	44.4	60.3	52.8
Black	41.3	68.1	53.2	26.4	27.2	27.0	41.5	50.5	45.4	31.3	54.2	41.4
Hispanic	45.2	69.7	57.3	27.6	26.0	26.8	43.5	54.8	49.1	37.4	57.8	47.4
Grade												
9th	61.6	79.9	71.5	27.0	24.8	26.0	62.1	62.2	62.1	49.6	64.0	57.4
10th	59.3	78.6	69.3	22.9	23.7	23.3	57.8	58.7	58.3	49.8	62.3	56.2
11th	47.2	72.3	60.3	19.6	21.0	20.3	45.5	50.9	48.3	37.1	56.8	47.3
12th	42.4	67.2	54.9	13.7	17.2	15.4	38.9	50.7	44.9	29.4	53.7	41.5
Total	52.1	74.4	63.7	20.5	21.6	21.1	50.4	55.5	53.0	41.0	59.1	50.3

Percent of high school students who participated in vigorous physical activity (activities that caused sweating and hard breathing for at least 20 minutes on ≥ 3 of the 7 days preceding the survey), moderate physical activity (walked or bicycled for at least 30 minutes on ≥ 5 of the 7 days), stretching exercises (such as toe touching, knee bending, or leg stretching on ≥ 3 of the 7 days) and strengthening exercises (such as push-ups, sit-ups or weight lifting on ≥ 3 of the 7 days), by sex, race/ethnicity and grade. From Youth Risk Behavior Survey 1995.

White girls also are most likely to be frequent smokers (smoking 20 or more cigarettes a month), with prevalence rates of 21 percent, compared with 18 percent of white boys. Rates for Hispanic boys and girls are, respectively, 11 and 9 percent, about half those of whites, and for black boys and girls, 9 and 1 percent, respectively.

Activity

Nearly two-thirds of students are active at the recommended level. This includes about 74 percent of boys and 52 percent of girls. For boys, these statistics are 76 percent of white, 70 percent of Hispanic, and 68 percent of black students. For girls, the figures are 57 percent of white, 45 percent of Hispanic, and 41 percent of black students who are sufficiently active (Table 4).

Activity drops with age. Thus, the study looking at age 12 to 21 reports somewhat lower activity. About half the young people in the United States in this age group are active at recommended levels. The percentages are double the 1990 figures, but represent a slight drop from 1993.

Half of all students play on at least one school sports team, with girls almost as likely to play on school teams as boys (42 vs 58 percent). This shows an increase from 1991 when 44 percent of all students were on school sports teams, with a significant increase for girls and older students in grades 11 and 12. But girls are much less likely to play on sports teams outside of school (27 vs 46 percent of boys).

About half of high school students do strengthening and toning activities at least 3 days a week. Boys are more likely to do these than girls, and white students are more likely than black students. As with most activities, freshman girls are more likely to do them than older girls.

Walking or biking for 30 minutes at least 5 days a week is used as a measure of moderate physical activity.

Table 5 Percentage of high school students with suicide thoughts and behavior			
	Thought seriously	Made a suicide plan	Attempted suicide one or more times
Female	30	21	12
Male	18	14	6

Self-reported suicide thoughts and behaviors of U.S. high school students during 12 months preceding the survey. From Youth Risk Behavior Survey, 1995; *Afraid to Eat*, 1997.

This declined from 26 percent of high school students to 21 percent between 1992 and 1995. Black and Hispanic students (27 percent), both boys and girls, are more likely than white students (18 percent) to walk or bicycle. Younger high school girls are much more likely to walk or bicycle than senior girls.

Nearly two-thirds of girls said the reason they exercised in the month before the survey was to lose weight or keep from gaining. This was true for one-third of the boys.

Nationwide, 60 percent of students are enrolled in physical education (PE) class, but only one-fourth attend PE class daily, in this survey. High school freshmen are much more likely to take PE than juniors and seniors. During an average class, 70 percent of students report being active for 20 minutes or more.

Measures of despair

Eating well, living actively, and having a healthy body-image contribute to feeling good about ourselves. But if suicidal thoughts and plans are an indication of how our youngsters are faring, they are not doing well. Girls especially may be in trouble (Table 5).

Nearly one-fourth of high school students nationwide report they seriously considered suicide during the 12 months before the survey, a slight increase over 1993.

Table 6 Median daily nutrient intake—percent of RDA recommended values												
	Female						Male					
	12–15 yr			16–19 yr			12–15 yr			16–19 yr		
Nutrient lack	White	Black	Mexican American	White	Black	Mexican American	White	Black	Mexican American	White	Black	Mexican American
Calcium	62	51	66	66	52	56	90	60	85	103	76	79
Iron	67	65	68	63	69	68	128	110	119	146	119	114
Copper	67	62	59	63	66	67	81	76	79	93	87	84
Vitamin A	63	64	59	73	60	54	85	55	70	77	55	67
Magnesium	64	70	74	62	58	66	103	85	97	78	68	70
Zinc	67	71	72	70	78	72	77	59	70	90	82	80
Vitamin E	70	85	63	72	78	76	68	74	67	93	92	77
Phosphorus	87	81	94	88	87	90	118	97	114	141	126	122
Vitamin B$_6$	78	96	83	75	83	87	110	92	95	104	93	83

Adapted from the Third report on nutrition monitoring, NHANES III, 1988–1991. *Afraid to Eat*, 1st Ed., 1997.

The rates are twice as high for girls, and highest of all for Hispanic girls. Of Hispanic girls, 34 percent reported seriously considering suicide, 26 percent made a suicide plan, 21 percent attempted suicide, and 7 percent made a suicide attempt that required medical attention, all during the previous 12 months. For white girls, the figures are 32 percent for those who considered suicide, 22, 10, and 3 percent, respectively; for black girls, 22 percent who considered suicide, 16, 11, and 4 percent, respectively.

For white boys the suicide behavior rates are: 19 percent reported seriously considering suicide, 15 percent made a suicide plan, 5 percent attempted suicide, and 2 percent made a suicide attempt that required medical attention. For black high school boys, the corresponding statistics are 17, 13, 7, and 3 percent; for Hispanic boys, 16, 13, 6, and 3 percent.

Third Report on Nutrition Monitoring

Adolescent girls in their younger teens, (12–15 yr), have the poorest diets of all Americans and are most at risk from nutrient deficiencies, as documented by the Third Report on Nutrition Monitoring in the United States. They are followed closely by the older group of teenage girls, (16–19 yr). Even at the median, most of these girls do not eat enough to avoid deficiencies in many important nutrients. Further, their food choices often increase the risk of nutrient deficiencies (Table 6).

At the same time, many children and adults apparently consume too many calories. There appears to be an increase in calorie intake, paralleling the national increase in obesity.

The Nutrition Monitoring report is published by the United States Department of Agriculture and the Depart-

ment of Health and Human Services and brings together information on nutrition from several surveys, analyses, and monitoring systems for the first phase of NHANES III (1988–1991). The following data are from 1-day 24-hour recall surveys, which the statisticians say may be more accurate than 3-day reports, yet tend to skew the data at the extremes by reporting fewer calories at the lower end and more calories at the higher end.[4]

Deficiencies for girls

The median intake for teenage girls is only about half or two-thirds of the recommended dietary allowance (RDA)

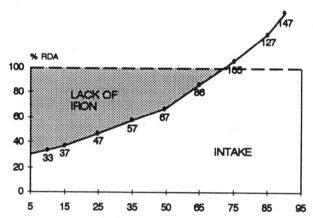

Figure 4. Iron intake for 12–15 year old white girls. Note: Most teenage girls are deficient in iron. At the 50th percentile white girls consume only 67% of recommended daily intake (RDA: 15 mg); at the 25th percentile, 47%; at the 10th percentile, 33%. This means all girls below these points are consuming less iron. Mexican-American girls get somewhat less iron, black girls somewhat more. Based on a 1-day 24-hour recall. Unpublished Data, NHANES III, phase 1, 1988–91; *Afraid to Eat*, 2nd Edition 1997.

for calcium, iron, vitamin A, magnesium, zinc, copper, and other critical nutrients.

The girls at the bottom one-fourth are much worse off than this. For the most part, these girls are undernourished or malnourished. When we look at the dietary intake of girls at the 25th and 10th percentiles, the severity of their nutrient deficiencies becomes clear.

For example, the recommended daily calorie intake is 2,200 for girls aged 12 to 15 years (range, 1,500 to 3,000). At the 10th percentile, white girls are consuming only 40 percent of the recommended calories (904 calories), Mexican-American girls somewhat less (833 calories), and black girls somewhat more (1,064 calories) (Fig. 3). At the 25th percentile, Mexican-American girls are still consuming only 1,300 calories; white girls, 1,358; and black girls, 1,400 calories. None of these meets the lowest recommended daily intake set in 1989.[5]

Two of the most critical nutrients for healthy growth and development are iron and calcium. Teenage girls at the

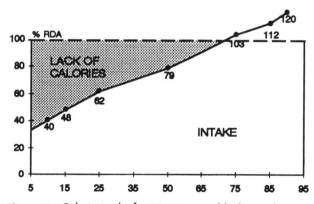

Figure 3. Calorie intake for 12–15 year old white girls. Note: The lower one-fourth of white girls aged 12–15 years consume 62% or less of the recommended daily calorie intake (RDA: 2,200). The lower one-tenth consume 40% or less. Mexican-American girls consume somewhat less, black girls somewhat more. Based on a 1-day 24-hour recall. Unpublished Data, NHANES III, phase 1, 1988–91; *Afraid to Eat*, 2nd Edition 1997.

10th percentile are getting only one-third of the iron they need, while at the 25th they are getting less than half the RDA (Fig. 4). The calcium situation is even worse. At the 10th percentile, girls are getting only 20 percent of what is considered essential to build strong bones and skeletal structure; at the 25th, slightly more than one-third (Fig. 5).

As can be expected, these girls also are deficient in many other nutrients. At the 10th percentile, they are getting barely 50 percent of the protein needed, 33 percent of the vitamin B_{12}, 25 percent of the zinc, and 15 percent of the vitamin A.

Teenage boys, too, may be low in calcium. At the 10th percentile they are getting only about 20 percent, and at the 25th percentile 33 percent of the calcium they need.

Overall, the younger group of girls and boys (age 6 to 11 yr) have more adequate nutrition. Yet even in this group, at

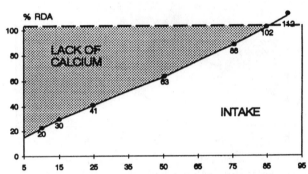

Figure 5. Calcium intake for 12–15 year old white girls. Note: Most teenage girls are severely deficient in calcium. At the 50th percentile white girls consume only 63% of recommended daily intake (RDA:1,200 mg); at the 25th percentile, 41%; at the 10th percentile, 20%. Mexican-American and black girls get less calcium at the 25th percentile, more at the 10th. Based on a 1-day 24-hour recall. Unpublished Data, NHANES III, phase 1, 1988– 91; *Afraid to Eat*, 2nd Edition 1997.

the lower percentiles, many are deficient. For example, at the 25th percentile, white girls in this age group are getting only about half the calories recommended. Their RDA is set at 2,400 calories (range, 1,650–3,300), somewhat higher than for older girls because of special growth needs at this age.

Adult nutrition

Overall, women also consume far less than the recommended number of calories at the median or 50th percentile. At the 25th percentile, most age groups are below the lowest desirable range, and at the 10 percentile, most get less than 1,000 calories a day (Table 7).

Men and boys consume close to the recommended daily allowance of calories at the median; at the 25th percentile, they are below the recommended range, and at the 75th percentile, above (Table 8).

Calcium levels are low for many people, especially women, black adult males, and elderly people across racial and ethnic groups. Iron intake is low for women to age 59, and anemia is correspondingly higher for them. Pregnant women tend to be low in several key nutrients (calcium, iron, folate, vitamin B_6, zinc, and magnesium).

Recommended calorie intake is determined for persons at average height and weight doing light work. Researchers suggest there may be under reporting (especially for overweight persons). The RDA provides an allowance for varied needs. In addition, intake does not include supplements taken.

Trends: Calories are up

Even though calorie intake is below recommended levels, there has been an increase in median calorie intake for adults since NHANES II (1976–1980). Methodology differs somewhat over the years, but the federal researchers

Table 7 Daily caloric intake for females in the United States					
			Age		
Percentile	12–15	16–19	20–29	40–49	60–69
5	803	842	844	824	668
10	904	1021	1015	970	768
25	1360	1335	1363	1328	1127
50	1800	1795	1838	1675	1494
75	2283	2400	2436	2147	1895
90	2695	3178	2939	2551	2340
95	3144	3860	3436	2948	2707
RDA*	2200	2100	2100	2000	1800
Range	1500–3000	1200–3000	1700–2500	1600–2400	1400–2200

*Recommended energy intake (U.S.) at mean heights and weights for persons doing light work. The customary range of daily energy output, shown in parentheses, is based on variations in energy needs of 400 calories at any one age, emphasizing the wide range of energy intakes appropriate for any group of people. Energy allowances for children through age 18 are based on median energy intakes of children in these age groups followed in longitudinal growth studies.[7] Unpublished data, NHANES III, phase 1, 1988–1991.

Table 8 Daily caloric intake for males in the United States					
	Age				
Percentile	*12–15*	*16–19*	*20–29*	*40–49*	*60–69*
5	1094	1287	1336	1146	870
10	1292	1620	1586	1426	1157
25	1831	2205	2111	1868	1511
50	2487	2919	2800	2351	1929
75	3024	3923	3699	3075	2584
90	3908	4637	4634	3779	3264
95	4707	5602	5436	4481	3679
RDA*	2700	2800	2900	2700	2400
Range	2000–3700	2100–3900	2500–3300	2300–3100	2000–2800

*See comments for Table 7.

believe the change is real since they also found an increase between phase 1 and phase 2.

Fat intake decreased to about 34 percent of total calories between 1988 and 1991, (36 percent, 1976–1980), but is still above the recommended level of 30 percent.

According to food disappearance data, between 1972 and 1992 people are now eating more flour, cereal, and prepared foods, more vegetable fats, and slightly more fruits and vegetables. Use of sugars and sweeteners increased to a high of 143 pounds per capita, an increase of 18 pounds, mostly in refined sugar and high fructose corn syrup. Use of low calorie sweeteners also tripled. Soft drink use rose from 26 to 44 gallons per person annually and far exceeds the consumption of milk, coffee, or fruit juices. From 1972, consumption of beer and wine is up, while distilled spirits are down. Overall, alcohol consumption is down from a high in the mid-1980s.

Consistent with this, the nationwide survey, conducted by the USDA in 1994, finds young people today are eating twice as much of foods such as crackers, popcorn, pretzels, and corn chips; more desserts and candy; more pasta with sauce, rice dishes, tacos, burritos, and pizza, the all time favorite. They eat less meat and eggs, and are still short on fruit and vegetables. They drink three times as much soda

pop as they did, but much less milk. Half of teenagers today drink no milk, compared with only one-fourth in the 1970s. Those who do, drink only about one-and-a-half to two cups a day on the average. The Dietary Guidelines for Americans recommend three servings a day from the milk group for teens, and the American Academy of Pediatrics is recommending that this be increased to five.[6]

References

1. Update: Prevalence of overweight among children, adolescents and adults U.S., 1988–1994. Morbidity and Mortality Weekly Report, March 7, 1997; 4:199–202.

2. CDC, unpublished data, 1997.

3. Youth Risk Behavior Surveillance–US, 1995. Morbidity and Mortality Weekly Report, CDC, US Public Health Service. Sept. 27, 1996: 45:SS-4:1–84.

4. Third Report on Nutrition Monitoring in the US, 1995, USDA. National Center for Health Statistics, NHANES III.

5. CDC, unpublished data NHANES III, phase 1, 1997.

6. What and where our children eat: 1994 Nationwide Survey results. USDA News release, Apr 18, 1996.

7. RDA information on calories from: Whitney EN, Hamilton EMN. Understanding nutrition, 4th Ed., 1987. St. Paul MN: West Publishing. 1–2 Appendix 1, Table 1–2.

The history of dieting and its effectiveness

by Wayne C. Miller, PhD

How effective have diets and dieting programs been in producing weight loss?

Throughout the years, dietitians and nutritionists have advocated moderate consistent weight loss through a balanced, energy controlled diet in conjunction with lifestyle changes. Although this may be the healthiest way to lose weight, it is not necessarily the way the public attempts to lose weight.

In the late 1950s and early 1960s, total fasting was used to reduce weight in the massively obese. Weight loss through fasting amounted to 1.0 kg per day the first month followed by 0.5 kg a day thereafter.[1] Although the desired outcome, weight loss, was achieved through fasting, serious side effects such as loss of lean body mass, depleted electrolytes, and death caused fasting to quickly wane in popularity.[1,2,3]

Next on the scene came the high-protein, low-carbohydrate diets of the 1960s and early 1970s. The theory of this epic, which still lingers today, was that carbohydrates (particularly starch) make you fat. Popular diets of that time (e.g. Stillman, Atkins) provided 1,200 to 2,000+ calories per day, with only 5 to 10 percent coming from carbohydrates.[4] On the other hand, 50 to 70 percent of the energy intake on these diets came from fat. The justification of this diet composition was that the high protein content prevented the loss of lean tissue, while the high fat content produced ketosis with its associated appetite suppression. Weight loss on these diets was rapid because of depleted glycogen stores and diuresis, but side effects included nausea, hyperuricemia, fatigue, and refeeding edema.[5]

VLCD liquids

During the mid 1970s very low calorie liquid diets became commercially available. These diets were known as protein-sparing-modified fasts or liquid protein diets. Their extremely low caloric content (300-400 calories per day) caused rapid weight loss. However, in spite of medical supervision, high quality protein, and potassium supplementation, several deaths due to ventricular arrhythmia occurred with prolonged use. These liquid protein diets were subsequently banned until research studies could assure their safety.[6]

A second generation of very low calorie formula diets became popular in the 1980s. These commercial formula products, such as Optifast and Health Management Resources, became part of a medical approach including patient counseling and support. Diets of 400 to 500 calories per day were offered as well as the option of an 800-calorie plan. At the same time, franchises like Nutri/System and Jenny Craig offered clients pre-packaged foods along with exercise and nutrition counseling. This second generation of very low calorie formula diets and pre-packaged foods has evolved to where many of these commercial programs now offer individualized approaches that emphasize exercise and behavior change.[7] These programs can cost up to $3,000 and/or $70 to $90 per week for food products.[7] Another problem is that these programs have not been well researched for safety and may be as detrimental to health as any other rapid weight loss regimen.[8]

Lowfat diets

Research related to the health risks of dietary fat in the 1970s and 1980s has spawned a fat-phobic society. Thus, the newest trend in the dieting realm is non-fat or low-fat diets. Fat-free and low-fat versions of foods have become popular while the Pritikin diet, which was first used in the 1970s to combat the risks of degenerative diseases, has been resurrected as a weight-loss diet. Other low-fat programs, like the T-Factor diet, promote counting fat grams rather than calories for weight control. Average weight loss due to reducing dietary fat alone is only 0.1 to 0.2 kg per week.[9,10] Moreover, there is some concern that the abundance of low-fat fat-free calorie-rich snack foods on the market will encourage overconsumption by would-be dieters who concern themselves only with dietary fat.

Diets challenged

Obesity researchers have been fighting an uphill battle ever since

❝ Long term weight loss following any type of intervention was limited to only a small minority of the obese people studied ❞
— NIH

Reprinted with permission from *Healthy Weight Journal* (formerly *Obesity & Health*), March/April 1997, pp. 28-29. © 1997 by Healthy Weight Journal, Research, News and Commentary Across the Weight Spectrum, 402 South 14th Street, Hettinger, ND 58639.

Stunkard and McLaren-Hume concluded that dieting was ineffective for 95 percent of those in a hospital nutrition clinic.[11] Since that time, the use of diets for weight control has been challenged by the public, a growing number of health care professionals, as well as some obesity researchers themselves.[8]

Hence, the National Institutes of Health (NIH) recently convened a Technology Assessment Conference to evaluate the effectiveness of voluntary methods for weight loss and control.

The report for very low calorie diets (VLCDs) revealed that weight loss following a 12-week VLCD totaled 20 kg, with a 35 to 50 percent weight regain after one year.[12,13] Furthermore, dropout rates in some VLCD programs can reach 80 percent. The less restrictive low calorie diets (LCDs) are even less effective. Following a 20-week LCD program, average weight loss is 8.5 kg, with a 33 percent regain after one year, and a 100 percent regain after five years.[14,15]

Nutrition education and behavior modification programs have become popular because they are supposedly self-empowering. However, success on these programs isn't any better than on VLCDs or LCDs. An 18-week behavior modification program will bring about a 10 kg weight loss, with a 95 percent relapse after two years.[15] Similarly discouraging is the finding that community programs, worksite interventions, and home correspondence programs show negligible success after one to three years.[16]

Weak data advanced

Data to support the effectiveness claims of commercial weight-loss programs was requested by the NIH and FDA at the time of the Technology Assessment Conference. Material was received from only five companies, three representing nonphysician-directed programs and two representing physician-directed programs. For the nonphysician-directed programs, one company submitted one research study and several abstracts. The study demonstrated reduced cardiovascular disease risk following short-term use of the program; the abstracts were judged scientifically inadequate. The second company representing nonphysician-directed programs submitted four research studies, but later withdrew the studies from the NIH review. The third company data was judged inadequate to evaluate.

For the physician-directed programs, one company submitted three research articles and several abstracts. Data from this company was evaluated as inconclusive. The other company representing a physician-directed program was the only company in the industry that submitted data that was scientifically sound. Although this company submitted 55 quality research reports, the NIH committee determined that long-term weight loss following this program was questionable.[17]

Odd conclusion

Surprisingly enough, even though only one commercial program in the whole industry provided data that could be seen as adequate, and that data provided no evidence for long-term success for weight control, the NIH assessment team concluded: *"Regardless of products used, successful weight loss and control is limited to and requires individualized programs consisting of restricted caloric intake, behavior modification and exercise.[17] "*

It is puzzling how the NIH could come to any effectiveness conclusion based on the paucity of data they received which they themselves judged to be inadequate, questionable, and inconclusive.[17] Only two conclusions seem possible to have been drawn, either 1) no conclusion can be made because there is no data upon which to base a conclusion, or 2) no commercial program is effective at producing long-term weight loss because no company could provide data to show otherwise.

It seems the NIH conclusion for commercial program effectiveness was based on an assumption or hope of what should be effective, not on the data evaluated.

The overall conclusion from NIH as to the effectiveness of any type of method for voluntary weight loss and control was more true to the facts than their conclusion for the commercial industry. The universal consensus of the conference was:

"Long term weight loss following any type of intervention was limited to only a small minority of the obese people studied.[18] "

Thus, it seems apparent that there is not enough data to support the claim that diet programs are effective in long-term weight control for a majority of the obese.

The question that is most relevant now is, *what intervention strategies should be used to promote health in the obese, if intervention is deemed appropriate at all?* This question will be addressed in the next issue of *Healthy Weight Journal*.

Wayne C. Miller, PhD, is Professor of Exercise Science and Nutrition at George Washington University Medical Center, Washington, DC.

REFERENCES
1. J Am Med Assoc 1964;187:100-106
2. J Am Diet Assoc 1990;90:722-726
3. J Nutr 1986;116:918-919
4. J Am Diet Assoc 1985;85:450-454
5. Clinical Nutrition and Dietetics. New York: Macmillan Publishing Co.; 1991.
6. Am J. Clin Nutr 1981;34:453-461
7. Environmental Nutr 1994;17:1,3
8. Health Risks of Weight Loss. Hettinger, ND: Healthy Weight Journal; 1995
9. Am J Clin Nutr 1991;53:1124-1129
10. Am J Clin Nutr 1991;54:821-828
11. J Am Diet Assoc 1991;91:1248-1251
12. Ann Int Med 1993;119:688-693
13. Ann Int Med 1993;119:764-770
14. Behav Ther 1987;18:353-374
15. Int J Obesity 1989;13:123-136
16. Ann Int Med 1993;119:719-721
17. Ann Int Med 1993;119:681-687
18. Ann Int Med 1993;119:764-770

Diet Pills
Are Millions of Women Playing Russian Roulette with Their Health?

Suddenly, diet pills seem to be everywhere. Prescriptions for "fen-phen"—the nickname for the unapproved combination of fenfluramine (Pondimin) and phentermine (Ionamin and others)—reached 18 million last year alone, and doctors wrote more than 3 million prescriptions for dexfenfluramine (Redux) during its first year.

Used along with calorie restriction and moderate exercise, fen-phen and Redux do appear to offer a weight-loss advantage over lifestyle changes alone. But the drugs are far from perfect—and for some unlucky women, they've proven to be deadly.

Handle with Care

To begin with, most people find that once they go off the drugs, the weight returns. "Everything we know indicates that when you stop the drug, you stop the effects," says James O. Hill, Ph.D., codirector of the Center for Human Nutrition at the University of Colorado Health Sciences Center in Denver. "If we're going to use drugs [to treat obesity], treatment is going to have to be chronic."

The catch is that no one has thoroughly studied either the safety or effectiveness of giving diet drugs over the long haul. Moreover, the risk of one very rare but deadly complication appears to rise with increased duration of use.

That complication is primary pulmonary hypertension (PPH), a disorder that permanently damages blood vessels in the lungs. Studies have linked both fenfluramine and dexfenfluramine to an increased risk of PPH.

PPH is exceedingly rare in the general population. It has few early symptoms, is difficult to diagnose, and has no consistently effective treatment. Half of those who develop the condition die of heart failure, usually within five years.

No one quarrels with the fact that PPH is deadly, and fenfluramine and dexfenfluramine now carry clear warnings about the disorder. The debate heats up over the degree of risk posed by the drugs and whether the benefits of the medications outweigh their risks.

A Looming Crisis?

Last year's approval of Redux seemed to signal a new era in the treatment of obesity. But shortly after the drug's approval, a study published in the *New England Journal of Medicine* found that people who took fenfluramine-based drugs for longer than three months were 23 times more likely to develop PPH than someone who had never used them (*WHA*, October 1996).

If those figures are correct—and not everyone agrees that they are—then 23 to 46 cases of PPH could be expected for every 1 million people who take a fenfluramine-based drug.

Those numbers have some observers worried that cases of the deadly disorder will increase dramatically as more and more people—primarily women—take fen-phen and Redux.

In the March *American Journal of Respiratory and Critical Care Medicine*, three lung specialists wrote that "physicians such as ourselves dealing with pulmonary hypertension are simply scared. We have little doubt that we will see new cases of PPH."

But many obesity experts believe the PPH risk has been overblown and that media coverage of the issue has been irresponsible. They caution against using one study as the basis for condemning potentially useful medications. Moreover, they point out that obesity is itself a risky condition, especially when potentially fatal complications such as heart disease and cancer are taken into account.

Disagreements over risk estimates aside, physicians on both sides of the issue worry about overuse and misuse of fenfluramine-based drugs. "These medications aren't for cosmetic weight loss. They're for people at serious risk of health problems," says Dr. Hill.

Unfortunately, far too many people aren't giving these drugs the respect they deserve. "People treat them as if they're 'just' diet pills—as in, 'It's no big deal, you don't have to worry about side effects,'" he says. "But these are serious medications. They really should be used only when we know that the patient will get some benefits and is already at some risk to begin with."

Food for Thought

If you're tempted to take fen-phen or Redux, here are some questions to ask yourself:

• How much do you want to lose? See the chart to see if you can even be considered a legitimate candidate for the drugs.

• How committed are you to making healthy long-term changes? Fen-phen and Redux may help you lose weight initially. However, they don't work for everyone—and even when they do, weight loss tends to plateau around the six-month mark.

Moreover, the rebound statistics are dismal. That doesn't mean it's impossible to keep the weight off once you stop taking the drugs, but be prepared to make major changes in your eating habits and a solid commitment to daily exercise.

• Who will be monitoring you? This isn't the time to take your prescription and run. You should be *closely* monitored by your personal physician or a reputable obesity specialist.

If you pursue long-term treatment, be aware that studies generally have been limited to one year. No one knows whether taking diet medications indefinitely is effective or safe.

As far as PPH is concerned, women in their 30s and 40s appear to be at highest risk, but there's no reliable way to predict who might develop the condition. Symptoms include shortness of breath, decreased exercise tolerance, fainting, chest pains, and swollen ankles.

In addition, other side effects can occur: Phentermine's side effects include nervousness, insomnia, and hypertension; side effects of fenfluramine and dexfenfluramine include drowsiness, lethargy, dry mouth, and diarrhea. In addition, about 15% of those who take fenfluramine-based drugs complain of short-term mental fuzziness or forgetfulness. Most of

these effects dissipate within a few weeks.

The issue of long-term brain toxicity with fenfluramine and dexfenfluramine was raised by studies of monkeys given dexfenfluramine. But differences in brain physiology lead to far higher levels of the drug in animal brains, says Richard L. Atkinson, M.D., professor of medicine and nutritional sciences at the University of Wisconsin in Madison. To date, there have been no reports of such toxicity in people, but the issue is being studied.

So, based on what's currently known, here's the bottom line: If you're significantly overweight and are already facing serious obesity-related health problems, these drugs may be worth a shot. But if you're slightly overweight and your biggest health problem is tight jeans, the drugs are an expensive shot in the dark—one that isn't worth the risk.

Weighing the Risk

Body mass index (BMI) is a standard used to measure obesity. If your BMI is 30 or greater (see the darker area), the benefits of treatment with diet drugs may outweigh the risks. The same is true if your BMI is between 27 and 30 and you also have diabetes, high cholesterol, or hypertension (see the lightly shaded area). But if your BMI is less than 27, don't even consider diet drugs.

Body Mass Index*

Height Weight	5'0"	5'2"	5'4"	5'6"	5'8"	5'10"	6'0"
140	27	26	24	22	21	20	19
150	29	27	26	24	23	21	20
160	31	29	27	26	24	23	22
170	33	31	29	27	26	24	23
180	35	33	31	29	27	26	24
190	37	35	33	31	29	27	26
200	39	36	34	32	30	28	27
210	41	38	36	34	32	30	28
220	43	40	38	35	33	31	30

* If your height or weight isn't shown on this chart, here's how to figure your BMI: Multiply your weight by 700, then divide that by the square of your height in inches.

Update '97

News and our views

'Fen-phen' therapy may be associated with heart problem

If you're taking a combination of the weight-loss medications fenfluramine and phentermine—commonly known as "fen-phen"—Mayo Clinic physicians recommend that you talk to your doctor. Mayo physicians have observed an unusual form of heart valve disease in 24 women taking fen-phen. In light of this finding, Mayo physicians suggest you discuss with your doctor the benefits and risks of continuing fen-phen therapy.

The heart valve damage was discovered during routine medical visits. Subsequent testing showed that the valves were thickened and blood was "leaking" backwards (regurgitating), making the heart work harder to pump blood through the body. In some of the women, more than one heart valve was affected. Five of the women needed heart surgery to repair or replace damaged valves.

The women, who were free of cardiovascular disease prior to taking fen-phen, had been using the medications for an average of one year. Eight were also found to have pulmonary hypertension, a serious disease of the heart and lungs. So far, none has died.

Mayo investigators say they don't know how the medications may cause heart valve damage, but the findings raise significant concern. More comprehensive study is needed and planned.

Fenfluramine and phentermine are each approved by the Food and Drug Administration for treatment of obesity. The combination of the two drugs is not FDA-approved, even though the medications are commonly prescribed that way. Last year, doctors wrote 18 million monthly prescriptions for the drugs.

From *Mayo Clinic Health Letter,* August 1997, p. 7.

Editor's note: On September 15, 1997, the U.S. Food and Drug Administration announced the withdrawal of dexfenfluramine and fenfluramine from the market. Studies appeared to indicate that up to 32% of individuals who were on dexfenfluramine or fenfluramine, with or without phentermine, may be afflicted with leaky heart valves.

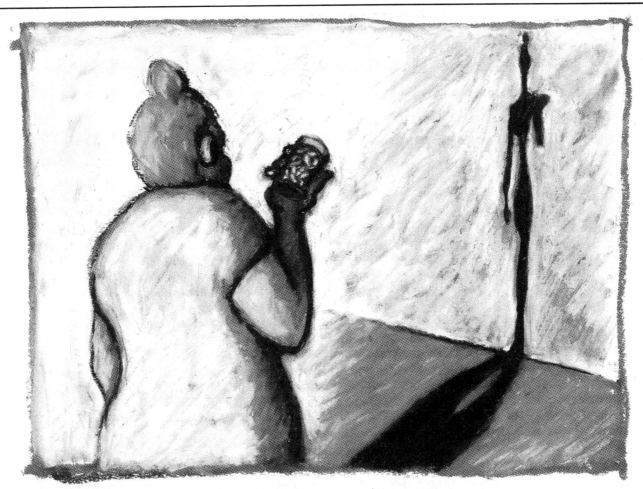

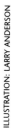

ILLUSTRATION: LARRY ANDERSON

OBESITY: NO MIRACLE CURE YET

KRISTINE NAPIER

People burdened with extra body fat know all too well that one size doesn't fit all—especially when it comes to weight loss. Many are hoping, though, that today's rapidly progressing research on the genetics of obesity will produce a one-size-fits-all approach to slimming down their bulging curves. But as exciting as this research is, the unfortunate reality is that most overweight people won't be able to squeeze a solution out of it.

Recently, U.S. health officials announced that the percentage of obese Americans—those packing 20 to 30 percent more than their ideal body weight—had grown from a decades-long level of a quarter of the population to a hefty third of the population. In everyday terms, that means that the average 5' 6" woman, who should weigh between 117 and 143 pounds (see box on page 134 to see how to figure your own healthy weight), is considered obese if her weight is above a range of 171 to 186 pounds.

Obesity. It's worse than a four-letter word. The condition ranks with the worst of physical afflictions. Obese people lug around enough extra weight to cause serious health problems. There is much evidence that obesity significantly increases a person's risk of developing high blood pressure, abnormal blood cholesterol levels, diabetes, gout and osteoarthritis. Indirectly, obesity is a major risk factor for dying too young. The collective impact of obesity on the nation's health—and on its health care costs—is enormous.

Americans express genuine concern about their excess weight. Of all their physical maladies, it's the one complaint that vast numbers of them focus on curing. But for all the talk there's very little action. Many Americans lose some weight with each dieting effort, but it's a paltry few that keep it off for more than a year. Repeated attempts at weight loss not only feed feelings of failure but also nurture tremendous frustration and negative self talk.

THE SKINNY ON ANTI-OBESITY DRUGS

People have long sought a "magic bullet" for obesity—a drink, injection or pill that would magically melt away those excess pounds. Cracking the obesity nut has also perplexed the scientists searching for an effective obesity cure. In the 50s and 60s many doctors prescribed amphetamines, also called "uppers." These drugs helped people lose weight by curbing their appetite, but they created more problems than they solved. Amphetamines were highly addictive; they also made users high or stimulated them to the point of euphoria and/or dangerous aggression.

Knowing that appetite could be controlled chemically, researchers began searching for a replacement for amphetamines—for a drug that could control appetite without producing amphetamines' harmful effects. Scientists today are still searching along three lines: They are investigating drugs that curb appetite, drugs that rev up the body's metabolic rate and burn fat faster and drugs that act like the body's own naturally occurring leptin (see main article).

The U.S. Food and Drug Administration (FDA) recently approved the first anti-obesity drug for long-term use. Dexfenfluramine, long available in Europe, will be sold in the U.S. later this year under the trade name Redux. This new drug is in the category of drugs that curb appetite.

Dexfenfluramine suppresses appetite—particularly carbohydrate cravings—by maintaining higher levels of serotonin, a so-called neurotransmitter, in the brain. Serotonin is a critical factor in mood control. Many antidepressant drugs work by controlling serotonin levels, and appetite control is linked to those mental processes that work to modulate mood and feelings of stress. High serotonin levels are desirable in people who need to lose weight because high serotonin levels help to reduce appetite. Dexfenfluramine works to keep serotonin levels high by preventing its breakdown and stimulating cells to produce even more.

There are concerns about using dexfenfluramine. Stopping it might cause a person to experience a sudden severe depression or might cause unpredictable, impulsive behavior. Rodent research has shown that serotonin levels can stay at abnormally low levels for months after the drug is discontinued—and normal serotonin levels are necessary for normal mood control. Another concern is whether it will be possible for a person to maintain weight loss without the drug. There is some speculation that indefinite, long-term use of dexfenfluramine may be necessary to prevent someone's regaining shed pounds.

Among the other drugs currently in use for weight loss are phentermine and fenfluramine. These two drugs are chemically related to amphetamines. Both phentermine and fenfluramine have been around for many years, but there has been a resurgence in their use as diet aids. Phentermine and fenfluramine are often prescribed together, and for a very good reason. "While fenfluramine can cause central nervous system depression, phentermine is more of a stimulant," says Mary Ann Stuhan, R.Ph., a clinical pharmacist at Cleveland's Mt. Sinai Medical Center.

Stuhan also points out that the FDA recommends that these two drugs be used for only a few weeks; among the reasons for this abbreviated use is that phentermine and fenfluramine are addictive. "Indeed, they are useful in appetite suppression short term, but the emphasis is on the short term. They should be used only in conjunction with education on how to change lifestyle. People have to remember that drugs alone will not cause any significant weight loss. Medications such as fenfluramine and phentermine should only be used in the first couple of weeks of weight loss effort when people are learning how to change their habits."

Some people have turned to what has been termed a natural weight loss aid—the mineral chromium. Its proponents claim that chromium, which is needed by the body in small amounts, can help overweight people shed excess pounds (this among other questionable health claims made for the mineral). But the studies conducted on chromium's weight-loss potential have themselves been questionable at best. In addition, preliminary research (and we stress *preliminary*) suggests that ingesting large quantities of chromium might cause chromosome damage. For now, experts say that chromium supplements simply cannot be recommended for weight loss or for any other condition.

What some people don't realize is that any weight-loss drug is only an aid. A drug must be accompanied by an intensive program of behavior modification—a program that helps define a healthier style of eating and exercising to be followed *forever*.

Editor's note: See note on page 130 for the latest action of the FDA concerning anti-obesity drugs.

That's precisely why news of advances in understanding the genetic underpinnings of obesity sends ripples of excitement through the country. News of the obesity (ob) gene, of the newly discovered hormone leptin and of new weight-loss drugs has captured headlines for months. But what's the news all about?

Exciting Discoveries

The first wave of news came with the December 1994 discovery by researchers at New York's Rockefeller University that the portliness of a strain of overweight mice can be explained by their having a defective version of the ob gene.

In normal mice, a properly working version of the ob gene tells fat cells to make a special protein—a hormone called leptin—but to make it only when the body's fat cells have stored enough fat. The leptin travels through the bloodstream to the brain and tells the brain the body has stored a healthy amount of body fat. The mice then regulate their food intake and maintain normal body weight.

Mice with an absent or defective ob gene don't make leptin when they've eaten enough food and stored enough fat. No leptin, no message to the brain. The mice overeat and plump up.

Six months after the discovery of the ob gene, three teams of researchers, including the Rockefeller team, reported injecting the ob mice with leptin—with dramatic results. The once obese rodents ate less, slimmed down and even revved up their metabolism to burn calories at an increased rate. Even normal-weight mice injected with leptin lost body weight.

Obese people were ready to line up for leptin injections. Their hopes were quickly dashed by the next discoveries, however. Unlike their rotund rodent friends, obese humans do not have a mutated ob gene. What's more, obese humans aren't even lacking leptin. Surprisingly, tests revealed that obese people actually have leptin levels some 20 to 30 times higher than the levels found in lean people.

Researchers speculated that the obese human body wasn't "hearing" the leptin's message. Like other body hormones, leptin can't do its job of curbing the appetite unless the body heeds the hormone's call. In a fascinating and intricate system, the body "hears" a hormone's message via receptors. Receptors are basically antennae—the connections through which the messages carried by the hormones are transmitted to the brain. When the receptors are faulty, a message cannot be relayed to the brain. Unheard by the brain, the message—such as the one contained in leptin—cannot bring about any change.

A further advance will help researchers discover if the deaf-to-leptin theory is true. In December 1995 researchers from Millennium Pharmaceuticals in Cambridge, Massachusetts, and Hoffman-LaRoche in Nutley, New Jersey, reported finding the location of the leptin receptor in the human brain. The researchers are now probing to find out if the leptin receptors in the brains of obese people are faulty. The scientists' hunch is that only a very small percentage of obese people have defective leptin receptors.

Americans have developed very poor health habits. We drop off dry cleaning, library books and mail at drive-up windows, then drive through a fast-food line to order a fat-laden, thousand-calorie lunch.

If any treatment is to result from this series of discoveries, it will probably come in the form of drugs devised to modulate or change the receptor to allow it to hook up with the leptin and receive its message. Scientists are engaged in promising research along these lines. Investigators in one line of research have discovered that when properly working leptin receptors in normal-weight mice are overstimulated, the mice eat less and become very thin. The investigators are hoping that overstimulating the properly functioning leptin receptors in obese humans will have the same effect—and will ultimately help those people to lose weight.

This solution would only work, however, if an obese person had enough properly working leptin receptors. Someone with severely abnormal leptin receptors or with very few normal receptors would need a far more complex type of therapy—therapy that could repair the severely defective gene responsible for making leptin receptors. This almost science-fiction solution is years away—probably even decades away. The first step is to identify leptin-receptor gene mutations in obese people—exactly what the researchers at Millennium are currently trying to do.

Other types of therapies would be necessary if an obese person's body produced normal amounts of leptin and had normal receptors—which might indeed be the case with some obese people. Such a person's brain cells might still be "deaf" to leptin's message. It's as if a television set had a normal antenna but a broken circuit board. This person would need a drug therapy that somehow could fix the broken circuit inside the cell to let leptin's message get through.

On still another front, investigators are conducting research they suspect will identify how leptin affects yet other genes to influence appetite and weight. One exciting research area involves a hormone called glucagon-like peptide-1 (GLP-1), a known appetite suppressant. It seems highly likely that leptin sends messages to genes that in turn signal cells to make more GLP-1.

It's Not All in the Genes

These discoveries have been reported well to a rapidly progressing scientific world. But a critical fact about these advances hasn't made it through the filter of the lay media to the consumer: These discoveries, however exciting, probably apply to only a small percentage of overweight Americans. Millennium researchers stress that very few obese Americans have a faulty leptin receptor or have cells deaf to leptin's message.

But how do scientists know this without having identified faulty leptin receptors yet? For one thing, they know that human genes haven't changed much for several generations—but the incidence of human obesity has. The researchers also know that we live in a world of caloric excess and activity deprivation. In short, Americans have developed very poor health habits. We drop off dry cleaning, library books and mail at drive-up windows, then drive through a fast-food line to order a fat-laden, thousand-calorie lunch. We replace too many home-cooked meals with higher fat frozen or carry-out versions. We snack in our easy chairs in front of the TV with remote in hand. A single convenience—an electric can opener or pencil sharpener, a garage-door opener, an extension phone in every room—doesn't make a huge difference in the number of calories burned, but taken together they turn us into sedentary blobs. Similarly, an occasional fast-food meal is perfectly fine; but the combination of a steady diet of fast food and convenience food with no regular exercise is deadly to the waistline.

Americans with 20 or 30 pounds to lose shouldn't wait for advancing obesity research to produce a magic pill. Instead, they should develop a lifestyle that focuses on fitness and health rather than on taste and convenience. They—and, indeed, most of us—need to eat less and exercise more. Even that small percentage of Americans whose obesity is due to genetic factors—and for whom new drugs may be developed one day—will have to eat less and exercise more. Some truths never change.

WHAT'S A HEALTHY WEIGHT?

Why does healthy weight vary so widely for people of the same height? Bone structure has a lot to do with it, as does the type of weight a person carries. Bigger boned people and people with dense muscle mass can safely carry around more weight than can people with large fat deposits.

The following is an easy, rule-of-thumb way to figure the range of normal body weight:

- For men: Figure 106 pounds for the first five feet of height and 6 additional pounds for each inch over five feet. Weights 10 percent over and 10 percent under this figure are within the normal range.

- For women: Figure 100 pounds for the first five feet and 5 additional pounds for each inch over five feet. Again, weights 10 percent over and 10 percent under this figure are normal

For example, for a woman 5' 6" tall (66 inches), the midpoint of healthy weight would be 130 pounds. That's 100 pounds plus the 6 additional inches times 5 pounds per inch, or 100 plus 30 pounds. This weight could be 10 percent lower (130 minus 13 pounds, or 117 pounds for a small-boned woman with low muscle) or 10 percent higher (130 plus 13 pounds, or 143 pounds for a large-boned woman who exercises and has a greater amount of muscle). A normal range of weight for a 5' 6" tall woman would thus be between 117 and 143 pounds.

KRISTINE NAPIER, M.P.H., R.D., IS A FREELANCE HEALTH AND SCIENCE WRITER AND EDITOR BASED IN CLEVELAND, OH. SHE CONTRIBUTES REGULARLY TO *PRIORITIES* AND OTHER ACSH PUBLICATIONS.

DIET AND EXERCISE: WHAT KIDS NEED TODAY

... INTRODUCTION

Health professionals are increasingly recognizing the synergistic beneficial health effects of diet and physical activity for all Americans (1). The U.S. Department of Health and Human Services' *Healthy People 2000* national health goals (2) will not be met until healthful eating habits and physical activity are merged into one lifestyle behavior. A recent survey indicates that children are beginning to understand this message (3). Most children surveyed expressed positive attitudes about food, nutrition, and physical activity. However, many children held nutrition misconceptions that could interfere with their enjoyment of healthful eating (3). And although 78% of children surveyed said that physical activity is fun and good for their health (3), many are inactive (4,5).

Obesity is the most prevalent disease of children and adolescents in the U.S. (4, 6a,7). Nearly one-quarter of the nation's youth are overweight despite public health efforts to reduce childhood overweight to less than 15% by the year 2000 (4,7). Although eating habits contribute to this major health problem, physical inactivity may play an even larger role (4,8,9).

This *Digest* reviews the problem of overweight among America's youth, examines reasons why they are becoming heavier, and provides lifestyle suggestions to promote healthful eating habits and regular physical activity patterns among children.

THE PROBLEM OF OVERWEIGHT IN YOUTH

Overweight in youth is a serious and growing public health problem in the U.S.

Today, nearly one-quarter of the nation's youth is overweight. Obesity in youth is associated with adverse health and psychosocial consequences. But the most negative effect may be the likelihood that it will persist throughout life.

(7,10). About 4.7 million children ages 6 to 17 years are overweight and the prevalence has increased significantly over the past three decades (7). Between 1963–65 and 1988–91, overweight in children more than doubled (i.e., increased from 5% to 10.9%). Most of this increase has occurred in the last 10 to 12 years (7). The prevalence of overweight may be even higher than 10.9%, depending on how overweight is defined. When overweight is defined at the 85th percentile of body mass for height and weight, instead of at the 95th percentile, 22% of the nation's children in 1988–91 were overweight, compared to 15% in 1963–65 (7).

Obesity in youth has both adverse medical and psychosocial consequences (6a,11). Obese children are at increased risk of high blood pressure, hypercholesterolemia, and glucose intolerance (6a). In addition, in obese teenagers, excess body fat in the abdominal area is associated with a variety of cardiovascular risk factors (12). The obese child also may suffer from teasing from other children, discrimination, and a poor self image (11). The most negative impact of obesity in youth is the likelihood that it will persist throughout the adult years (6a). Research indicates that the more overweight a child and the later the onset of overweight during childhood, the greater the risk of increased obesity-related morbidity and mortality in adulthood (6a,7,13–16).

WHY ARE CHILDREN BECOMING HEAVIER?

Overweight is caused by energy imbalance, or energy (calorie) intake in excess of energy expenditure. Multiple factors, both genetic and environmental, contribute to this imbalance. Among environmental factors, most attention is focused on diet and physical activity.

The Role of Genetics. Genetics contributes to obesity (6b,17,18). Recent studies of humans have identified at least six genes linked to increased body fatness and/or susceptibility to obesity and five other genes linked to a disproportionate storage of fat in the abdominal region (18). Studies of twins, adoptees, and families support the heritabil-

ity of obesity (17). In identical twins, heritability may account for about 70% of the variability in body mass index (17).

A child's risk of becoming obese is influenced by the weight of his or her parents (17). In about 30% of cases of childhood obesity, both parents of obese children are obese. However, despite the fact that a child's risk of becoming obese is higher if both parents are obese, about 25% to 35% of obese children are from families with normal weight parents (17). Although heredity accounts for about one-third of individual differences in body weight (6b,17), genetics is unlikely to explain the dramatic rise in childhood overweight in recent decades, a period of time too short to alter the frequency of obesity genes (18).

Is Overconsumption of Energy and Fat the Cause of the Rise in Overweight in Youth? Societal and environmental factors favor a positive energy balance in children and adolescents (7,19). Because more mothers are working outside the home, children and adolescents today are assuming increased responsibility for their food decisions, including buying foods and preparing meals (10). The increased availability and heavy advertising of relatively inexpensive high calorie, high fat foods (e.g., sugared cereals, candy, soft drinks) may steer many children away from healthful food choices (19). Also, the trend of eating away-from-home (20), often at fast food restaurants where high calorie, high fat foods are abundant, may increase children's intake of energy and fat.

Despite the environmental influences supporting a more positive energy balance in children, findings from food intake surveys indicate that children and adolescents are consuming about the same or slightly fewer calories than in previous decades (21–23), or as recommended (24). These findings are inconsistent with the increasing prevalence of overweight among youth.

Because dietary fat is a concentrated source of energy, supplying more than twice the number of calories as either carbohydrate or protein, excess intake of this nutrient may contribute to childhood overweight. However, the rise in overweight among youth has not been accompanied by an

Both genetic and environmental factors contribute to overweight. Sedentary behavior, at home and at school, is a key factor contributing to the recent rise in overweight among the nation's youth.

increase in the percent of calories from dietary fat. On the contrary, total fat intake among children has decreased from about 38% of total calories in the 1960s to 34% in 1988–91 (21,25,26).

Contribution of a Sedentary Lifestyle to Overweight in Youth.

Although a potential role for diet in the etiology of obesity cannot be ignored, researchers primarily attribute the current rise in childhood overweight to physical inactivity or a sedentary lifestyle (16,27,28).

Findings from national studies indicate that many youth are leading sedentary lifestyles (4,5,29,30). Fewer students are participating in regular physical education classes, more schools are having problems providing adequate physical education classes, playgrounds, and after-school sports programs because of financial constraints, and many students who do attend physical education classes spend most of their time being inactive (4,31). Nationwide, only approximately one-half of all high school students are enrolled in physical education classes (5).

Both inside and outside of school, opportunities for children to be physically active have declined. Safety concerns, parents' work habits, the increased availability of video and computer games, and television viewing have all contributed to children's sedentary behavior (32). As children grow older, girls become less active than boys, and children of both gender become less physically active as they go through adolescence (30).

Television viewing is a major contributor to youth's sedentary lifestyle and risk of overweight (9,33–36). A recent study of 746 youths aged 10 to 15 years found that those who watched more than 5 hours of television a day were 4.6 times more likely to be overweight than youth who watched zero to 2 hours of television a day (9). Researchers contend that children spend more time watching television than they spend in school (9). Television viewing may contribute to overweight in youth by both taking time away from physical activities, thereby reducing daily energy expenditure, and increasing energy intake. Because television viewing time potentially affects the prevalence of overweight among children, the American Academy of Pediatrics (36) recommends that children spend no more than 1 to 2 hours a day watching television.

PROMOTING HEALTHFUL EATING HABITS AND PHYSICAL ACTIVITY PATTERNS FOR CHILDREN

Stemming the rising tide of overweight among American youth requires a concerted effort by parents, schools, the community, the media, health care professionals, and public policy makers (37a). To prevent overweight and promote normal growth and development, children must be provided with an environment conducive to healthful lifestyles. While it is important that children adopt healthful lifestyles, it is even more important that such lifestyles be maintained throughout life (37b,38).

Healthful Eating Habits.

Regardless of their weight, all children should be encouraged to consume sufficient food to achieve appropriate growth and development (1). To prevent or treat overweight, health professionals advise children to consume foods from all the major food groups and be physically active (1). For overweight children, dietary treatment is complicated by possible interference with growth (1,7). Although overconsumption of energy and fat can increase a child's risk of overweight, restrictive dieting is discouraged (16,37b). Extremely low fat diets may jeopardize children's nutritional status and adversely affect their growth (37a). Dieting and an obsession with food and weight also may predispose children to developing eating disorders such as anorexia nervosa and bulimia nervosa (16,37a). Approximately 40% of children, especially girls, are trying to lose weight (39).

Children's energy needs vary as a result of their physical growth, stage of development, physical activity, and metabolic rate (24). Therefore, regular monitoring of children's growth by a health professional is needed to determine whether energy

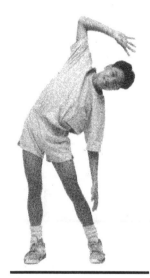

Parents, other care providers, schools, and the community need to work together to create an environment in which children and adolescents can adopt healthful eating and physical activity habits.

intake is sufficient to maintain weight or reduce the rate of weight gain (16).

To prevent or treat overweight, the focus should be on normalizing children's eating behavior by emphasizing healthful food selections, not dieting. Recognizing the unique challenges of preventing and treating overweight in children, the American Institute of Nutrition Steering Committee on Healthy Weights recommends that separate guidelines for "healthy weights" be developed for children and adolescents (40).

Children's major sources of nutrition and health information are parents and schools, according to a recent survey of over 400 children between the ages of 9 and 15 years (3). Parents and other care providers can help children adopt healthful diets by being positive role models by consuming healthful diets themselves; by making healthful food choices including snacks readily available to children; by involving children in the selection of foods and preparation of meals; by encouraging a "play" approach to eating which enables children to learn to make choices and assume responsibility for their choices (38); and by avoiding making weight and food an issue.

Parents/care providers also should encourage children not to skip meals such as breakfast and to make healthful food choices when eating out. Consuming breakfast helps children establish a regular eating pattern, meet their nutrient needs, control body weight, regulate appetite, and discourage snacking or overeating. In addition, consuming a healthful breakfast can help children perform better in school by increasing their problem-solving ability, memory, verbal fluency, and creativity (41).

Because 6- to 11-year old and 12- to 19-year old children obtain 25% and 33%, respectively, of their total calories away from home (42), encouraging children to choose a healthful diet at fast food restaurants and school cafeterias is just as important as at home. Schools are an important site for the development of healthful habits through classroom activities, school lunch/breakfast programs,

and physical education classes. Schools are currently offering more healthful food choices to comply with recent regulations updating the nutrition standards for federally reimbursable school meals (43).

Achieving normal growth and development and a healthy weight is the primary goal for all children. For children who participate in organized/competitive sports, it is especially important that they consume sufficient energy and nutrients to support their growth and development, as well as meet the increased energy needs imposed by the sport (44–47).

Children and adolescents involved in organized sports should be discouraged from following unhealthful nutrition practices such as rapid weight loss methods (e.g.,fasting), fluid restriction, and misuse of dietary supplements (44,45, 48). Health professionals and parents should promote the key messages of variety, moderation, and balance in food choices to all children (49).

Physical Activity. Although children view physical activity as fun and enjoyable, many children are not physically active (3,8). Experts encourage all children to engage in 30 minutes or more of moderate intensity physical activities (such as brisk walking or running) on most and preferably all days (1,30). Regardless of the type of activity chosen, it should be performed regularly and at a level of exertion sufficient to increase the metabolic rate about fivefold for a total of 30 minutes (30). Time spent on the activity can be continuous or in 10 minute segments provided that these segments total 30 minutes or more each day.

The health benefits associated with a physically active lifestyle in children include a reduction in body fat, weight control, lower blood pressure, and favorable blood lipid levels (37b,50–52). Increasing physical activity allows children to use more calories and have more food choices. Several studies indicate that regular, moderate, weight-bearing activity during childhood increases peak bone mass, an important determinant of

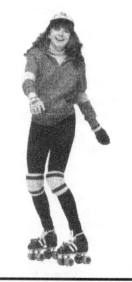

Appealing to children's zest for play and fun can help them choose a healthful diet and be physically active.

osteoporosis (53–58). Although exercise benefits bones, it cannot compensate for the adverse effects of a low calcium intake. Consuming an adequate intake of calcium during childhood—800 to 1,000 mg/day (equivalent to 3 to 4 servings of milk or other dairy foods)—is not only critical to bone formation, but also helps to protect bones against osteoporosis in later years (59).

In addition to its numerous health benefits, exercise provides children with opportunities for fun, social interaction, and skill development, which in turn can increase self-esteem and confidence (47). Regular physical activity may even improve children's cognitive function and academic performance (60).

The observed health benefits of regular physical activity are temporary, lasting only as long as the activity is maintained (37a). One of the most important benefits of physical activity during childhood may be its potential to persist throughout adult life (37c). Some evidence indicates that physical activity tracks during childhood and early adulthood (61–63).

Parents/care providers can play a key role in encouraging children to be physically active by:

- Being a positive role model and making physical activity a part of everyday life by instituting family-based recreational activities.
- Limiting television viewing to no more than 1 to 2 hours a day, as recommended by the American Academy of Pediatrics (36), and promoting active play as a substitute for television, computer, and video activities.
- Providing children with a safe, supportive environment to play actively (1).
- Lobbying schools for physical education and after-school programs that promote fitness.
- Making physical activity fun (38) thereby appealing to children's primary reason for being physically active (3).
- Encouraging physical activities that are appropriate to the age-specific abilities and interests of the child (37c).

Schools should support children's physical activity (30). They can provide opportunities for children to be physically active that are not limited to competitive sports; that appeal to girls as well as boys and to children from diverse backgrounds; that can serve as a foundation for lifelong activities; and that are offered daily (30).

Success in developing a lifelong healthy lifestyle depends on introducing children to good nutrition and physical activities that they enjoy. Reducing children's access to sedentary behaviors and encouraging everyday physical activities such as walking, climbing stairs, and active play, instead of a regimented exercise program, can lead to more sustainable weight control and, potentially, a lifelong healthy lifestyle (64).

REFERENCES

1. U.S. Department of Agriculture and U.S. Department of Health and Human Services. *Nutrition and Your Health: Dietary Guidelines for Americans*. 4th edition. Home and Garden Bulletin No. 232. Washington, DC: U.S. Government Printing Office, December 1995.

2. U.S. Public Health Service. *Healthy People 2000. National Health Promotion and Disease Prevention Objectives: Full Report with Commentary*. PHS 91-50212. Washington, DC: USDHHS, 1991.

3. The American Dietetic Association National Center for Nutrition and Dietetics, International Food Information Council, and the President's Council on Physical Fitness and Sports. *Food, Physical Activity, & Fun. What Kids Think*. Chicago, IL: The American Dietetic Association, January 1995.

4. U.S. Department of Health and Human Services, Public Health Service. *Healthy People 2000. Midcourse Review and 1995 Revisions*. Hyattsville, MD: National Center for Health Statistics, 1995.

5. Kann, L., C.W. Warren, W.A. Harris, et. al. MMWR *44*: SS-1, 1995.

6. Brownell, K.D., and C.G. Fairburn (Eds). *Eating Disorders and Obesity. A Comprehensive Handbook*. New York: The Guilford Press, 1995, a) Dietz, p.438; b) Bouchard, p.21.

7. Troiano, R.P., K.M. Flegal, R.J. Kuczmarski, et. al. Arch. Pediatr. Adolesc. Med. *149*: 1085, 1995.

8. Borra, S.T., N.E. Schwartz, C.G. Spain, et. al. J. Am. Diet. Assoc. *95*: 816, 1995.

9. Gortmaker, S.L., A. Must, A.M. Sobol, et. al. Arch. Pediatr. Adolesc. Med. *150*: 356, 1996.

10. Centers for Disease Control and Prevention. MMWR *43*: 818, 1994.

11. Gortmaker, S.L., A. Must, J.M. Perrin, et. al. N. Engl. J. Med. *329*: 1008, 1993.

12. Caprio, S., L.D. Hyman, S. McCarthy, et. al. Am. J. Clin. Nutr. *64*: 12, 1996.

13. Serdula, M.K., D. Ivery, R.J. Coates, et. al. Prev. Med. *22*: 167, 1993.

14. Clark, W.R., and R.M. Lauer. Crit. Rev. Food Sci. & Nutr. *33(4/5)*: 423, 1993.

15. Guo, S.S., A.F. Roche, W.C. Chumlea, et. al. Am. J. Clin. Nutr. *59*: 810, 1994.

16. Schlicker, S.A., S.T. Borra, and C. Regan. Nutr. Rev. *52(1)*: 11, 1994.

17. Bouchard, C. Nutr. Rev. *54(4)*: S125, 1996.

18. Roberts, S.B., and A.S. Greenberg. Nutr. Rev. *54(2)*: 41, 1996.

19. Crockett, S.J., and L.S. Sims. J. Nutr. Educ. *27(5)*: 235, 1995.

20. Manchester, A., and A. Clauson. Food Review *18(2)*: 12, 1995.

21. McDowell, M.A., R.R. Briefel, K. Alaimo, et. al. Energy and macronutrient intakes of persons ages 2 months and over in the United States: Third National Health and Nutrition Examination Survey, Phase 1, 1988–91. Advance Data From Vital and Health Statistics, No. 255. Hyattsville, MD: National Center for Health Statistics, 1994.

22. Federation of American Societies for Experimental Biology, Life Sciences Research Office. Prepared for the Interagency Board for Nutrition Monitoring and Related Research. *Third Report on Nutrition Monitoring in the United States: Executive Summary*. Washington, DC: U.S. Government Printing Office, 1995.

23. Riddick, H. Family Economics and Nutrition Review *9(3)*: 21, 1996.

24. Food and Nutrition Board, Commission on Life Sciences, National Research Council. *Recommended Dietary Allowances, 10th ed.* Washington, DC: National Academy Press, 1989.

25. Nicklas, T.A. J. Am. Diet. Assoc. *95*: 1127, 1995.

26. McPherson, R.S., D.H. Montgomery, and M.Z. Nichaman. J. Nutr. Educ. *27(5)*: 225, 1995.

27. Moore, L.L., U.-S.D.T. Nguyen, K.J. Rothman, et. al. Am. J. Epidemiol. *142*: 982, 1995.

28. Davies, P.S.W., J. Gregory, and A. White. Int. J. Obesity *19*: 6, 1995.

29. Heath, G.W., M. Pratt, C.W. Warren, et. al. Arch. Pediatr. Adolesc. Med. *148*: 1131, 1994.

30. National Institutes of Health Consensus Development Conference Statement. *Physical Activity and Cardiovascular Health*. December 18–20, 1995.

31. American Medical Association. *Healthy Youth 2000. A Mid-Decade Review*. Chicago, IL: American Medical Association, Department of Adolescent Health, 1995.

32. Gutin, B., and T.M. Manos. Ann. N.Y. Acad. Sci. *699*: 115, 1993.

33. Dietz, W.H., and S.L. Gortmaker. Pediatrics *75*: 807, 1985.

34. Klesges, R.C., M.L. Shelton, and L.M. Klesges. Pediatrics *91*: 281, 1993.

35. Kotz, K., and M. Story. J. Am. Diet. Assoc. *94*: 1296, 1994.

36. American Academy of Pediatrics, Committee on Communications. Pediatrics *96*: 786, 1995.

37. Cheung, L.W.Y., and J.B. Richmond. *Child Health, Nutrition, and Physical Activity*. Champaign, IL: Human Kinetics, 1995, a) Cheung, p.301; b) Bar-Or & Malina, p.79; c) Pate, p.139.

38. Rickard, K.A., D.L. Gallahue, G.E. Gruen, et. al. J. Am. Diet. Assoc. *95*: 1121, 1995.

39. Schreiber, G.B., M. Robins, R. Striegel-Moore, et. al. Pediatrics *98*: 63, 1996.

40. Report of the American Institute of Nutrition (AIN) Steering Committee on Healthy Weight. J. Nutr. *124*: 2240, 1994.

41. Pollitt, E. J. Am. Diet. Assoc. *95*: 1134, 1995.

42. Anonymous. Nutr. Rev. *54(5)*: 159, 1996.

43. U.S. Department of Agriculture, Food and Consumer Service. Fed. Regist. *60(113)*: 31188, 1995.

44. The American Dietetic Association. J. Am. Diet. Assoc. *96*: 610, 1996.

45. The American Dietetic Association. J. Am. Diet. Assoc. *96*: 611, 1996.

46. Jennings, D.S., S.N. Steen, and The American Dietetic Association. *Play Hard Eat Right*. Minneapolis, MN: Chronimed Publ., 1995.

47. Steen, S.N. Sports Med. *17(3)*: 152, 1994.

48. American Academy of Pediatrics, Committee on Sports Medicine & Fitness. Pediatrics *97(5)*: 752, 1996.

49. The American Dietetic Association. J. Am. Diet. Assoc. *95*: 370, 1995.

50. Obarzanek, E., G.B. Schreiber, P.B. Crawford, et. al. Am. J. Clin. Nutr. *60*: 15, 1994.

51. Klesges, R.C., L.M. Klesges, L.H. Eck, et. al. Pediatrics *95*: 126, 1995.

52. Shea, S., C.E. Basch, B. Gutin, et. al. Pediatrics *94*: 465, 1994.

53. Slemenda, C.W., J.Z. Miller, S.L. Hui, et. al. J. Bone Miner. Res. *6(11)*: 1227, 1991.

54. Grimston, S.K., N.D. Willows, and D.A. Hanley. Med. Sci. Sports Exerc. *25(11)*: 1203, 1993.

55. Matkovic, V., T. Jelic, G.M. Wardlaw, et. al. J. Clin. Invest. *93*: 799, 1994.

56. Cooper, C., M. Cawley, A. Bhalla, et. al. J. Bone Miner. Res. *10(6)*: 940, 1995.

57. Teegarden, D., W. Proulx, M. Kern, et. al. Med. Sci. Sports Exerc. *28(1)*: 105, 1996.

58. Vuori, I. Nutr. Rev. *54(4)*: S11, 1996.

59. Optimal Calcium Intake. NIH Consensus Statement June 6–8; *12(4)*: 1–31, 1994.

60. Shephard, R.J. Nutr. Rev. *54(4)*: S32, 1996.

61. Kelder, S.H., C.L. Perry, K.I. Klepp, et. al. Am. J. Public Health *84*: 1121, 1994.

62. Raitakari, O.T., K.V.K. Porkka, S. Taimela, et. al. Am. J. Epidemiol. *140(3)*: 195, 1994.

63. Pate, R.R., T. Baranowski, M. Dowda, et. al. Med. Sci. Sports Exerc. *28(1)*: 92, 1996.

64. Epstein, L.H., K.J. Coleman, and M.D. Myers. Med. Sci. Sports Exerc. *28(4)*: 428, 1996.

Dysfunctional eating: A new concept

by Frances M. Berg, MS

Children are growing up with twisted attitudes toward food, eating and weight because of our cultural fear of fat. They are turning away from normal eating and mealtimes with family to restrained and chaotic eating. Dieting and restricting food often starts as early as age 9, and by age 11 is so common that some researchers have called it the norm.

If abnormal eating is becoming so prevalent, we need to know more about it. What is abnormal, restrictive eating? What are its effects? How can it be measured, and should it be prevented?

Dysfunctional eating is a new, inclusive term to describe the kinds of abnormal, inappropriate eating which are becoming widely prevalent in the developed world, especially among girls and women. It is a disruption of normal eating and, too often, starvation in the midst of plenty.

What is dysfunctional eating?

Dysfunctional eating is eating which is separated or disjoined from its normal function and normal internal controls.

Normal eating nourishes the body for health, energy and strength, enhancing feelings of well-being, and results in "feeling good." Dysfunctional eating is often focused on eating for thinness, body shaping, or using food for comfort or emotional reasons.

Normal eating is controlled by an internal system that regulates the balance of energy intake with expenditure, through hunger, appetite and satiety signals, so that a person eats when hungry and stops when full and satisfied. Normal eating is flexible and includes eating for pleasure and social reasons. In normal eating a person usually follows regular habits, such as eating three meals and snacks to satisfy hunger.

Dysfunctional eating exists on a continuum between normal eating and eating disorders. It may be of mild, moderate or severe intensity. Individuals may move back and forth across the continuum, returning to normal eating after unsuccessful bouts of dieting, or restricting food so severely they develop debilitating eating disorders from which they cannot recover alone.

Dysfunctional eating includes variations of chaotic eating and chronic dieting as well as both persistent undereating and overeating. There are at least three general patterns: irregular or chaotic eating, consistent undereating, and consistent overeating of much more than the body wants or needs, eating past satiety.

Dysfunctional eating encompasses restrained eating, disordered eating and chronic dieting syndrome. It is also being called disturbed, disruptive, abnormal and emotional eating. The broader focus has the advantage of providing a coherent framework for concerns which have been nebulous and incompletely defined.

Reprinted with permission from *Healthy Weight Journal* (formerly *Obesity & Health*), September/October 1996, pp. 88-92, 99. © 1996 by Healthy Weight Journal, Research, News and Commentary Across the Weight Spectrum, 402 South 14th Street, Hettingger, ND 58639.

In contrast to normal eating, dysfunctional eating most often serves functions other than nourishment, such as to shape the body, improve body image, to seek comfort or pleasure, to numb pain or unhappy memory, or to relieve stress, anxiety, anger, loneliness or boredom.

Dysfunctional eating is regulated by inappropriate external and internal controls, such as "will power," a planned diet, calories or fat grams, or sensory or emotional cues.

Though often the internal function is to relieve stress, it does not do this well. Instead of relieving pain, eating often makes the situation worse, or relief may be fleeting, followed by remorse. It is common to feel guilty, ashamed, uncomfortably full, to regret or berate oneself for having eating or, if unsatisfied, to feel ravenously hungry and fear or anticipate an onrushing eating binge.

Studies suggest that dysfunctional eating is prevalent among girls and women. It appears to be increasing and striking at younger ages as cultural pressures to be thin continue to increase. It may include at times as many as the 50 to 80 percent of girls and women in the U.S., age 11 and up, who report they are trying to lose weight. Increasingly, it includes teenage boys and men, who are re-

---

A definition

Dysfunctional eating is eating that is separated or disjoined from its normal function and normal regulation.

Normal eating nourishes the body for health, energy and strength, enhancing feelings of well-being, and is regulated by hunger, appetite and satiety. Dysfunctional eating is often focused on eating for thinness, body shaping, or using food to comfort, numb pain, relieve stress, anxiety, anger or loneliness. It is regulated by inappropriate external and internal controls such as "will power," planned diets, or sensory and emotional cues.

Dysfunctional eating includes irregular or chaotic eating, consistent undereating, and consistent overeating of more than the body wants or needs. It exists on a continuum between normal eating and eating disorders, and may be of mild, moderate or severe intensity.

---

sponding to new advertising pressures to reshape their bodies.

Dysfunctional eating is unlikely for infants, small children and others who don't diet or have not learned to interfere with the normal eating process.

Undereating and overeating

The consistent undereating pattern may have the purpose of shaping the body, or may be because of depression, alcoholism, or other mental or physical factors.

Consistent overeating, which is eating more than the body wants or needs, eating past satiety, is less understood and scarcely researched. Prevalence is unknown.

Overeating patterns may develop for emotional reasons, or from family or peer group habits of eating large amounts of food, or eating more because abundant, good tasting foods are readily available.

In the U.S. today, studies suggest that overeating is being encouraged. People are eating out more, and they favor fast food chains and restaurants where they perceive they are getting more for their money. In response, studies show restaurants are offering larger servings and larger meals.

Body size is not to be taken as an indicator of dysfunctional eating. It cannot be assumed that large persons are eating abnormally, or past the point of satiety. Persons of any size may be eating normally, or they may have eating disorders or dysfunctional eating patterns.

Conditions such as Prader-Willi syndrome, which involves a disruption of hunger, appetite and satiety regulation, may or may not fit into this category.

Physical effects

The person with dysfunctional eating may often feel tired and lacking in energy, especially when undernourished. There is risk of stunted growth and reduced brain development in children and teens. Bone development may be decreased for youth; for women increased bone demineralization may occur, leading to bone fractures. Puberty may be delayed and sexual interest decreased.

Dysfunctional eating affects weight, yet in its various forms it is associated with a wide range of weights as genetic potential interacts with environmental lifestyle factors. Associated with chaotic eating and dieting, weight often cycles up and down in "yo-yo" fashion. Consistent undereating can be expected to result in a weight lower than normal for that person. Overeating will likely result in a higher weight than might be normal for that individual, perhaps increasing year by year.

Mental focus

One of the most dramatic effects of dysfunctional eating may be its impact on the thinking process.

As dysfunctional eating becomes more severe, the individual often loses mental focus, mental alertness and the ability to concentrate. Her interests may narrow, turning inward, and she loses ambition. As interest in food heightens the individual tends to lose interest in school work, career, family and friends, and pulls back from social activities.

This increase in food preoccupation is clear in the wartime Minnesota Human Starvation study, and more recently has been researched by Dan Reiff, MPH, RD, and Kim Lampson Reiff, PhD, of Mercer Island, Wash.[4]

Dysfunctional eating: a description

Contrasted and compared with normal eating and eating disorders

	Normal eating	Dysfunctional eating *mild* · *moderate* · *severe*	Eating disorders
Eating pattern	Regular eating habits and patterns. Typical pattern in U.S. is to eat three regular meals and snacks to satisfy hunger.	Irregular, chaotic eating — often overeat or undereat, skip meals, fast, binge, diet. Or usual pattern is of overeating or undereating much more or much less than body wants or needs.	Patterns typical of anorexia nervosa, bulimia nervosa, binge eating disorder, other eating disorders.
Function, purpose of eating	Eat for nourishment, health, energy. Also for pleasure and social reasons. Eating enhances feelings of well-being, makes one "feel good."	Eating often for reasons other than nourishment: to shape body, improve body image, seek comfort or pleasure, numb pain, relieve stress, anxiety, anger, loneliness or boredom. May feel uncomfortable after eating, or have feelings of remorse, guilt, shame.	Eating almost entirely for purposes other than nourishment or energy, as for body shaping, to numb pain, relieve stress.
Use of hunger, appetite and satiety to regulate eating	Eating regulated by internal signals of hunger, appetite and satiety. Eat when hungry, stop when full and satisfied; usually hungry at mealtime.	Eating often separated from normal controls of hunger, appetite and satiety. May be regulated by "will power," a planned diet, calories or fat grams, emotional or sensory cues, such as sight or smell of food.	Eating regulated predominantly by external and internal controls other than hunger and satiety.
Prevalence	Infants, small children, persons who don't diet or interfere with normal eating. At this time, higher rates among males, fewer among females.	Chaotic eating and undereating affect many girls and women in U.S., perhaps at times as many as the 50 to 80 percent age 11 and over who say they are trying to lose weight; also increasing numbers of boys and men. Consistent overeating may occur for both genders.	Estimated prevalence is 10% of high school and college students; 90-95% female, 5-10% male.

Reprinted from *Children and Teens in Weight Crisis*, by Frances M. Berg. Copyright 1996. All rights reserved. Publisher's written permission required for reproduction. Published by Healthy Weight Journal, 402 South 14th Street, Hettinger, ND 58639 (701-567-2646; Fax 701-567-2602).

Dysfunctional eating: effects and relationships

	Normal eating	Dysfunctional eating mild · moderate · severe	Eating disorders
Physical	Promotes health, energy, strength, and the healthy growth and development of children and youth. WEIGHT: Normal weight for the individual, expressing genetic and environmental factors. Any weight within wide range; usually stable.	May typically feel tired, apathetic, lacking in energy, chilled. Increased risk of stunted growth and reduced brain development with undernutrition. Decreased bone development or bone demineralization and higher risk of fractures. Delayed puberty, decrease in sexual interest. WEIGHT: Any weight within wide range depending on genetic potential. Eating pattern may cause weight to decrease, cycle up and down, remain stable, or increase.	Physical effects may be severe. Mortality reportedly as high as 18% for anorexia nervosa and bulimia nervosa. WEIGHT: Any weight within wide range, depending on genetic potential and the disorder and its expression.
Mental focus	Promotes clear thinking ability to concentrate. FOOD THOUGHTS: low key, usually at mealtime. For women, 10-15% of time awake may be spent thinking of food, hunger, weight.	Risk of decreased mental alertness and ability to concentrate, narrowing of interests, loss of ambition, and a turning inward. FOOD THOUGHTS: Increased preoccupation with food. Thoughts often focused on eating, weight, planning when and what to eat, counting calories or fat grams. Thoughts of food, hunger, weight may occupy 20-65% of time.	Diminished capacity to think, memory loss, extreme narrowing of interests. FOOD THOUGHTS: Thoughts focused most of time on food, hunger, weight. For untreated anorexia about 90-110%, bulimia 70-90% of time awake (extra 10% includes dreaming).
Emotional	Promotes mood stability.	Potentially greater mood instability — highs and lows. May be easily upset, irritable, anxious, have lowered self-esteem. Increasing preoccupation and concern with body image. Increased risk of eating disorders.	Greater risk of mood instability and functional depression.
Social	Social integration; promotes healthy relationships with family, peers and community.	Less social integration, more risk of feeling isolated, self-absorbed and self-focused, stigmatized, disconnected from society, lonely. May have less interest in values of generosity, sharing, volunteer activities; less sense of community.	Social withdrawal, isolated from family and friends, avoidance of and by peers, alienation, often eating alone; worsening family relations.

In their book, *Eating Disorders: Nutrition Therapy in the Recovery Process*, the Reiffs provide a food preoccupation scale. Individuals are asked to indicate total conscious time spent thinking about food, weight and hunger at three times in their lives: currently, at its highest, and at its lowest, and to give their age and weight for each. This includes time spent in shopping, preparing food, eating, thinking about eating or food cravings, purging, weighing, reading diet books, suppressing feelings of hunger, using strategies such as smoking or chewing gum to distract from hunger, and thinking about or discussing weight.

The researchers tested more than 500 eating disordered patients on this scale. They found that for untreated anorexia nervosa patients, 90 to 110 percent of waking time is spent thinking about food, weight and hunger. The extra 10 percent comes from dreams of food or weight, or having their sleep disturbed by hunger. Bulimic patients report about 70 to 90 percent.

From the testing he has done, Dan Reiff suggests that for women with normal eating, who are buying and preparing food for the family, the amount of time spent thinking about food, weight and hunger may be about 10 to 15 percent of waking time. In dysfunctional eating, this may occupy about 20 to 65 percent of waking hours, he reports.

In his studies, preoccupation with food is directly related to body weight and the degree and duration of semi-starvation. In the Minnesota study, it appeared to be most closely related to the drop in body weight, as the men consumed a fairly adequate diet of 1,500 to 1,700 calories for six months, but lost one-fourth of their weight.

Dysfunctional eating can have severe physical and emotional effects. The individual may become moody, easily upset, irritable, anxious, apathetic and increasingly concerned about body image. She is often self-absorbed and self-focused. Self-esteem may be low, or focused on appearance.

The girl with dysfunctional eating may isolate herself socially, feeling lonely, alienated, and disconnected from society. She may focus less than others on the values of generosity, sharing, caring, and participate less in volunteer and community activities.

Eating disorder risk

A major concern with the current high prevalence of dysfunctional eating is whether it will increase eating disorders.

A recent review reports that several one- and two-year longitudinal studies find that up to 35 percent of normal dieters progress to pathological dieting, and of pathological dieters, 20 to 25 percent progress to partial or full syndrome disorders. The report also says that 15 to 45 percent of those with partial syndrome progress to full syndrome eating disorders within one to four years.[5]

Survival traits

Can some of these effects and relationships be explained as natural survival traits?

Early humans must have frequently feasted weeks on the carcass of a mammoth or beached whale, followed by a famine of seven months or seven years.

In deprivation, their bodies would have shut down to conserve fuel, not just with slowed heart rate and metabolism, but in every activity. Growth stopped or was severely stunted. Nearly all fat consumed was routed to storage to replace what was lost, instead of being used normally. Sexual activity and fertility shut down; as starvation progressed it was more critical to care for the young than to procreate. Ultimately, even children were abandoned, as Colin Turnbull reports so vividly in "The Mountain People."

At the same time, starvation causes high stress.

There is no peace for starving people. They crave food and focus all attention on this need. A useful survival trait, this kept our ancestors out hunting food despite weakness or danger, instead of lying listless in the cave, awaiting death. Without this complex internal regulation, the human race could hardly have survived.

But this ancient legacy haunts the dysfunctional eater today.

Research needed

The adverse factors associated with dysfunctional eating and its high prevalence make further study imperative. Much research is needed in these areas.

How can we identify and measure the various patterns of dysfunctional eating? What causes the related adverse effects: is it abnormal eating habits, insufficient calories, iron or other nutrient deficiencies, weight loss, depleted fat cells, or psychological factors?

If dysfunctional eating is unhealthy, how can it be prevented? And how can normal eating be restored for children and adult women?

Normal eating itself needs study. What is normal eating and does it have its own range of patterns? How can it be measured?

A note of caution: The case made here for normal eating is not meant to imply that nutrition is the primary factor in good mental and physical health, but rather, that each person has a baseline of adequate nutrition, and perhaps an upper level, as well, and when this is disrupted there may be severe disruption of normal life and a diminishing of the mind, body and spirit.

Only when food supply is stable can people eat and live normally, as we interpret this today. With adequate nutrition and regular eating habits, they are able to focus on developing their full potential through a wide range of interests. They can afford the luxury of being generous, sharing, caring, and reaching out to others.

Research basis

The concepts of dysfunctional eating presented here are based on the insights and research of numerous leaders in obesity, eating disorders and size acceptance fields. Among the important resources are: the early work on restrained eating by Janet Polivy and Peter Herman[6]; writings by Susan Wooley[7]; the work of Ellyn Satter on normal eating and "dieting casualties"[8]; Linda Omichinski's nondiet leadership and program development[9]; work on food preoccupation by Dan and Kim Reiff; starvation studies, including the Minnesota Experiment[10], United Nations reports on world malnutrition[11], and Colin Turnbull's description of starvation pressures on the African Ik tribe in "The Mountain People"[12]; national and local studies showing the high prevalence of dieting and disordered eating among children and adolescents[13]; research revealing the mental and physical effects of eating disorders, and their association with dieting[14]; writings on dieting risks and need to treat chronic dieting syndrome[15]; and the No Diet Day movement, led by Mary Evans Young,[16] and Eating Disorder Awareness Week, sponsored by eating disorder organizations.[17]

Most of this information has been reviewed in *Healthy Weight Journal* over the past 11 years, and is discussed extensively and referenced in the journal's special report "Health Risks of Weight Loss."

REFERENCES:

Berg F. Health Risks of Weight Loss, 1995. Chapter 1. General treatment risks, 14-26; Ch 7. Eating disorders, 56-62; Ch 8. Psychological risks, 63-69; Ch 9. Weight cycling, 70-79; Ch 11. Thinness: a cultural obsession, 89-99; Ch 13. To treat or not to treat, 108-113.

1. Niven C, D Carroll. The Health psychology of women. Harwood Academic Publ., Chur, Switzerland. 1993:115.

2. JADA 1992;92;92:7:851-53; Healthy Weight J/O&H 1993;7:3:46.

3. Third report on nutrition monitoring in the US, Life Sciences Research Office, Dec 1995. Interagency Board for Nutrition Monitoring and Related Research, US Gov Printing Office.

4. Reiff D, KK Lampson Reiff, Eating Disorders: Nutrition Therapy in the Recovery Process, 1992. Aspen, Gaithersburg, MD; Personal communication with Dan Reiff, 1996.

5. Estes L, M Crago, C Shisslak. Eating disorders prevention. The Renfrew Perspective, 1996;2:1:3-5.

6. Herman P, J Polivy. Eating and its disorders, edit Stunkard and Steller, 1984, 141-56. Raven Press; Healthy Weight J Mar/Apr 1996;10:2:32-33.

7. Wooley S, W Wooley. Eating and its disorders, edit Stunkard and Steller, 1984. Raven Press.

8. Satter, Ellyn. How to get your kids to eat — but not too much, Bull Publ, Palo Alto, CA; Workshops, "Treating the dieting casualty," Satter Assoc., Madison, WI.

9. Omichinski L. You Count, Calories Don't, 1992; HUGS facilitator programs, HUGS International, Box 102A, Rt3, Portage la Prairie, Manitoba, R1N 3A3, Canada; Teens & Diets — No Weigh, Healthy Weight J 1996;10:3:49-52; Berg F. Nondiet movement gains strength HWJ/Obesity & Health Sep/Oct 1992;6:5:82-90.

10. Keys A, et al. Biology of human starvation, 1950. U of Minn Press, Minneapolis, MN; Berg F, Starvation stages in weight loss patients similar to famine victims, HWJ/Obesity & Health Apr 1989;3:4:27-30.

11. Berg F. World starvation: weight may be best tool to measure malnutrition, Healthy Weight J May/Jun 1995;9:3:47-49; Body Mass Index: FAO, A measure of chronic energy deficiency in adults, 1994, United Nations report.

12. Turnbull, Colin. The Mountain People, 1972. Simon and Schuster, NY.

13. CDC USHHS, Behavioral Risk Survey; Calorie Control Council, 1991 National Survey; Berg F. Who is dieting in the U.S. Healthy Weight J/Obesity & Health 1992;6:3:48-49; Dieting and purging behavior in black and white high school students, JADA 1992;92:3:306-312; Adolescents dieting; JAMA 1991;266:2811-2812; Berg F. Harmful weight loss practices among adolescents, HWJ/O&H Jul/Aug 1992;6:4:69-72.

14. Fallon P, Katzman M, Wooley S. Feminist perspectives on eating disorders 1994, Guilford Press, NY; Baker D, R Sansone, Overview of eating disorders, 1994:1-10, NEDO; Kaplan A, P Garfinkel. Medical issues and the eating disorders, 1993, Brunner/Mazel, NY; Berg F. Eating disorders: physical and mental effects, Healthy Weight J Mar/Apr 1995;9:2:27-30; Smolak L, M Levine. Toward an empirical basis for primary prevention of eating problems with elementary school children, Eat Disorders 1994;2:4:293-307

15. Andersen A. The last word, Eating Disorders 1994;2:1:81-82; Bowers M. The last word. Eating Disorders 1994;2:4:375-377.

16. Young, Mary Evans. Diet Breaking, 1996, Hodder & Stoughton, London.

17. Biely J. Eating Disorder Awareness Week '96, EDAP Matters Winter 1996;2.

REDUCED-FAT FOODS: DIETER'S DREAM OR MARKETER'S PLOY?

Reduced-fat foods do have a place in a low-fat diet. But they're not a magic wand for weight loss.

'Total indulgence, zero guilt," Weight Watchers claimed in ads for its reduced-fat desserts. That's typical of what marketers would like you to believe about low- or no-fat foods. While such foods can help you reduce the fat in your diet, they will not necessarily help you lose weight and, under certain circumstances, they may even lead to weight gain.

The skinny on fat

Fat imparts a variety of tastes, textures, and aromas to food. It makes steak flavorful and tender, piecrust flaky, and ice cream creamy. In addition, most fatty foods are high in calories, so the body digests them more slowly than leaner foods, with their typically lower calorie content. That's why you feel full longer after eating a well-marbled steak than a lean piece of fish. And the taste of fatty foods lingers in the mouth, since the chemicals in fat that provide flavor emerge gradually as you chew.

The most widely used fat replacers are carbohydrates, which show up on food labels as dextrins, maltodextrins, modified food starches, polydextrose, cellulose, and various gums. These add bulk to replace the lost fat, hold up to 100 times their weight in water to provide moistness, and thicken the ingredients, making them creamier. Fat can also be replaced by protein. Microparticulated protein, for example, is made by heating and blending proteins to create tiny round particles that slip and slide over the tongue to simulate the feel of fat.

Neither carbohydrates nor proteins capture the elusive flavor and texture of fat. Carbohydrates, for example, keep baked goods moist, but not necessarily light or flaky. And neither carbohydrates nor protein can be used for cooking methods that require high temperatures, such as frying.

Where reduced-fat foods fall short

Eating less fat is clearly a good idea. Studies have linked dietary fat with an increased risk of numerous health problems, including obesity, coronary heart disease, and certain cancers. And cutting fat intake, even without cutting calories, does seem to help people lose weight, apparently because the body creates stored fat much more readily from dietary fat than from dietary protein or carbohydrates.

But calories still count. Recent research has confirmed that people who cut calories as well as fat lose more weight and body fat than those who cut fat alone. While foods that are naturally low in fat tend to be low in calories, the same is not true of many foods manufactured to be low in fat. *Fat-Free Fig Newtons*, for example, have almost as many calories as regular *Fig Newtons*, in part because the no-fat cookies contain more sugar. Strawberry *Light-N-Lively Free Yogurt* has no fat, but it contains 63 percent more sugar—and 9 percent more calories—than *Stonyfield Farm's* full-fat strawberry yogurt.

Sticking with low-fat products that do have fewer calories doesn't guarantee effortless weight loss, either. Studies suggest that people tend to compensate for lower-fat, lower-calorie meals and snacks by eating more at other times. In part, that's because the lack of fat and calories simply makes them hungrier. But a recent study from Pennsylvania State University demonstrated another reason: Just knowing that they're eating a low-fat food may make some people feel they're entitled to indulge their appetite later. The researchers gave volunteers either of two different yogurts—one low in fat and the other high in fat—that contained the same number of calories. Only half the volunteers knew which yogurt they were eating. Among those who did not know, the

Reprinted with permission from *Consumer Reports on Health,* July 1995, pp. 78-80. © 1995 by Consumers Union of U.S., Inc., Yonkers, NY 10703-1057.

SELECTED REDUCED-FAT AND FULL-FAT PRODUCTS

Products	Serving size [1]	Fat (g)	Calories	Sugar (g)	Sodium (mg)
PASTRIES AND SNACKS					
Better Cheddars Snack Crackers (22 crackers)	30 g	8	150	<1	290
Reduced Fat Better Cheddars Snack Crackers (24)	30 g	6	140	<1	350
Wheatsworth Stoned Ground Wheat Crackers (5)	16 g	3.5	80	1	170
SnackWell's Fat Free Wheat Crackers (5)	15 g	0	60	2	170
Chips Ahoy! cookies (3)	32 g	8	160	10	105
Reduced Fat Chips Ahoy! cookies (3)	32 g	6	150	10	150
Fig Newtons (2)	31 g	2.5	110	13	120
Fat Free Fig Newtons (2)	29 g	0	100	15	115
Marshmallow Puffs Fudge Cookies (1)	21 g	4	90	11	45
SnackWell's Devil's Food Cookie Cakes (1)	16 g	0	50	9	25
Oreo cookies (3)	33 g	7	160	13	220
Reduced Fat Oreo cookies (3)	32 g	5	140	13	190
Hostess Chocolate Cup Cakes (1)	46 g	5	170	16	260
Hostess Chocolate Cup Cakes Light (1)	39 g	1.5	120	17	170
Pop-Tarts, cherry (1)	52 g	5	200	16	220
Low Fat Pop-Tarts, cherry (1)	52 g	3	190	18	220
DAIRY					
Regular Swiss cheese, average (1 slice)	1 oz	8	107	1	74
Kraft Singles Swiss Flavor (1.3 slice)	1 oz	3	67	1	362
Weight Watchers Fat Free Swiss (1.3 slice)	1 oz	0	40	1	375
Regular vanilla ice cream	½ cup	7	133	15	53
Weight Watchers Oh! So Very Vanilla	½ cup	2.5	120	16	65
Healthy Choice Premium Low Fat Ice Cream, vanilla	½ cup	2	100	17	50
Stonyfield Farm Yogurt, strawberry (1 container)	1 cup	8	220	27	115
Breyer's Lowfat Yogurt, strawberry (1 container)	1 cup	2.5	250	46	110
Light N'Lively Free Nonfat Yogurt, strawberry (1.3 containers)	1 cup	0	239	44	140
Light N'Lively Free Nonfat Yogurt with Aspartame, strawberry (1.3 containers)	1 cup	0	93	11	113
CONDIMENTS					
Hidden Valley Ranch salad dressing	2 tbsp	14	140	1	260
Hidden Valley Ranch Light salad dressing	2 tbsp	7	80	1	270
Hidden Valley Fat Free Ranch salad dressing	2 tbsp	0	45	8	320
Kraft Mayonnaise	1 tbsp	11	100	0	75
Kraft Light Mayonnaise	1 tbsp	5	50	0	110
Kraft Free Mayonnaise	1 tbsp	0	10	<1	105
MEATS					
Hillshire Farms Smoked Sausage	2 oz	17	190	2	460
Hillshire Farms Lite Smoked Sausage	2 oz	8	120	2	510
Healthy Choice Low Fat Smoked Sausage	2 oz	1.5	70	2	590
Ground beef, regular	4 oz	22	331	0	105
Ground beef, extra lean	4 oz	18	300	0	93
Swift 95 Supreme Extra Lean ground beef	4 oz	5	140	0	330
Oscar Mayer Wiener (1 link)	45 g	13	150	<1	450
Oscar Mayer Light Wiener (1 link)	57 g	9	110	<1	590
Oscar Mayer Free Hot Dog (1 link)	50 g	0	40	2	460

[1] Serving-size portions (containers or slices, for example) of a few comparable items differ in order to yield equal weights. In certain cases, portion sizes are the same but weights differ.

Sources: Product labels, manufacturers' data, and ESHA Research, Salem, Ore.

type of yogurt they ate made no difference in the number of calories they consumed at a subsequent lunch. But among those who did know, the ones who had eaten the low-fat yogurt consumed significantly more than those who had eaten the high-fat item.

People who stick with low-fat foods, without frequent lapses of discipline, may eventually start losing their "fat tooth"—the lust for fatty foods. But one recent study has raised the possibility that the best way to retrain your palate is to acquire a taste for naturally low-fat foods, not the artificial versions. Researchers at the Monell Chemical Senses Center in Philadelphia divided 27 people into three groups. One group cut their fat intake by eating a diet that included reduced-fat substitutes for foods such as salad dressing, butter, and desserts. Another cut their intake by the same amount without those fat substitutes. The third group stuck with their usual diet. After three months, only the group that had avoided all fat substitutes rated fatty foods less tasty than they did at the start of the study.

Whether or not further research confirms that finding, a diet rich in naturally low-fat foods, notably fruits, vegetables, grains, and beans, does have one clear benefit: It provides a wealth of vital nutrients. In contrast, many of the new reduced-fat snacks and desserts offer little except empty calories and an increased risk of tooth decay from the extra sugar.

Where reduced-fat foods fit

While the ideal diet should be based on naturally lean foods, reduced-fat products can still play a significant role. Eating an occasional low-fat snack or dessert may help people stick with a low-fat regimen. Switching from regular salad dressing to low- or no-fat dressing can substantially cut both fat and calories. And reduced-fat dairy products provide the calcium that would be lost to the body if you merely cut dairy products from your diet. (Our nutritional consultants say that many dairy products taste unusually good for reduced-fat foods.) You'll even find low- and no-fat alternatives to such meat products as luncheon meat, sausage, hot dogs, and ground beef, although they may contain even more sodium than their full-fat counterparts.

Few reduced-fat products taste as good as their high-fat counterparts. You'll probably miss the fat least in products with strong flavors; in fat-free ice creams, for example, chocolate may taste richer than vanilla. Likewise, you probably won't notice a difference between reduced-fat and regular ground meat when you use it with other ingredients.

THE NEW FAKE FATS

Food engineers are trying to reproduce the taste and texture of fat without all the calories and other unhealthy features by changing the chemical structure of fat itself. The U.S. Food and Drug Administration allows manufacturers to begin marketing products made with three of the altered fats described below, *Caprenin*, *SALATRIM*, and *Appetize*, although the FDA has not formally approved any of them. Here's a rundown of what's coming:

Caprenin. This fat substitute is designed to simulate the rich taste and feel of cocoa without all the calories. Since *Caprenin* is made from poorly absorbed fats, it supplies about 40 percent fewer calories than cocoa butter, although you get roughly the same amount of saturated fat.

SALATRIM. *Nabisco* makes this product from various fats that either have fewer calories or are harder to absorb than other fats. For both reasons, *SALATRIM*, like *Caprenin*, supplies about 40 percent fewer calories than unaltered fats do. The main drawbacks: *SALATRIM* is high in unhealthful saturated fat, and it doesn't stand up to frying.

Appetize. Manufacturers combine vegetable oils with hydrogen gas to make them more solid and more stable. But "hydrogenation" creates trans fats, which can raise blood-cholesterol levels. To create a healthier solid shortening, researchers at Brandeis University removed the cholesterol from animal fats and combined them with vegetable oils. In theory, the modest amount of saturated fats in that combination may be less harmful for the arteries than the fats in either margarine or butter. But *Appetize* contains as many calories as regular fat, so it's no better for the waistline.

Olestra. The best known of a group of compounds known as sucrose polyesters, *Olestra* seems to mimic fat better than any product developed so far. The fat in *Olestra* is firmly bound to molecules of sugar, so it travels through the body undigested. What you get is essentially a nonfat fat that can be used for all types of cooking. Researchers who have tasted fat-free potato chips made with *Olestra* told us that they taste like the real thing. . . .

Food Safety

> The dichotomization of risk distorts the reality that nothing is absolutely safe or absolutely dangerous.
> —Peter Sandman, quoted in "Determining Risk," *FDA Consumer*, June 1990.

In 1906, with the passage of the first Food and Drug Act, the federal government began to assume some responsibility for food safety. Increased governmental involvement has been an inevitable trend ever since. With the 1950s came a fear that chemicals in the food supply, especially additives, might be carcinogenic. Congress responded with tighter control on the use and testing of additives. In 1958, the Delaney Clause prevented the use of any additive found to induce cancer in man or experimental animals, and the GRAS (Generally Recognized as Safe) list identified those believed by scientists to be safe for human consumption. This list is periodically revised, and the testing and retesting of additives continues. The Food and Drug Administration (FDA) governs all of these procedures, and books of regulations cover all aspects of food production and service.

The concept in the quote at the top of this page is not new. A sixteenth-century physician, Paracelsus, said, "All things are poison. Nothing is without poison." Yet, many of today's consumers frequently fail to assess risk and benefit rationally. With little knowledge to draw upon, they do not understand that even an essential nutrient can be both life-giving and life-threatening. Sodium, for example, is absolutely necessary for life, but if put into an infant's formula instead of sugar, it can (and has) resulted in death. Likewise, arctic explorers have become very ill from eating a small portion of polar bear liver due to its excessive vitamin A content.

Given the complexity of biological interactions, the uniqueness of each human organism, and the multitude of chemicals that could potentially interact, few knowledgeable people would contend that the absolute safety of anything can be ensured. Yet activist groups demand just that and have become experts at escalating a minor or nonexistent issue into a major catastrophe. It has been argued that if it takes programs like *60 Minutes*, or a partisan political group such as the National Resources Defense Council, or a self-appointed watchdog group such as Food and Water, Inc., to create a public issue, then it probably isn't a safety issue at all. Alar—a growth regulator used in apple orchards—is a good example. The scare in 1989 over Alar's safety appears to have been nothing more than media hype, but it seriously hurt the apple industry and shook parents' confidence in apple juice for their children.

Some current surveys show that safety has become the primary concern of consumers about their food supply. The perception of more and more food-borne illness is fueled by media coverage of outbreaks traced to large quantities of contaminated beef, apple cider, raspberries, and other products, both in retail markets and restaurants. News of "mad cow" disease in Europe has tended to make us feel vulnerable as well, even though no cases have been found in the United States and steps are being taken to ensure that it cannot happen here. Even more recently, fear of Pfiesteria has caused a dramatic drop in purchases of Chesapeake Bay seafood—even though the organism has been found in only a few of the bay's tributaries and no evidence of linkage between food fish and human illness exists. That bacteria-laden foods do result in significant numbers of ill people cannot be denied. In a recent year, the Council for Agricultural Science and Technology reported 33 million cases and 9 thousand deaths. Other sources suggest the figures may be even higher. On a yearly basis, total costs of these illnesses are estimated at $3 to $10 billion.

Some of the most prevalent food-borne organisms today were not public health issues 20 years ago, a sign that conditions and lifestyles have changed. One of these is *E. coli* 0157:H7, which became infamous for causing a 1991 outbreak of food poisoning from undercooked hamburger in Washington State. Repeated outbreaks later, it is clear that this is truly serious. We have learned that illness from *E. coli* can be carried, not just by undercooked hamburger, but by raw vegetables, unpasteurized cider, mayonnaise, and other food products as well. Reports indicate that this organism will have to be aggressively controlled both in the processing industry and in the kitchen.

Many people blame the packing industry or the government's food inspection procedures for the presence of illness-producing organisms in the food supply. And, indeed, government agencies are responding to the challenge. The National Food Safety Initiative was launched in April 1997 by the U.S. Department of Agriculture (USDA), the FDA, the Centers for Disease Control and Prevention (CDC), and the Environmental Protection Agency (EPA). Their combined efforts are expected to reduce morbidity and mortality due to food-borne diseases by improving the inspection system, initiating better ways to track and contain outbreaks of illness, and waging a national education campaign to improve food handling practices at home and in stores and restaurants.

All of us must learn about safe food handling. While many people assume that food-borne illness is contracted primarily in restaurants, it is revealing to discover that each of us is his or her own worst enemy. Food properly handled in home kitchens could reduce the incidence of disease significantly. This always includes conformance with rules governing bacterial growth, time, and temperature. A case in point is undercooked ground meat and

UNIT 5

the *E.coli* organism discussed above. Even more likely is the very common bacterium, salmonella, which is the most common cause of food-borne illness and is found in a high percentage of raw poultry and which may also be in raw eggs. Three articles in this unit discuss the food-borne illnesses and food handling practices that should be of interest to the consumer.

In assessing risk and safety, it is appropriate for critics to question the continued usefulness of the Delaney Clause. When this law was passed, they argue, only about 50 carcinogens were known. Today thousands are known, and advances in analytical methods enable the detection of amounts with no biological or toxicological significance, causing useful products to be banned needlessly. That pesticides are no longer subject to the Delaney Clause is certainly a step in the right direction. This replaces a "zero risk" policy with a standard of "reasonable certainty of no harm." The National Academy of Sciences (NAS), in response to public concern over a possible connection between pesticides and cancer, points out that the incidence of lung cancer alone is really rising. A major NAS report on pesticides in the diets of infants and children finds no current cause for concern and certainly no reason to reduce the consumption of fresh produce. In "How Much Are Pesticides Hurting Your Health?" the mythology surrounding the values and dangers of pesticides is discussed.

Food irradiation, as addressed by Alan Morton in "After the Glow," is both a food safety issue and a political issue. There is word that a 3-year-old petition to permit irradiation of red meat will now be expedited, as irradiation will destroy pathogenic bacteria but does not produce radioactive food. Irradiation also helps to maintain high-quality produce over a prolonged shelf life, both of which are advantages to the consumer. Yet, some activist groups, such as Food and Water, Inc., have used very aggressive scare tactics to delay its use in the United States. Despite Food and Water's considerable efforts, however, irradiation has been approved for a number of products, including fresh fruits and vegetables, poultry, and pork.

Related articles can be found in other units. An article on genetic engineering is in unit 1, an article on fluoridation is in unit 2, and two articles on the risks and benefits of supplements and herbals are in unit 6.

All would agree that it is appropriate to raise questions about the safety of our food supply. Sometimes there is disagreement on the extent of the problem and on how to solve it. As consumers, we must accept personal responsibility for safe food handling. We must also continue to expect our regulatory agencies to do their best. Problems arising over the safety of food supplies can be documented throughout history. Clearly, solutions are not easy.

Looking Ahead: Challenge Questions

Rank-order three issues of food safety that you think are the most important and justify your selection.

What measures would you suggest to counteract misinformation about food safety and the tactics used by activist organizations?

Observe yourself when you handle food. In what ways might you be the vector of food-borne illness?

Read Upton Sinclair's muckraking novel *The Jungle* (R. Bentley, 1971 [© 1946]). Compare conditions and problems described in this book with today's procedures for ensuring a safe food supply.

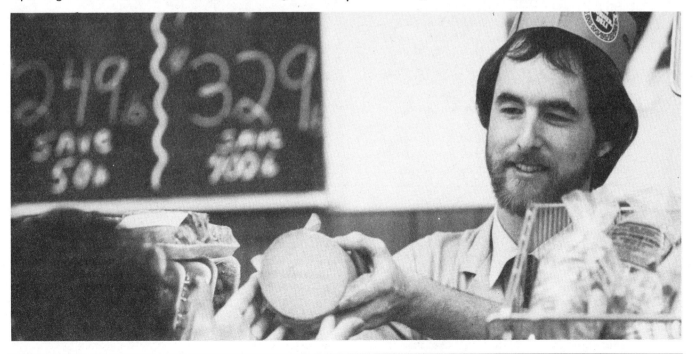

FOODBORNE ILLNESS:
ROLE OF HOME FOOD HANDLING PRACTICES

The Principal author of this Scientific Status Summary was S. J. Knable, Ph.D., The Pennsylvania State University

Outbreaks of foodborne illness, such as the highly publicized outbreaks of *Escherichia coli* O157:H7 in the western United States in early 1993 that led to the tragic deaths of four children (CDC, 1993), remind us that under certain circumstances, familiar foods can lead to serious consequences, even death. Despite progress in improving the overall quality and safety of foods produced in the U.S., significant foodborne illness and death due to microbial pathogens still occur. . . .

FACTORS CONTRIBUTING TO NEW MICROBIOLOGICAL CHALLENGES

Several interrelated factors contribute to new microbiological challenges and risks throughout the food system.

Demographics and lifestyles. Demography and lifestyle of U.S. consumers have changed dramatically during the past two decades. The U.S. population has increased and family size has decreased. There are more families with both parents working outside the home and more single-parent households than previously. More children are shopping for and preparing their own food because no parent is home during the day (Goldman, 1990). In addition, the proportion of elderly individuals in the population has also increased and the number of people at increased risk for foodborne illness has grown.

Preference for quick methods of food preparation, convenience foods, fresh and "fresh-like foods," minimally processed foods, and foods that meet specific health/dietary needs has increased. To meet these preferences and the needs of a growing population, new processing, preservation, and packaging techniques have been incorporated into the manufacturing of food products. Distribution networks have become large, centralized, and complex. Changes such as these affect the epidemiology of foodborne illnesses and present new microbiological risks.

Minimally processed foods, for example, are designed for convenience, "fresh-like" state, and extended shelf life. Minimally processed foods present concerns to food manufacturers in maintaining product safety. These foods may receive a lower heat treatment than required for commercial sterility. They may be vacuum packaged or packaged in atmospheres modified by the addition of nitrogen and/or carbon dioxide. Such processing and packaging conditions alter the microbial ecology of foods. The heat treatment may destroy some microorganisms but not others, e.g., bacterial spores. The modified atmospheres may inhibit the growth of some microorganisms surviving the heat treatment, but may enhance the growth of others, even at refrigeration temperatures. The extension of shelf life may allow time for growth of undesirable, harmful microorganisms. This is of particular concern in ready-to-eat products not requiring cooking before consumption. . . .

Several microorganisms that were not previously recognized as important foodborne pathogens have emerged during the past two decades, adding to our microbiological challenges. These pathogens include Norwalk virus, *Campylobacter jejuni*, *E. coli* O157:H7, *Listeria monocytogenes*, *Vibrio vulnificus*, *Vibrio cholera*, and *Yersinia enterocolitica* (IOM, 1992; Doyle, 1991; Doyle, 1985). Some of these microorganisms, *Campylobacter*, for example, may have come to our attention through investigative surveillance and ability of laboratories to identify them (Hedberg et al., 1994). *E. coli* O157:H7 appears to be a new pathogen that acquired genetic determinants for new virulence factors (Whittam et al., 1993; Griffin and Tauxe, 1991). *E.coli* O157:H7 was first recognized as a foodborne pathogen in 1982 and is now known as an important cause of the diarrheal form of hemorrhagic colitis (painful bloody diarrhea) and renal failure in humans (Padhye and Doyle, 1992; Griffin and Tauxe, 1991; Doyle, 1985). In its report on a small outbreak in California, the CDC noted that many unrecognized sporadic cases and small outbreaks of *E. coli* O157:H7 due to

From *Food Technology: Scientific Status Summary*, April 1995, pp. 119-131. Reprinted by permission of *Food Technology: Scientific Status Summary*, a publication of the Institute of Food Technologists' Expert Panel on Food Safety and Nutrition.

Table 1—Common Foodborne Diseases Caused by Bacteria. *From Cliver (1993)*

Disease (causative agent)	Latency Period (duration)	Principal Symptoms	Typical Foods	Mode of Contamination	Prevention of Disease
(*Bacillus cereus*) food poisoning, diarrheal	8–16 hr (12–24 hr)	Diarrhea, cramps, occasional vomiting	Meat products, soups sauces, vegetables	From soil or dust	Thorough heating and rapid cooling of foods
(*Bacillus cereus*) food poisoning, emetic	1–5 hr (6–24 hr)	Nausea, vomiting, sometimes diarrhea and cramps	Cooked rice and pasta	From soil or dust	Thorough heating and rapid cooling of foods
Botulism; food poisoning (heat-labile toxin of *Clostridium botulinum*)	12–36 hr (months)	Fatigue, weakness, double vision, slurred speech, respiratory failure, sometimes death	Types A&B: vegetables; fruits; meat, fish, and poultry products; condiments; Type E: fish and fish products	Types A&B: from soil or dust; Type E: water and sediments	Thorough heating and rapid cooling of foods
Botulism; food poisoning infant infection	Unknown	Constipation, weakness, respiratory failure, sometimes death	Honey, soil	Ingested spores from soil or dust or honey colonize intestine	Do not feed honey to infants —will not prevent all
Campylobacteriosis (*Camplyobacter jejuni*)	3–5 days (2–10 days)	Diarrhea, abdominal pain, fever, nausea, vomiting	Infected food-source animals	Chicken, raw milk	Cook chicken thoroughly; avoid cross-contamination; irradiate chickens; pasteurize milk
Cholera (*Vibrio cholerae*)	2–3 days hours to days	Profuse, watery stools; sometimes vomiting, dehydration; often fatal if untreated	Raw or undercooked seafood	Human feces in marine environment	Cook seafood thoroughly; general sanitation
(*Clostridium perfringens*) food poisoning	8–22 hr (12–24 hr)	Diarrhea, cramps, rarely nausea and vomiting	Cooked meat and poultry	Soil, raw foods	Thorough heating and rapid cooling of foods
(*Escherichia coli*) foodborne infections enterohemorrhagic	12–60 hr (2–9 days)	Watery, bloody diarrhea	Raw or undercooked beef, raw milk	Infected cattle	Cook beef thoroughly pasteurize milk
(*Escherichia coli*) foodborne infections entroinvasive	at least 18 hr (uncertain)	Cramps, diarrhea, fever, dysentery	Raw foods	Human fecal contamination, direct or via water	Cook foods thoroughly; general sanitation
(*Escherichia coli*) foodborne infection enterotoxigenic	10–72 hr (3–5 days)	Profuse watery diarrhea; sometimes cramps, vomiting	Raw foods	Human fecal contamination, direct or via water	Cook foods thoroughly; general sanitation
Listeriosis (*Listeria monocytogenes*)	3–70 days	Meningoencephalitis; stillbirths; septicemia or meningitis in newborns	Raw milk, cheese and vegetables	Soil or infected animals, directly or via manure	Pasteurization of milk; cooking
Salmonellosis (*Salmonella* species)	5–72 hr (1–4 days)	Diarrhea, abdominal pain, chills, fever, vomiting, dehydration	Raw, undercooked eggs; raw milk, meat and poultry	Infected food-source animals; human feces	Cook eggs, meat and poultry thoroughly; pasteurize milk; irradiate chickens
Shigellosis (*Shigella* species)	12–96 hr (4–7 days)	Diarrhea, fever, nausea; sometimes vomiting, cramps	Raw foods	Human fecal contamination, direct or via water	General sanitation; cook foods thoroughly
Staphylococcal food poisoning (heat-stable enterotoxin of *Staphylococcus aureus*)	1–6 hr (6–24 hr)	Nausea, vomiting, diarrhea, cramps	Ham, meat, poultry products, cream-filled pastries, whipped butter, cheese	Handlers with colds, sore throats or infected cuts, food slicers	Thorough heating and rapid cooling of foods
Streptococcal foodborne infection (*Streptococcus pyogenes*)	1–3 days (varies)	Various, including sore throat, erysipelas, scarlet fever	Raw milk, deviled eggs	Handlers with sore throats, other "strep" infections	General sanitation, pasteurize milk
Vibrio parahaemolyticus foodborne infection	12–24 hr (4–7 days)	Diarrhea, cramps; sometimes nausea, vomiting, fever, headache	Fish and seafoods	Marine coastal environment	Cook fish and seafoods thoroughly
Vibrio vulnificus foodborne infection	In persons with high serum iron: 1 day	Chills, fever, prostration, often death	Raw oysters and clams	Marine coastal environment	Cook shellfish thoroughly
Yersiniosis (*Yersinia enterocolitica*)	3–7 days (2–3 weeks)	Diarrhea, pains mimicking appendicitis, fever vomiting, etc.	Raw or undercooked pork and beef; tofu packed in spring water	Infected animals especially swine; contaminated water	Cook meats thoroughly, chlorinate water

undercooking of hamburger in the home probably occur throughout the U.S. (CDC, 1994a).

Listeria monocytogenes has been recognized as a human pathogen for several decades but the importance of food as a vehicle for transmission has only recently been identified (Doyle, 1985). *L. monocytogenes* is widely distributed in the environment and carried in the intestinal tracts of a variety of animals and humans (Doyle, 1985). Of significance to food safety, the microorganism can grow, although slowly, at refrigeration temperatures. *Listeria monocytogenes* causes illness primarily in individuals at increased risk for foodborne illness. Infection with *L. monocytogenes* may result in meningitis, miscarriage, and perinatal septicemia (Doyle, 1985). *S. enteriditis* can contaminate whole shell eggs when infected hens transmit the pathogen to the egg when it is produced. The global incidence of this serotype increased dramatically from 5% of all isolates in the U.S. in the 1970s to 20% of isolates in 1989 (St. Louis et al., 1988).

Emergence of these microbial health threats (diseases and their causative agents) may be due to several factors. These include: emergence of new microorganisms, recognition of existing diseases previously undetected, and changes in the environment that provide an epidemiologic "bridge" (IOM, 1992). The potential for foods to be involved in the emergence or reemergence of microbial threats to humans is great, largely because there are many points in the food system at which food safety can be compromised (IOM, 1992). . . .

FACTORS CONTRIBUTING TO FOODBORNE ILLNESS IN THE HOME

The extent of the hazards associated with pathogenic microorganisms and the risk of acquiring foodborne illness depend on several factors. These include type of pathogen, number of microorganisms ingested, and the consumers' susceptibility to the pathogen.

Pathogens. Pathogenic bacteria, viruses, fungi, parasitic protozoa, other parasites, and marine phytoplankton may cause foodborne illness. One way foodborne illness may arise is from infection by microorganisms and parasites. Infection occurs when pathogens, such as *Campylobacter* or *Salmonella*, in the ingested food, grow in the host's intestine. The infection may involve subsequent growth in other tissues or the production of toxin, in which case the illness is classified as a toxicoinfection. Foodborne illness may also stem from intoxication. Intoxication occurs when pathogens, such as *S. aureus*, produce toxin in a food or when a toxic chemical occurs in food before consumption. Common foodborne diseases caused by pathogenic microorganisms or their toxins are described in Tables 1–4. Depending on host susceptibility, foodborne illness may be mild to severe or lead to serious chronic complications such as arthritis, carditis, Guillain-Barre' syndrome, and hemolytic anemia (CAST, 1994; Smith, 1994; Archer and Young, 1988; Mossel, 1988; Archer 1985) or death. The complications that may be associated with certain foodborne illnesses are listed in Table 5.

Among outbreaks of known etiology reported to the Centers for Disease Control and Prevention (CDC) between 1973 and 1987, bacterial pathogens were responsible for most of the outbreaks (66%) and cases (92%; Bean et al., 1990). . . .

About 60% of the foodborne illnesses reported to CDC from 1973–1987 were of unknown etiology. The inability to determine the etiologic agent in reported outbreaks may be attributable to late or incomplete laboratory investigations, lack of recognition of the pathogen as a disease agent, or inability to identify the pathogen with available laboratory techniques (Bean and Griffin, 1990; Bean et al., 1990). . . .

The ability of several bacterial pathogens to multiply rapidly to dangerous levels in foods allowed to warm up or to remain warm for an extended period is responsible for their frequent implication in foodborne illness. Some pathogens, however, such as *L. monocytogenes*

> *"The potential for foods to be involved in the emergence or reemergence of microbial threats to humans is great ... (IOM, 1992)."*

Table 2—Common Foodborne Diseases Caused by Viruses. *From Cliver (1993)*

Disease (causative agent)	Onset (duration)	Principal Symptoms	Typical Foods	Mode of Contamination	Prevention of Disease
Hepatitis A (Hepatitis A virus)	15–20 days (weeks to months)	Fever, weakness, nausea discomfort; often jaundice	Raw or undercooked shellfish; sandwiches, salads, etc.	Human fecal contamination, via water or direct	Cook shellfish thoroughly; general sanitation
Viral gastroenteritis (Norwalk-like viruses)	1–2 days (1–2 days)	Nausea, vomiting, diarrhea, pains, headache, mild fever	Raw or undercooked shellfish; sandwiches, salads, etc.	Human fecal contamination, via water or direct	Cook shellfish thoroughly, general sanitation
Viral gastroenteritis (rotaviruses)	1–3 days (4–6 days)	Diarrhea, especially in infants and young children	Raw or mishandled foods	Probably human fecal contamination	General sanitation

and *Y. enterocolitica*, can grow at refrigeration temperatures and others, such as *E. coli* O157:H7, and viruses, can cause illness at very low levels in foods.

Certain pathogens may be a greater problem in the home than in foodservice establishments or in commercially prepared foods. Approximately 92% of the 231 outbreaks of botulism from 1973–1987 were associated with food prepared in the home, especially home-canned foods (Bean and Griffin, 1990)....

Foods. A variety of foods are associated with foodborne illnesses, including foods of animal origin, such as fish and shellfish, red meats, poultry, fruits and vegetables, eggs, and dairy products (CAST, 1994; Bean and Griffin, 1990; Bryan, 1988a). In recent years, foodborne illnesses have been associated with novel substrates, such as potatoes, sauteed onions, garlic-in-oil mixtures, cooked rice, and sliced fruits. Vegetables grown in the ground or close to it are likely to be contaminated by

the spore-forming bacteria *C. botulinum*, *C. perfringens*, and *B. cereus* (Bryan 1988a). Outbreaks of botulism have been associated with foil-wrapped baked potatoes left at room temperature, sauteed onions, and garlic-in-oil mixtures. Outbreaks of *B. cereus* food poisoning have been associated with cooked rice held at room temperature.

Mishandling Factors. From 1973–1987, 7,458 outbreaks and 237,545 cases of foodborne illness were reported to the CDC. Among the 7,219 outbreaks in which it was reported, the site of preparation of the implicated food was a commercial or institutional establishment in 79% of outbreaks and the home in 21%, with variations for different illness etiologies (Bean and Griffin, 1990). Sporadic cases and small outbreaks in homes, however, are considered far more common than cases constituting recognized outbreaks and comprise most of the foodborne illness cases in the U.S. (Schuchat et al. 1992; Tauxe, 1992, 1991; Bean and

Table 3—Common Foodborne Diseases Caused by Protozoa and Parasites. *From Cliver (1993)*

Disease (causative agent)	Onset (duration)	Principal Symptoms	Typical Foods	Mode of Contamination	Prevention of Disease
(PROTOZOA) Amebic dysentery (*Entamoeba histolytica*)	2–4 weeks (varies)	Dysentery, fever, chills; sometimes liver abscess	Raw or mishandled foods	Cysts in human feces	General sanitation; thorough cooking
Cryptosporidiosis (*Cryptosporidium parvum*)	1–12 days (1–30 days)	Diarrhea; sometimes fever, nausea, and vomiting	Mishandled foods	Oocysts in human feces	General sanitation; thorough cooking
Giardiasis (*Giardia lamblia*)	5–25 days (varies)	Diarrhea with greasy stools, cramps, bloat	Mishandled foods	Cysts in human and animal feces, directly or via water	General sanitation; thorough cooking
Toxoplasmosis (*Toxoplasma gondii*)	10–23 days (varies)	Resembles mononucleosis fetal abnormality or death	Raw or undercooked meats; raw milk; mishandled foods	Cysts in pork or mutton, rarely beef; oocysts in cat feces	Cook meat thoroughly; pasteurize milk; general sanitation
(ROUNDWORMS, Nematodes) Anisakiasis (*Anisakis simplex, Pseudoterranova decipiens*)	Hours to weeks (varies)	Abdominal cramps, nausea, vomiting	Raw or undercooked marine fish, squid or octopus	Larvae occur naturally in edible parts of seafoods	Cook fish thoroughly or freeze at -4° F for 30 days
Ascariasis (*Ascaris lumbricoides*)	10 days –8 weeks (1–2 years)	Sometimes pneumonitis, bowel obstructions	Raw fruits or vegetables that grow in or near soil	Eggs in soil from human feces	Sanitary disposal of feces; cooking food
Trichinosis (*Trichinella spiralis*)	8–15 days (weeks, months)	Muscle pain, swollen eyelids, fever; sometimes death	Raw or undercooked pork or meat of carnivorous animals (e.g., bears)	Larvae encysted in animal's muscles	Thorough cooking of meat; freezing pork at 5° F for 30 days; irradiation
(TAPEWORMS, Cestodes) Beef tapeworm (*Taenia saginata*)	10–14 weeks (20–30 years)	Worm segments in stool; sometimes digestive disturbances	Raw or undercooked beef	"Cysticerci" in beef muscle	Cook beef thoroughly or freeze below 23°F
Fish tapeworm (*Diphyllobothrium latum*)	3–6 weeks (years)	Limited: sometimes vitamin B-12 deficiency	Raw or undercooked fresh-water fish	"Plerocercoids" in fish muscle	Heat fish 5 minutes at 133°F or freeze 24 hours at 0°F
Pork tapeworm (*Taenia solium*)	8 weeks–10 years (20–30 years)	Worm segments in stool; sometimes "cysticercosis" of muscles, organs, heart, or brain	Raw or undercooked pork; any food mishandled by a *T. solium* carrier	"Cysticerci" in pork muscle; any food —human feces with *T. solium* eggs	Cook pork thoroughly or freeze below 23°F; general sanitiation

Table 4—Common Foodborne Diseases Caused by Toxins in Seafood. *Adapted from Cliver (1993)*

Disease (causative agent)	Onset (duration)	Principal Symptoms	Typical Foods	Mode of Contamination	Prevention of Disease
(TOXINS IN FINFISH) Ciguatera poisoning (ciguatoxin, etc.)	3–4 hr (rapid)	Diarrhea, nausea, vomiting, abdominal pain	"Reef and island" fish: grouper, surgeon fish, barracuda, pompano, snapper, etc.	(Sporadic); food chain, from algae	Eat only small fish
	12–18 hr (days–months)	Numbness & tingling of face; taste & vision aberrations, sometimes convulsions, respiratory arrest, and death (1–24 hrs)			
Fugu or pufferfish poisoning (tetrodotoxin, etc.)	10–45 min to ≥ 3 hr	Nausea, vomiting, tingling lips and tongue, ataxia, dizziness, respiratory distress/arrest, sometimes death	Pufferfish, "fugu" (many species)	Toxin collects in gonads, viscera	Avoid pufferfish (or their gonads)
Scombroid or histamine poisoning (histamine, etc.)	minutes to few hours (few hours)	Nausea, vomiting, diarrhea, cramps, flushing, headache, burning in mouth	"Scombroid" fish (tuna, mackerel, etc.); mahimahi, others	Bacterial action	Refrigerate fish immediately when caught
(TOXINS IN SHELLFISH) Amnesic shellfish poisoning (domoic acid)		Vomiting, abdominal cramps, diarrhea, disorientation, memory loss; sometimes death	Mussels, clams	From algae	Heed surveillance warnings
Paralytic shellfish poisoning (saxitoxin, etc.)	≤ 1 hr (≤ 24 hr)	Vomiting, diarrhea, paresthesias of face, sensory and motor disorders; respiratory paralysis, death	Mussels, clams, scallops, oysters	From "red tide" algae	Heed surveillance warnings

Reprinted with permission from the American Council on Science and Health, New York, NY

Table 5–Medical Complications Associated with Certain Foodborne Infections. *From CAST (1994)*

Bacterial Infections Transmitted by Foods	Complications/sequelae
Aeromonas hydrophila enteritis[a]	Bronchopneumonia, cholecystitis
Brucellosis	Aortitis, epididymo-orchitis, meningitis, pericarditis, spondylitis
Campylobacteriosis	Arthritis, carditis, cholecystitis, colitis, endocarditis, erythema nodosum, Guillain-Barre' syndrome, hemolytic-uremic syndrome, meningitis, pancreatitis, septicemia
Escherichia coli (EHEC-types) enteritis	Erythema nodosum, hemolytic uremic syndrome, seronegative arthropathy, thrombotic thrombocytopenic purpura
Q-fever	Endocarditis, granulomatous hepatitis
Salmonellosis	Aortitis, cholecystitis, colitis, endocarditis, epididymoorchitis, meningitis, myocarditis, osteomyelitis, pancreatitis, Reiter's disease, rheumatoid syndromes, septicemia, splenic abscesses, thyroiditis, septic arthritis (sickle-cell anemic persons)
Shigellosis	Erythema nodosum, hemolytic-uremic syndrome, peripheral neuropathy, pneumonia, Reiter's disease, septicemia, splenic abscesses, synovitis
Vibrio parahaemolyticus enteritis	Septicemia
Yersiniosis	Arthritis, cholangitis, erythema nodosum, liver and splenic abscesses, lymphadenitis, pneumonia, pyomyositis, Reiter's disease, septicemia, spondylitis, Still's disease
Parasitic Infections Transmitted by Foods	Complications/sequelae
Cryptosporidiosis[b]	Severe diarrhea, prolonged and sometimes fatal
Giardiasis[b]	Cholangitis, dystrophy, joint symptoms, lymphoidal hyperplasia
Taeniasis	Arthritis, cysticercosis (*T. solium*)
Toxoplasmosis	Encephalitis and other central nervous system diseases, pancarditis, polymyositis
Trichinosis	Cardiac dysfunction, neurologic sequelae

[a]Suspected to be foodborne or waterborne.
[b]Waterborne.

Griffin, 1990; Schwartz et al., 1988). Foodborne illness in the home is reported much less frequently than institutional outbreaks because fewer people are typically involved. Additionally, sporadic cases of mild illnesses are less likely than more serious illnesses to result in medical attention, reporting, and investigation.

Bryan (1988b) reviewed the handling errors leading to foodborne illness outbreaks in the U.S. reported to CDC between 1961 and 1982. The top 12 factors contributing to 345 outbreaks resulting from mishandling/mistreatment of foods in the home are listed in Table 6. Use of contaminated foods or raw ingredients, inadequate cooking/canning/heat processing, and obtaining food from an unsafe source were the three leading factors contributing to foodborne illness in the home. Raw animal products may contain low levels of pathogenic microorganisms and cause illness if not properly cooked. For example, poultry may contain various species of *Salmonella* and *Campylobacter*; shell eggs may contain species of *Salmonella,* especially *S. enteritidis;* and ground beef may contain various pathogens, including *E. coli* O157:H7. Shellfish from sewage-polluted waters, raw milk, and wild mushrooms are foods obtained from unsafe sources. Microorganisms associated with these foods may be spread during preparation and may survive inadequate heating. Bacterial spores may be present on soil-grown cereals, vegetables, and fruits and may survive heating that is less severe than heating in a pressure cooker.

The fourth and fifth factors, improper cooling and lapse of time between preparation and eating, are time and temperature violations. The sixth factor is contamination of food by food handlers. People who carry foodborne pathogens in their intestinal tracts or touch fecally contaminated surfaces and fail to completely remove traces of fecal contamination by proper hand washing may contaminate any food they touch.

Bean and Griffin (1990) listed the mishandling factors thought to contribute to 1,678 foodborne illness outbreaks occurring during 1973–1987 with corresponding etiologies. Improper storage or holding temperature was the factor most often reported in *B. cereus* (94%), *C. perfringens* (97%), *Salmonella* (84%), *S. aureus* (98%), and group A *Streptococcus* (100%) outbreaks. Inadequate cooking was the factor most often reported in outbreaks due to *C. botulinum* (91%), *V. parahaemolyticus* (92%), and *Trichinella spiralis* (100%). Food from an unsafe source was the factor most often cited for outbreaks due to *Brucella* (100%), *Campylobacter* (67%), ciguatoxin (83%), mushroom poisoning (98%), and paralytic shellfish poisoning (100%). Personal hygiene was most frequently reported in *Shigella* (91%), Hepatitis A (96%), Norwalk virus

(78%), and *Giardia* (100%) outbreaks. For each year from 1983–1987, Bean et al. (1990) reported that the most common practice that contributed to foodborne disease was improper

Table 6–Top Twelve Factors Contributing to 345 Outbreaks of Foodborne Disease Caused by Mishandling and/or Mistreatment of Foods in Homes in the U.S., 1973-1982. From Bryan (1988b)

Rank	Contributing Factor	Percent[a]
1.	Contaminated raw food/ ingredient	42.0
2.	Inadequate cooking/ canning/heat processing	31.3
3.	Obtained food from unsafe source	28.7
4.	Improper cooling	22.3
5.	Lapse of 12 or more hours between preparing and eating	12.8
6.	Colonized person handling implicated food	9.9
7.	Mistaken for food	7.0
8.	Improper fermentations	4.6
9.	Inadequate reheating	3.5
10.	Toxic containers	3.5
11.	Improper hot holding	3.2
12.	Cross-contamination	3.2

[a]Percentage exceeds 100 because multiple factors contribute to single outbreaks.

storage or holding temperature, followed by poor personal hygiene of the food handler.

Usually several sequential factors result in foodborne illness (Bryan, 1988b). These are: (1) a pathogen must reach the food, (2) it must survive there until ingested, (3) in some cases, it must multiply to reach infectious levels or produce toxins, and (4) the person ingesting the food must be susceptible to the levels ingested. For example, in staphylococcal food poisoning, *S. aureus* typically reaches cooked food during handling. With sufficient time at room temperature or during inadequate cooling in too large a container in the refrigerator, the pathogen produces enterotoxin. The first six of the top 12 factors contributing to foodborne illness outbreaks (listed in Table 6) are either contamination and/or time and temperature-related errors. These errors account for the vast majority of foodborne illnesses in the home.

PREVENTING FOODBORNE ILLNESS IN THE HOME

Everyone in the food system, from those

"Everyone in the food system, from those who produce food to those who prepare it, has a role in food safety."

who produce food to those who prepare it, has a role in food safety. People in each segment of the food system need to understand the compelling reasons for proactive control of food safety. These reasons include: (1) microorganisms are ubiquitous in the environment and are found on raw agricultural products, (2) pathogens may survive minimal preservation treatments, (3) humans may introduce pathogens into food products during production, processing, distribution and/or preparation just before consumption, (4) depending on individual susceptibility, foodborne illness can range from mild to severe and life-threatening, with chronic complications.

People need to be aware of the control they have in their own kitchen for foodborne illness. They also need to understand how important food handling practices—acquisition, storage, preparation, serving, and dealing with leftovers—affect food safety. The top four mishandling factors cited in Table 6 are the most critical food handling practices to stress in food safety programs (Bryan, 1988b). Messages to the public about handling practices important in maintaining the safety of new unfamiliar food products may also be useful.

Messages and Educational Strategies. The most effective and practical strategy for controlling hazards and assuring food safety throughout the food system is the Hazard Analysis and Critical Control Points (HACCP) concept (Bauman, 1990). Successful application of the HACCP concept requires monitoring the points, processes, or practices that are critical for food safety and then actively controlling them to prevent problems from occurring. The food processing industry has effectively applied HACCP to the control of foodborne pathogens since the 1970s (Bauman, 1990). HACCP is relevant to all stages of the food system, from production to consumption. Education and training of people in each segment of the food system—from producers, retailers, foodservice operators, to preparers—should be an integral part of HACCP. Educational efforts, varying appropriately for different target audiences, should be proactive and messages should be HACCP-based, clear, consistent, and persuasive.

The U.S. Dept. of Agriculture (USDA, 1989) applied the HACCP concept in developing educational material for consumers. The agency identified five "educational critical control points" defined as the points most important in preventing foodborne illness but least understood by consumers. The points identified were: acquisition, storage, preparation, service, and handling leftovers. For example, in "A Quick Consumer Guide to Safe Food Handling" the agency provides the following advice based on the five critical control points:

- When you shop, buy cold food last, get it home fast.
- When you store food, keep it safe, refrigerate.
- When you prepare food, keep everything clean, thaw in refrigerator.
- When you're cooking, cook thoroughly.
- When you serve food, never leave it out over two hours.
- When you handle leftovers, use small, shallow containers for quick cooling.
- When in doubt, throw it out.

Similarly, the agency's safe food handling labels, shown in Fig. 1, required in July 1994 on packages of raw and partially cooked meat and poultry products, provide advice based on critical control points.

Some foodborne pathogens present few risks to most individuals but life-threatening risks to others, e.g., those with immunosuppression due to illness or medications, infants, pregnant women, and elderly individuals. Special educational emphasis should be given to these "at risk" groups. These individuals need to understand that they are more susceptible to foodborne illness even if they consume very low levels of foodborne pathogens, and therefore, must vigilantly use proper food handling practices. They must understand the need to avoid eating raw or undercooked animal foods, such as unpasteurized milk, avoid eating raw or undercooked seafood, particularly molluscan shellfish, and prevent cross-contamination between raw and cooked foods during preparation and storage. Individuals in these "at risk" groups and those who serve them need to understand that they should thoroughly cook raw animal foods to at least 160°F to kill any pathogens that may be present, promptly refrigerate leftovers in small shallow containers, and reheat leftovers to 165°F before consumption. Because outbreaks involving many deaths have occurred in nursing homes as a result of consumption of undercooked eggs or products made from raw eggs, the CDC recommends use of pasteurized eggs for institutions such as nursing homes and hospitals (CDC, 1990). The CDC recommends that, to avoid listeriosis, people at high risk use proper food handling practices and thoroughly wash raw vegetables before eating, avoid eating soft cheeses (e.g., Mexican-style and feta) and reheat ready-to-eat foods (e.g., hot dogs) thoroughly to at least 165°F. The CDC also said that these individuals may choose to avoid foods from delicatessen counters and to thoroughly reheat cold cuts to at least 165°F before eating (CDC, 1992; Schuchat et al., 1992).

Caregivers of infants younger than age one must understand the need for close attention to their use of sanitary containers, potable water (safe drinking water), good personal hygiene

"Education and training of people in each segment of the food system—from producers, retailers, foodservice operators, to preparers— should be an integral part of HACCP."

(hand washing), and sanitary practices in the preparation of infant formula. If possible, individuals who change diapers in institutional day care centers should refrain from preparing foods for infants. Because microorganisms may be introduced into the formula from the infant during feeding, leftover infant formula should be discarded after each feeding and a new container should be prepared immediately before the next feeding.

The CDC (1994b) suggested that because messages about behaviors that prevent or foster emerging infections are often most effective before unsafe behaviors develop, educational efforts targeting children and adolescents should be emphasized. Similarly, the National Advisory Committee on Microbiological Criteria for Foods (NACMCF), formed in 1988 by agencies of the U.S. Depts. of Agriculture, Health and Human Services, Commerce, and Defense, recommended the development of a basic food safety curriculum and specific lesson plans with accompanying audiovisual materials for public and private school systems (Rhodes, 1991). The NACMCF also advised that training be provided for teachers of children, initially, in grades 4–6. Further, the committee said that public service announcements were needed to foster the awareness of food safety principles (Rhodes, 1991). Additional strategies for reaching consumers include providing information in leaflets at retail markets, in recipes, in computer programs, and on computer networks. Safe food handling educational programs for national television audiences similar to those targeted at preventing AIDS and automobile injuries would be helpful.

As new innovative foods, such as minimally processed foods, are developed, clear, HACCP-based information about the importance of refrigeration and other handling practices would be useful. The NACMCF recommended the development of a mandatory, uniform logo, to read "*Important* Must Be Kept Refrigerated," for perishable refrigerated items for which temperature is the key element of safety (Rhodes, 1991). Because temperature maintenance can be extremely important, the committee also recommended that manufacturers use time/temperature indicators where possible to show product mishandling. Sherlock et al. (1992) suggested that consumer education may be necessary to ensure the success of time/temperature indicators. Incorporation of food handling information into product labels may be useful to actively and continuously educate consumers about new food products and the necessary safe food handling practices.

Resources for Consumers and Educators. A variety of information about food safety, including food handling tips, is available for

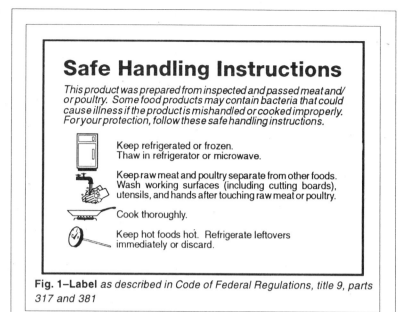

Fig. 1–Label *as described in Code of Federal Regulations, title 9, parts 317 and 381*

consumers and educators from several sources including: federal agencies (Food and Drug Administration, USDA, CDC), food industry trade organizations, scientific societies, food science and nutrition departments at land grant colleges and universities, and other organizations. Information formats include printed materials and videos for educators, other professionals, and the public. Much of the material is free or available for a nominal cost. Some material is written specifically for certain groups of people, such as people at high risk for foodborne disease. Information published by federal agencies may also be available from the local offices of these agencies.

As part of a national campaign to reduce the risk of foodborne illness and to increase knowledge of food-related risks from food production through consumption, the FDA and USDA established in 1994 the Foodborne Illness Education Information Center (Beltsville, MD). The Center is developing an educational database that will be made available to educators, trainers, and organizations producing educational and training materials for food workers and consumers. The database is accessible through a variety of electronic networks such as Internet, the National Agriculture Library electronic bulletin board, and PENpages' International Food and Nutrition Database.

The USDA's Food Safety and Inspection Service also operates a Meat and Poultry Hotline (1-800-535-4555) to answer questions about safe handling of meat and poultry. The number of consumer calls to the Hotline has grown steadily since 1985. Journalists, cookbook authors, and extension agents also use the Hotline for the latest information about food safety (USDA, 1994, 1991a,b). Similarly, the FDA operates a Seafood Hotline (1-800-FDA-4010) to answer questions about seafood safety.

CONCLUSION

Because microorganisms are ubiquitous in the environment they naturally occur on plants and animals. A small percentage of these microorganisms are pathogenic and, therefore, require control measures. Humans may also introduce pathogens into foods during production, processing, distribution, and/or preparation. Everyone in the food system, from people who produce food to those who prepare it, has a significant role in food safety, including activities broadly defined as food handling.

Surveys have found that some people consider homes the least likely place for food safety problems to occur. In contrast, epidemiologic studies indicate that sporadic cases and small outbreaks in homes comprise most of the foodborne illness cases in the U.S. Botulism, campylobacteriosis, and listeriosis are often caused by mishandling of foods in the home. Additional epidemiologic studies on sporadic cases of *Salmonella* and *E. coli* O157:H7 are urgently needed to help determine the magnitude of problems associated with these pathogens and to determine common causes and sites of preparation of implicated foods.

Several changes in society contribute to microbiological challenges. People have expressed concern about food safety, but some appear to be unaware of the home food handling practices that can affect their risk of acquiring a foodborne illness. Education, with specific programs targeted at individuals at high risk, is the key means for increasing public awareness of foodborne disease risks and preventing foodborne illness. To enable the public to make informed food safety decisions affecting their health, educational efforts must provide compelling reasons for the need for vigilance in proper food handling practices. Information about the means for preventing, controlling, or eliminating microbial hazards must be clear, consistent, and science-based.

REFERENCES

Archer, D.L. 1985. Enteric microorganisms in rheumatoid diseases: Causative agents and possible mechanisms. J. Food Protect. 48: 538-545.

Archer, D.L. and Kvenberg, J.E. 1985. Incidence and cost of foodborne diarrheal disease in the United States. J. Food Protect. 48: 887-894.

Archer, D.L. and Young, F.E. 1988. Contemporary issues: Diseases with a food vector. Clin. Microbiol. Rev. 1: 377-398.

Bauman, H. 1990. HACCP: Concept, development, and application. Food Technol. 44(5): 156-158.

Bean, N.H. and Griffin, P.M. 1990. Foodborne disease outbreaks in the United States,1973-1987: Pathogens, vehicles, and trends. J. Food Protect. 53: 804-817.

Bean, N.H., Griffin, P.M., Goulding, J.S., and Ivey, C.B. 1990. Foodborne disease outbreaks, 5-year summary, 1983-1987. J. Food Protect. 53(8): 711-728.

Bennett, J.V., Holmberg, S.D., Rogers, M.F., and Solomon, S.L. 1987. Infectious and parasitic diseases. In "Closing the Gap: The Burden of Unnecessary Illness," Oxford University Press, New York.

Bryan, F.L. 1988a. Risks associated with vehicles of foodborne pathogens and toxins. J. Food Protect. 51: 498-508.

Bryan, F.L. 1988b. Risks of practices, procedures and processes that lead to outbreaks of foodborne diseases. J. Food Protect. 51: 663-673.

Buchanan, R.L. and Deroever, C.M. 1993. Limits in assessing microbiological food safety. J. Food Protect. 56(8): 725-729.

CAST. 1994. Foodborne Pathogens: Risks and Consequences. A report of a Task Force of the Council for Agricultural Science and Technology, Ames, Iowa.

CDC. 1990. Update: *Salmonella enteritidis* infections and shell eggs-United States, 1990. Morbid. Mortal. Wkly. Rept. 39: 909-912, Centers for Disease Control and Prevention, Atlanta, Georgia.

CDC. 1992. Update: Foodborne listeriosis—United States, 1988-1990. Morbid. Mortal. Wkly. Rept. 41(15): 251-258, Centers for Disease Control and Prevention, Atlanta, Georgia.

CDC. 1993. Update: Multistate outbreak of *Escherichia coli* O157:H7 infections from hamburgers-Western United States, 1992-1993. Morbid. Mortal. Wkly. Rept. 42: 258-263, Centers for Disease Control and Prevention, Atlanta, Georgia.

CDC. 1994a. *Escherichia coli* O157:H7 outbreak linked to home-cooked hamburger—California, July 1993. Morbid. Mortal. Wkly. Rept. 43: 213-215, Centers for Disease Control and Prevention, Atlanta, Georgia.

CDC. 1994b. Addressing Emerging Health Threats: A Prevention Strategy for the United States. Centers for Disease Control and Prevention, Atlanta, Georgia.

Cliver, D.O. 1990. Organizing a safe food supply system. IV. Consumer's role in food safety. In "Foodborne Diseases," ed. D.O. Cliver, pp. 361-367. Academic Press, New York.

Cliver, D.O. 1993. "Eating Safely: Avoiding Foodborne Illness," ed. A. Golaine, American Council on Science and Health, New York.

Cousin, M.A., Jay, J.M., and Vasavada, P.C. 1992. Psychrotrophic microorganisms. In "Compendium of Methods for the Microbiological Examination of Foods," ed. C. Vanderzant and D.F. Splittstoesser, 3rd ed., pp. 153-168. American Public Health Association, Washington, D.C.

Doyle, M.P. 1985. Food-borne pathogens of recent concern. Ann. Rev. Nutr. 5: 25-41.

Doyle, M.P. 1991. A new generation of foodborne pathogens. Contemp. Nutr. 16(6), General Mills Nutrition Department, General Mills, Stacy, Minn.

FMI. 1994. Trends in the U.S.: Consumer Attitudes and the Supermarket 1994. Food Marketing Inst. Washington, D.C.

Goldman, D. 1990. The new consumer, superbrands 1990. Adv. Weekly Suppl., Sept. 17, pp. 25-32.

Griffin, P.M. and Tauxe, R.V. 1991. The epidemiology of infections caused by *Escherichia coli* O157:H7, other enterohemorrhagic *E. coli*, and the associated hemolytic uremic syndrome. Epidemiol. Rev. 13: 60-98.

Hauschild, A.H.W. and Bryan, F.L. 1980. Estimate of cases of food- and waterborne illness in Canada and the United States. J. Food Protect. 43: 435-440.

Hedberg, C.W., MacDonald, K.L., and Osterholm, M.T. 1994. Changing epidemiology of food-borne disease: A Minnesota perspective. Clin. Infect. Dis. 18: 671-682.

IOM. 1992. "Emerging Infections: Microbial Threats to Health in the United States," ed. J. Lederberg, R.E. Shope, and S.C. Oaks, Jr., Institute of Medicine, National Academy Press, Washington, D.C.

Jay, J.M. 1992a. Microbiological food safety. Crit. Rev. Food Sci. Nutr. 31(3): 177-190.

Jay., J.M. 1992b. "Modern Food Microbiology," 4th ed. Van Nostrand Reinhold, New York.

Jones, J.M. 1992. "Food Safety." Eagan Press, St. Paul, Minn.

Lechowich, R.V. 1988. Microbiological challenges of refrigerated foods. Food Technol. 42(12): 84-89.

Lee, L.A., Gerber, A.R., Lonsway, D.R., Smith, J.D.,

Carter, G.P., Puhr, N.D., Parrish, C.M., Sikes, R.K., Finton, R.J., and Tauxe, R.V. 1990. *Yersinia enterocolitica* O:3 infections in infants and children, associated with the household preparation of chitterlings. N. Engl. J. Med. 14: 984-987.

Ollinger-Snyder, P. and Matthews, E. 1994. Food safety issues: Press reports heighten consumer awareness of microbiological safety. Dairy, Food, Environ. Sanita. 14(10): 580-589.

Mossel, D.A.A. 1988. Impact of foodborne pathogens on today's world, and prospects for management. An. Hum. Health. 1: 13-23.

Padhye, N.V. and Doyle, M.P. 1992. *Escherichia coli* O157:H7: Epidemiology, pathogenesis, and methods for detection in food. J. Food Protect. 55: 555-565.

Penner, K., Kramer, C., and Frantz, G. 1985. Consumer food safety perceptions. MF774. Kansas State Univ. Ext. Service, Manhattan, Kansas.

Potter, J.E. 1994. The role of epidemiology and risk assessment: A CDC perspective. Dairy, Food, Environ. Sanita. 14(12): 738-741.

Rhodes, M.E. 1991. Educating professionals and consumers about extended-shelf-life refrigerated foods. Food Technol. 45(4): 162-164.

Roberts, T. 1993. Cost of foodborne illness and prevention interventions. In "Proceedings of the 1993 Public Health Conference on Records and Statistics. Toward the year 2000 - Refining the Measures," pp. 514-518. U.S. Dept. of Health and Human Services, Washington, D.C.

Schuchat, A., Deaver, K.A., Wenger, J.D., Plikaytis, B.D., Mascola, L., Piner, R.W., Reingold, A.L., and Broome, C.V. 1992. Role of foods in sporadic listeriosis: I. Case-control study of dietary risk factors. J. Am. Med. Assn. 267(15): 2041-2045.

Schwartz, B., Broome, C.V., Brown, G.R., Hightower, A.W., Ciesielski, C.A., Gaventa, S., Gellin, B.G., and Mascola, L. 1988. Association of sporadic listeriosis with consumption of uncooked hot dogs and undercooked chicken. Lancet 2: 779-782.

Sherlock, M., Fu, G., Taoukis, P.S., and Labuza, T.P. 1992. Consumer perceptions of consumer type time-temperature indicators for use on refrigerated dairy foods. Dairy, Food, Environ. Sanita. 12: 559-565.

Smith, J.L. 1994. Arthritis and foodborne bacteria. J. Food Protect. 57(10): 935-941.

St. Louis, M.E., Morse, D.L., Potter, M.E., DeMelfi, T.M., Guzewich, J.J., Tauxe, R.V., and Blake, P.A.

1988. The emergence of grade A eggs as a major source of *S. enteritidis* infections: New implications for the control of salmonellosis. J. Am. Med. Assn. 259: 2103-2107.

Tauxe, R.V. 1991. Salmonella: A postmodern pathogen. J. Food Protect. 54: 563-568.

Tauxe, R.V. 1992. Epidemiology of *Campylobacter jejuni* infections in the United States and other industrialized nations. In "*Campylobacter jejuni*—Current Status and Future Trends," eds. I. Nachamkim, M.J. Blaser, L.S. Tompkins, p. 9-19. American Society for Microbiology, Washington, D.C.

Tauxe, R.V. 1995. Personal communication. Centers for Disease Control and Prevention, Atlanta, Georgia.

Todd, E.C.D. 1989. Preliminary estimates of the cost of foodborne disease in the United States. J. Food Protect. 52: 595-601.

USDA. 1989. A margin of safety: The HACCP approach to food safety education. Project Report. U.S. Dept. of Agriculture, U.S. Government Printing Office, Washington, D.C.

USDA. 1991a. The Meat and Poultry Hotline. A retrospective, 1985-1990. U.S. Dept. of Agriculture, U.S. Government Printing Office, Washington, D.C.

USDA. 1991b. USDA's Meat and Poultry Hotline links scientists and consumers. Food News for Consumers 7(4): 4-5. U.S. Dept. of Agriculture, Food Safety and Inspection Service, Washington, D.C.

USDA. 1994. Making the connection: An update - USDA's Meat and Poultry Hotline, 1993. U.S. Dept. of Agriculture, U.S. Government Printing Office, Washington, D.C.

USDA/FDA. 1991. Results of the Food and Drug Administration's 1988 health and diet survey—Food handling practices and food safety knowledge for consumers, U.S. Dept. of Agriculture and Food and Drug Administration, Washington, D.C.

Whittam, T.S., Wolfe, M.L., Wachsmuth, K., Orskov, F., Orskov, I., and Wilson, R.A. 1993. Clonal relationships among *Escherichia coli* strains that cause hemorrhagic colitis and infantile diarrhea. Infect. Immunol. 61(5): 1619-1629.

Williamson, D.M. 1991. Home Food Preparation Practice: Results of a National Consumer Survey. M.S. thesis. Cornell University, Ithaca, New York.

Williamson, D.M., Gravani, R.B., and Lawless, H.T. 1992. Correlating food safety knowledge with home food-preparation practices. Food Technol. 46(5): 94-100.

For Safety's Sake: Scrub Your Produce

THE STORY

Any savvy traveller knows the rules: On trips to a developing country, avoid the local fruits and vegetables. If you eat salads, juices, or produce that isn't peeled or cooked, you risk a bout of nasty stomach upset.

Now it seems the same rules apply even to trips to your local supermarket and favorite hometown restaurant. Over and over, Americans are hearing about local outbreaks of gastrointestinal disease traced to raw fruits or vegetables contaminated with dangerous microorganisms.

Several months ago, nearly 200 Michigan schoolchildren developed stomach pains and jaundice and were found to have hepatitis A. Epidemiologists traced their illness to a school treat of strawberry shortcake. The dessert was made from frozen strawberries that had been grown in Mexico, processed in southern California, and contaminated with the hepatitis A virus somewhere in their travels.

Last summer, an outbreak of infectious diarrhea also was caused by imported berries: Raspberries from Guatemala were identified as the vehicle that infected North Americans from New York to Texas to Toronto with an unusual diarrhea-causing parasite called *Cyclospora cayetanensis*. Again this year, cases in five states seem linked to raspberries from Guatemala.

But produce need not be imported to be dangerous. Last fall in the Western US, dozens of cases of bloody diarrhea — and one death — were traced to a batch of organic apple juice made from California apples that had somehow been contaminated with the virulent bacteria *E. coli* 0157:H7.

E. coli 0157:H7 is the same microbe that contaminated undercooked hamburger meat in the infamous Jack-in-the-Box outbreak of 1993 that resulted in the deaths of four children. It also caused illness traced to contaminated lettuce in 1995.

What may appear to be an increase in produce-related outbreaks has been ascribed to a number of factors, including far more produce from around the world entering the US, more widespread use of national-brand packaged and processed foods, and scientific techniques that enable better tracking of outbreaks. The outbreaks have concerned not only consumers but also federal officials, who now estimate that up to 33 million cases of food-borne illness occur in the US yearly, resulting in about 9,000 deaths and an annual expense of some $3 billion.

President Clinton recently proposed that $43 million of the 1998 budget be used to improve food safety by expanding surveillance and diagnosis networks. Proposals for reorganizing food-protection agencies are also afoot. Until such steps have an impact on the safety of your supermarket produce section, how can you ensure that you and your family will not become part of the worrisome statistics?

— *The Editors*

THE PHYSICIAN'S PERSPECTIVE

Abigail Zuger, MD

It seems like the ultimate paradox. Just as medical science announces that fruits and vegetables can protect you from everything from cancer to heart disease, you learn that your gastrointestinal health may suffer severely for your efforts.

In fact, it is easy enough to reap the benefits of raw fruits and vegetables while avoiding their risks by taking just a little extra care with your food-buying and preparation habits.

The produce-associated outbreaks described above may appear all quite different — they involved different kinds of organisms (parasites, viruses, bacteria) contaminating different kinds of fruits and vegetables (berries, apples, lettuce) that were grown in different parts of the world and prepared in different ways.

Even so, these incidents have enough in common to easily deduce a set of rules for avoiding similar disasters. Plainly speaking, all the outbreaks occurred because of fecal contamination. At some point in the growth and processing of the implicated fruit or vegetable, human or animal feces contaminated its surface. It may have been contaminated water used to irrigate a berry patch in Guatemala, or manure from a California cow infected with *E. coli* 0157:H7 that was spread underneath an apple tree and touched the falling fruit. It may have been the dirty hands of a worker ill with hepatitis A, picking fruit in a Mexican berry patch without adequate bathroom facilities. However it happened, the microbe grew whole colonies on the surface of the fruit or vegetable, which may have traveled thousands of miles and arrived on someone's plate without being washed clean.

Thus the first and most important rule for preventing foodborne disease: Scrub your produce carefully. Then scrub your cutting board with soap and water, and then scrub your hands. Even without soap, a good rinse can rid fruit and vegetable skins of most harmful organisms. It may not completely eliminate the risk of cyclospora in the tiny crevices of berries, but it should decrease the risk. If the skin of a piece of produce is broken, toss it out: Organisms may have crawled into the pulp beyond the reach of your scrubbing. After washing, refrigerate all cut or peeled fruits and vegetables.

What about liquids like the tainted California apple juice? That question perplexed French scientist Louis Pasteur in the 19th century when he was trying to eradicate milk-borne disease. Pasteurization was his solution — and it still is today.

Briefly heating beverages and then rapidly cooling them can kill most feces-associated bacteria and make even contaminated drinks safe. The California juice was unpasteurized: Some raw food aficionados eschew pasteurization, arguing that it detracts from taste and nutritional content. While these issues are certainly debatable, the health benefit of pasteurization is not. Avoid unpasteurized foods. If you feel like buying raw cider at a roadside stand, go right ahead — but if you want to be certain of its safety, boil it before drinking.

Finally, what to do about produce served in a restaurant or at a party or mass-prepared school lunches? These answers are less clear. Any item that is clearly the worse for wear (slimy lettuce or gritty, dirty fruit) should be avoided, as should any item that has been implicated in a current outbreak.

Fruits and vegetables are essential to a healthy diet and needn't be shunned. But if you want to be absolutely sure to steer clear of produce-associated illness, you might elect to do most of your raw fruit and vegetable eating at home, where you can make sure that thorough washing precedes serving and eating. HN

Abigail Zuger, MD, a specialist in infectious diseases, is an attending physician at Beth Israel Medical Center in New York.

New risks in ground beef revealed

It looked as though the government acted effectively. Less than a year after undercooked, bacteria-laden hamburgers led to hundreds of illnesses and four deaths in the infamous Jack-in-the-Box incident of 1993, the U.S. Department of Agriculture declared the offending strain of bacteria—*E. coli* 0157:H7—an "adulterant." The legal implication: meat containing the bug is not considered fit for sale and is subject to federal seizure.

Nevertheless, illness-producing bacteria have become the leading cause of acute kidney failure among children in the United States, causing some 40,000 illnesses and 250 to 500 deaths each year. According to a team of Tufts University researchers, the government may be missing the forest for the trees by focusing primarily on *E. coli* 0157:H7. Judging by a new report from the group, as much as 25 percent of ground meat sold in supermarkets may contain other types of bacteria that are just as capable of causing kidney failure and related complications.

For a closer look at the state of the meat supply and some answers on how you can protect yourself and your loved ones, we spoke with the lead researcher of the new study, David W. Acheson, MD, of the Division of Geographic Medicine and Infectious Diseases at the Tufts New England Medical Center.

Q: *Ever since the Jack-in-the-Box story hit the media, fingers have been pointed at* E. coli *0157:H7 as the emerging culprit in food-borne illness. Why are you saying it's not the only one that's so lethal?*

Dr. Acheson: To answer that, let me roll back a bit. Bacteriologists discovered *E. coli* 0157:H7 back in 1982. It caused two very unusual outbreaks of grossly bloody diarrhea—one in Oregon and the other in Michigan. That was really when it got on the scientific map. By the mid to late '80s, it was determined that *E. coli* 0157 was making a toxin that was essentially identical to a toxin that had been discovered about a hundred years ago, called Shiga toxin.

Over the past ten years it has become very clear that Shiga toxin, not the bacteria themselves, is causing the problems associated with *E. coli* 0157:H7. It has also become clear that many other strains of bacteria are capable of producing Shiga toxin. What's happened is that the toxin genes have been moving around the world. Particles called bacteriophages are able to jump from one strain of bacteria and land in another. The bacteriophages then give the bacteria the genes that enable them to produce Shiga toxin.

Q: *So shouldn't the government be looking for Shiga toxin rather than* E. coli *0157:H7?*

Dr. Acheson: Yes, that's where the logic is. Look for the toxins, or look for *all* the toxin-producing bacteria and get away from the dogma of just checking for 0157. That's what has led us down this track here at Tufts.

Q: *How many types of bacteria can make Shiga toxin?*

Dr. Acheson: So far in North America more than 50

From *Tufts University Diet & Nutrition Letter*, June 1996, pp. 3-6. © 1996 by Tufts University Diet & Nutrition Letter. Reprinted by permission.

different types of *E. coli* have been linked to illness caused by Shiga toxin. The same numbers are coming out of Europe, South America, and Australia. In fact, in Australia there's almost no 0157:H7. But in January of last year there was a really nasty outbreak of illness due to an 0111 strain of *E. coli* in sausage. About two dozen people ended up with serious kidney complications, and one child died.

We've been trying to get Australians to realize that they need to move away from 0157. They test for it, even though they don't have it, and what they don't routinely test for is 0111.

Ironically, the United States imports a lot of beef from Australia, and according to my colleagues in Australia, the USDA makes the Australian meat companies test their beef for 0157 before they export it. There's evidence that 0111 is killing people in Australia, and it's in Australian cattle. But do we look for it in our imported Australian meat? No—we test for the bug they *don't* have in Australia. It's like a head-in-the-sand mentality.

Q: *It sounds like* E. coli *is the big problem, and we should try to get rid of all strains of it.*

Dr. Acheson: Actually, most strains of *E. coli* are "good" bacteria. We've all got millions of them in our guts, and we'd be a mess without them. It's just the toxin-producing strains that are a problem.

In the last couple of years it has also come out that Shiga toxin genes seem to be able to jump into bacteria other than *E. coli*. There was an outbreak in Europe in 1994 linked to a bacterium called *Citrobacter freundii*. It's part of the same general family as *E. coli*, but it's somewhat different. The outbreak occurred among a group of kids who had eaten something known in Germany as green butter, which is regular butter mixed with parsley. It turned out the parsley had been grown with cow manure or hadn't been washed properly. When these kids got sick, the illness was traced to Shiga toxin genes in the *Citrobacter*.

A similar thing was reported in Australia this year. A 5-month-old girl got sick from a strain of bacteria called *Enterobacter cloacae*, which had Shiga toxin genes in it.

Q: *Is there a test on the market that labs can use to check for Shiga toxin rather than just 0157?*

Dr. Acheson: Yes, we've been working on the Shiga toxin for years, and one of the things we developed was a rapid, accurate test that detects its presence. Following the Jack-in-the-Box outbreak, we decided we should try to do something to get the test out there where it could be useful. So Meridian Diagnostics in Cincinnati took it and made it suitable for use in hospital clinics. This way when a patient presents with diarrhea or bloody diarrhea, you're not just looking

for 0157. You can also use a variation of the test to check for toxins in, say, ground beef.

Q: *Are many people using the test?*

Dr. Acheson: No, not routinely. Many labs don't even check for 0157 in the stools of potentially affected patients. The Centers for Disease Control and Prevention published a survey this year showing that only about 50 percent of labs are looking for 0157. It's really quite scary how little attention is being paid to this.

Q: *What about the meat industry? Why isn't it testing for Shiga toxin or for bacteria other than 0157?*

Dr. Acheson: According to our research, 25 percent of ground beef is contaminated. If the results of our study are borne out with larger studies, I can see why the meat industry doesn't want to test for the toxin. It's going to cost them to do the test, and it's going to cost them to deal with the meat that comes up positive for Shiga toxin.

Still, it's only fair that consumers know that it's not just 0157 that's a problem, and the meat they're buying off their supermarket shelves is potentially as deadly as the half-cooked meat served in Jack in the Box in 1993.

Q: *What led you to conclude that 25 percent of ground beef may be contaminated with Shiga toxin?*

Dr. Acheson: We wanted to see whether the test we had developed to check for Shiga toxin in human stool was able to identify it in ground beef. So we bought ground beef and spiked it with different strains of toxin-producing bacteria. But we found that some of our "controls," non-spiked beef samples used for comparison, were kicking over positive for the toxin.

Of course, that set us all wondering what was going on here. So we mounted a very small scale study in which various members of the lab just went to supermarkets and bought ground beef, both here in Boston and in Cincinnati. We used several different tests and found that 25 percent of the samples contained toxin-producing bacteria. And none of it was *E. coli* 0157:H7.

Q: *It's enough to make a person never want to eat another hamburger. Is it safe to eat ground beef?*

Dr. Acheson: Yes, so long as it's thoroughly cooked and properly handled. [See box on next page.] You know, I think people have learned to be very careful with chicken because of *Salmonella* bacteria. They've woken up to the fact that if they prepare chicken on the countertop, they get out the bleach and make sure that everything is washed. But they may not do the same with ground beef. And it's fun to play with. The kids will come in and say, "Oh, let's make hamburgers." But in reality beef with toxin-producing bacteria is potentially as deadly, if not more so, than chicken with *Salmonella*.

Q: *Why are Shiga toxin-producing bacteria so harmful?*

Dr. Acheson: One of the things is that the infectious dosage seems to be really small. From studying the Jack-in-the-Box incident, scientists reckon that some of the hamburgers they rescued from the distributors contained only 100 or 200 toxin-producing bacteria per quarter-pound burger. That's much different than *Salmonella* food poisoning, in which it might take a million bacteria to get sick. This probably explains why person-to-person transmission is such a big deal. In fact, about 20 percent of U.S. outbreaks of 0157:H7 occurred in daycare settings and nursing homes and were caused by relatively few bacteria spread, for example, by not washing hands after changing diapers.

Another reason Shiga-producing bacteria are so harmful is that they are likely to make you much sicker than you would be with *Salmonella*. Roughly 5 to 10 percent of people who get sick enough to seek the attention of a physician end up with hemolytic uremic syndrome (HUS), a serious illness that often leads to kidney failure. Of those who get HUS, about 5 percent

die during the acute stages of the disease, and 5 percent suffer major medical complications such as stroke or permanent kidney damage requiring transplant or dialysis. Of the remainder, 2 or 3 years later, probably half of them will still have significant kidney damage. So although it's not a frightfully common problem, it's not just like your regular food poisoning where you spend a couple of days in the bathroom and it's all over.

Q: *Most of the media coverage of hemolytic uremic syndrome seems to focus on children as the victims. Can, say, a middle-aged person suffer serious illness from Shiga toxin?*

Dr. Acheson: It can hit at any age, but it seems that children and the elderly are the most vulnerable. If you want to put numbers on it, I'd say that consumers under 10 and over 75 are the two populations that are hardest hit. We don't know exactly why, but it's probably related to the immune system. In young children, immunity hasn't fully kicked in yet, and in the elderly it's waning.

Q: *How can a parent tell if a child is sick with Shiga toxin?*

Bacteria busters: Tips for keeping food safe

To prevent illness from *E. coli* 0157:H7 and other Shiga toxin-producing bacteria, heed the following advice.

- At the supermarket, make sure meat and poultry are bagged separately from fruits and vegetables or that the meat is wrapped in a small plastic bag. Produce bagged along with meat can become contaminated with bacteria if the meat's juices seep out of the package and onto the fruits and vegetables. And since fruits and many vegetables are not cooked, any toxin-producing bacteria that reach them will not be destroyed.

- Rinse fruits and vegetables thoroughly with cold water before serving. Toxin-producing bacteria reside in animal feces rather than produce. But some outbreaks of illness due to *E. coli* 0157:H7 have been linked to lettuce and other produce that apparently had been exposed to fecal matter during growing or transport to the supermarket. Even cantaloupe and other melons with inedible skins should be rinsed carefully. The knife used to cut the fruit can carry bacteria lurking on the exterior into the fleshy inside of the fruit.

- During cooking, flip steaks with tongs or a spatula rather than a fork. Unlike ground beef, in which bacteria are mixed throughout the meat during the grinding process, steak harbors bacteria only on the surface. Sticking a fork into the

meat, however, injects the interior with bacteria from the outside.

- Cook all meat and poultry to 160 degrees Fahrenheit. The meat should not look pink, and the juices should run yellow, with no trace of pink or red.

- Wash with hot soapy water hands, utensils, cutting boards, and countertops that have come into contact with raw meat or poultry. Also wash sponges and dishcloths used to wipe surfaces exposed to raw meat.

- When dining out, order hamburgers and other ground beef items well-done.

- Buy pasteurized apple cider or heat fresh cider to 160 degrees Fahrenheit. In 1991, about two dozen people were infected with *E. coli* 0157:H7 after drinking fresh cider at a mill in Massachusetts. Public health officials suspect that the contaminated cider was made with unwashed apples that had fallen off the tree and come into contact with animal feces on the ground.

- Do not drink raw milk.

- Wash hands thoroughly after changing diapers. If your child is in a daycare setting, make sure the staff does the same.

Dr. Acheson: That's one of the big problems, because its initial presentation is like any other illness a kid gets. Symptoms usually start 1 or 2 days after exposure. There isn't much of a fever, and about half the kids have vomiting and generalized abdominal pain, and they just feel bad. Often, they will have non-bloody diarrhea, which may or may not progress to bloody diarrhea.

Then, typically, the gut part of the disease—the abdominal pain, vomiting, and diarrhea—begins to get better. But as the gut part is improving or is even gone altogether, the child re-presents with a stroke, seizure, or kidney failure. One thing we're working on in our lab is figuring out how the toxin gets from the inside of the gut, where the bacteria produce it, across the gut wall and to the brain and kidneys. We don't know whether it is actually getting into the bloodstream or whether something else is going on.

Of course, the important thing for parents is that you're not going to want to run and have a checkup done every time your child gets diarrhea. But if the child has *bloody* diarrhea, unquestionably ask for a Shiga toxin test.

Q: *If parents start talking Shiga toxin, won't some pediatricians think they're crazy? Are physicians even aware of this problem?*

Dr. Acheson: Probably not as aware as they should be. We've got a real education job to do. There have been multiple cases in the literature of kids going to a doctor with these kinds of symptoms and then having their appendixes taken out or, in adults, having surgery to check for intestinal disease. In the meantime, somebody sends a stool sample off for a test, and then 3 days after the surgery they find toxin-producing bacteria. Some poor kid has gone through an operation and general anesthesia just because people don't think of Shiga toxin.

But consumers can go into the physician's office with an article like this and say, "Look, it may be Shiga toxin."

Q: *Once someone is diagnosed with Shiga toxin, what kind of treatment is available?*

Dr. Acheson: There is a drug called Synsorb-Pk being tested in Canada that mops up Shiga toxin in the gut. It looks moderately promising, but it's not a panacea. Unfortunately, there isn't a wonder drug.

But for me both as a physician and a parent, I'd want to know if my child had Shiga toxin. I mentioned the two phases: the diarrhea, vomiting, and fever that seem to get better; and the second stage where a child presents with a seizure or stroke. If you know that a child is infected with toxin-producing bacteria, you can at least watch for signs of kidney failure and for the other things we know happen. And you can be in there with supportive therapy. Being aware, watching fluid balance and other vital signs, can help avoid dialysis and may prevent strokes.

How much are pesticides hurting your health?

Pesticides. Just the word conjures up images of ruined cropland and diseased wildlife. For many consumers, even scarier than those images are the things they can't see: potentially cancer-causing chemical residues tainting otherwise healthful-looking fruits and vegetables.

It's a catch-22. At the same time that health experts keep pushing for more consumption of fruits and vegetables to lessen cancer risk, alarming headlines and news stories warning of the risks of dietary pesticide residues constantly leach into the public stream of consciousness.

Are pesticides the cancer threat many are afraid of? Should you spend the extra money on organically grown produce? What about children? Should they be given anything but pesticide-free food? Following is a look at some of the common beliefs about pesticides in the food supply—and the realities behind them.

Myth: Pesticides and other chemicals rank as the most significant diet-related cancer threat.

Reality: In the United States, diets too rich in calories, fat, and alcohol pose a far greater cancer threat than pesticides and other chemical residues, according to a 400-plus page report just released by the National Research Council, which scrutinized the data on more than 200 known carcinogens in food. What's more, a wealth of research indicates that a diet rich in fruits and vegetables protects against cancer. Thus, the risks incurred by avoiding fruits and vegetables for fear of ingesting pesticide residues far outweigh any risks that come from eating a produce-rich diet.

Myth: The only cancer-causing compounds found in produce and grains are synthetic chemicals added during farming and processing.

Reality: The number of naturally occurring chemicals found in the food supply probably exceeds a million, and some of these are known to be potent carcino-

gens. For example, a class of substances called mycotoxins, which are produced by fungal growth on food crops either in the field or during harvesting, are highly toxic and play a role in liver cancer. Many countries, including the United States, impose strict limits on the levels of mycotoxins allowed in foods.

Myth: To determine the amount of pesticide residues allowed in foods, the Environmental Protection Agency finds out what dose of the chemical is toxic and then sets the legal limit slightly below that level.

Reality: To come up with limits, the EPA looks at animal studies that help project the maximum amount of a pesticide residue that a person could consume daily during a 70-year life span without suffering any harm. Once they determine this level, they set the legal limit at just a small fraction of that amount—generally 100 times lower—just to be on the safe side.

Myth: Pesticides are more toxic to children than to adults.

Reality: While most people assume that children's small size leaves them much more vulnerable than adults to the effects of pesticides and other chemicals, that's not necessarily the case. The ability of a child's rapidly developing body to metabolize, detoxify, and excrete chemicals is profoundly different from that of adults and plays a major role in their vulnerability to pesticides. Children's metabolic rates are much higher than adults', which may allow youngsters to excrete certain pesticides and other chemicals much more quickly.

That's not to say pesticides do not pose a problem for youngsters. Infants and children eat a far less varied diet than adults and so consume much more of certain foods for their body weight, which could boost their exposure to certain pesticide residues. This difference and others are not considered thoroughly when the government determines what levels of pesticides will be allowed in the food supply, according to a major report from the National Research Council issued in 1993.

Still, the report concluded that when it comes to pesticide exposure and physiologic responses, differences between children and adults are usually less than 10-fold. Given that the EPA typically factors in a 100-fold margin of safety, the problem certainly doesn't warrant keeping fruits and vegetables out of a child's diet.

Myth: All fruits and vegetables should be washed in detergent and peeled carefully to eliminate all traces of pesticide residues.

Reality: All fresh fruits and vegetables should be

To find out everything from how to dispose of an insect repellent used in your garden to whether the chemicals your exterminator is using are safe, call the National Pesticide Telecommunications Network's toll-free hotline at 1-800-858-7378. Operators are available from 9:30 a.m. to 7:30 p.m. Eastern time, Monday through Friday.

rinsed thoroughly with water to remove any dirt, bacteria, and surface chemicals that may have come into contact with the food. Fruits and vegetables with edible peels should also be scrubbed thoroughly with a brush, and the outer leaves of lettuce, cabbage, and other greens should be removed. Most experts advise against cleaning produce with detergents, however, because soapy products may leave behind traces of other chemicals not intended for consumption.

As for peeling, it does help rid produce of pesticides, since some chemicals tend to remain on or just under the skin of fruits and vegetables. That's particularly true of waxed products, like cucumbers; the wax that gives the fruit or vegetable its shiny appearance sometimes contains fungicides. On the other hand, you might not want to make a habit of peeling every vegetable and fruit you eat; much of the fiber and cancer-fighting nutrients in produce concentrate in or just beneath the skin.

Myth: Media reports that caution consumers about pesticide residues in certain foods should be taken as warnings to avoid those foods.

Reality: Headlines and news bites alarming consumers about pesticide residues should be viewed with a skeptic's eye. Scientists have developed sophisticated techniques that enable them to detect residues of pesticides so minute as to be virtually meaningless in many cases. In other words, the mere presence of a pesticide doesn't mean it's concentrated in a large enough dose to do any harm. The real question to ask is whether the pesticide level exceeds federal limits.

Keep in mind that residues are expressed in parts per million (ppm), parts per billion (ppb), and parts per trillion (ppt). Just what does that mean in practical terms?

    1 ppm = 1 cent in $10,000, or
            1 pancake in a stack four miles high

    1 ppb = 1 second in 32 years, or
            1 inch in 16,000 miles

    1 ppt = 1 second in 32,000 years, or
            1 square foot of tile in a floor the size
            of Indiana

Myth: Once the government determines that a pesticide is unsafe for the public in any amount, its production in the United States is prohibited.

Reality: Unfortunately, between 1991 and 1994 alone, U.S. companies exported some 58 million pounds of pesticides banned for use in this country to other nations with more lax pesticide laws. This practice creates what has been dubbed "the circle of poison." Pesticides prohibited in the United States can travel the globe, boomeranging back to us through wind, rain, waterways, even imported food products. The scenario raises numerous ethical questions and highlights the necessity of considering the global, rather than just the national, impact of pesticides and other environmental contaminants.

Myth: Foods labeled organic must meet strict federal standards.

Reality: The federal government has yet to set a legal definition of "organic." Granted, 11 states currently have their own organic certification programs in place, as do 33 private organizations. Nevertheless, these programs vary in their definition of "organic" as well as in the degree to which the standards are enforced. As a result, consumers have no assurance what an organic label means.

The major roadblock to an all-encompassing federal definition has been financial. While the 1990 Farm Bill called for establishment of a national "organic" standard, funding for a staff to work out the details was not allocated until 1994. Officials at the National Organic Standards Board, the group of experts assigned to the issue, are still working away at a set of proposals to present to the governmental powers-that-be. Once a proposal has been made, it will likely be critiqued and revised before finally being set in stone—a process that could easily take another year or two.

Not in my backyard

Most people think farmers are the only people who need to take responsibility for pesticide use, but many suburbanites regularly dabble with lawn and garden chemicals that affect the environment as well. In fact, 64 million pounds of pesticides were spread on lawns and golf courses last year—amounting to 10 percent of all pesticides used in the United States. Keeping lawns green also wreaks havoc with the environment in other ways. Running a power lawn mower for one hour spews as much smog as driving a car 50 miles. And watering lawns regularly can contribute to water shortages.

Homeowners who want to care for their lawns in an eco-friendly manner can apply some of the same integrated pest management techniques currently used by farmers. The Environmental Protection Agency offers an excellent, free 18-page primer on the subject: *Healthy Lawn, Healthy Environment*. Write or call the National Center for Environmental Publications and Information, P.O. Box 42419, Cincinnati, OH 45242-2419; phone: (513) 489-8190.

While you're at it, you also might want to request another free publication, the *Citizen's Guide to Pest Control and Pesticide Safety*. This comprehensive 49-page resource covers everything from steps to control pests in and around your home; alternatives to chemical pesticides available to homeowners; ways to use, store, and dispose of pesticides safely; how to choose a pest control company; and what to do if someone is accidentally poisoned by pesticide exposure. Since pesticides are in everything from kitchen and bath disinfectants to pet collars to swimming pool chemicals, it's a booklet worth having.

AFTER THE GLOW

Irradiation is gaining new acceptance as a possible defense against foodborne contaminants like E. coli

ALAN MORTON

THIRTY NATIONS HAVE BANNED IT. CHAINS LIKE McDonald's and Boston Chicken won't have anything to do with it. Respected consumer-advocacy groups have blasted it as a serious health hazard and nutritional menace.

Yet concerns about food safety have kindled new interest in irradiation, the little-used process that kills foodborne pathogens with a burst of radiation. Proponents are touting the technology as one more safeguard against food contaminants, particularly the deadly E. coli bacterium. And their argument seems to be winning guarded support from regulators, foodservice suppliers and industry trade groups.

Influential opponents are still convinced the side effects of irradiation may be harmful even if the process itself is not. Still, advocates say the question is no longer whether food should be irradiated, but how it should be done. "It's inevitable," says Roy Martin, vice president of science and technology for the National Fisheries Institute.

That's good news for restaurants, says Robert Harrington, director of technical services for the National Restaurant Association. "We'd like to see irradiation added to the list of things available to be used" against food pathogens, he notes.

Consumers' demand for a more wholesome food supply has been repeatedly chronicled in repeated media flashbacks to the deaths two years ago of four children in the northwest U.S. who are fast-food hamburgers tainted with E. coli. One result: a petition for government approval for the irradiation of ground beef, with an estimated annual consumption of 7 billion pounds.

The public has already reacted favorably to the marketing of some irradiated foods, notably chicken treated to combat salmonella contamination. And some legislators who led efforts to ban the sale of irradiated products in their states are now rethinking their positions, particularly with the advent of new technology that would use electricity—rather than radioactive isotopes—to produce the irradiation.

But, Harrington is quick to point out, "it's definitely not a panacea." Health authorities stress that even irradiated foods can be contaminated through subsequent mishandling. "Food irradiation, like pasteurization of milk, can prevent countless infections," Dr. Phillip R. Lee, director of the U.S. Public Health Service, wrote last summer in the *Journal of the American Medical Association*. Yet "irradiation would neither replace good manufacturing practices nor provide the sole answer to foodborne illnesses."

A new push for safety at the point of production came in October when the U.S. Department of Agriculture reclassified E. coli O157:H7 as an illegal adulterant instead of a natural contaminant. Meat suppliers would be subject to hefty penalties if the bacteria were found in their products, and the USDA said it would conduct 5,000 sampling tests a year to enforce the regulation.

The American Meat Institute and other associations went to court to stop the USDA, claiming that the agency didn't have the authority to promulgate such a rule. But their request for an injunction was denied.

And so, says Dr. Joe Borsa, head of radiation applications for AECL Research in Canada, "The pressure is building" to make irradiation more widespread. "As far as I know there's only one effective technique for cleaning up meat with pathogens and that's irradiation," Borsa says.

The USDA's plan carries heavy economic implications for meat processors because E. coli O157:H7 is hard to detect without a comprehensive and costly effort. But even a few of the bacteria can be deadly if the screening isn't thorough.

"It takes millions of, say, salmonella organisms to cause disease," says Dennis Olson, meat irradiation researcher at Iowa State University, "but it takes just 10 of O157:H7 to cause illness and death."

Cooking to the well-done stage—at least 155°F.—kills E. coli, though some consumers stubbornly insist on having

Regulators are already considering proposals to permit the irradiation of ground beef and seafood

Reprinted with permission from *Restaurant Business,* February 10, 1995, pp. 42, 44, 48, 53. © 1995 by Bill Communications, Inc.

their meat cooked rare. But if other stringent safety measures are in place, the risk of contamination may be insignificant for most beef cuts.

Hamburger is another story. As a recent TV news report noted, a ground-beef patty could contain meat from 100 animals, any one of which may have harbored the deadly bacterium. Because irradiation would be used on whole patties prior to shipping, an E. coli bug would be destroyed regardless of its source.

So even though the American Meat Institute opposes USDA meat-sampling plans, the AMI is throwing its weight behind research to develop irradiation techniques to produce disease-free ground beef with acceptable taste and odor.

FOR STARTERS, THE AMI IS SUPPORTING A PETItion that the Food and Drug Administration approve the sale of irradiated ground beef and other meat products. The petition was written by a well-known irradiation consultant, Dr. George Giddings, and presented on July 6 by Isomedix, a New Jersey-based company with a string of irradiation plants dedicated mainly to sterilizing medical supplies.

In November the petition appeared well on the road to approval although the FDA itself, as is its practice, would not predict a date for it. "We're in touch with the FDA every couple of weeks," says Isomedix senior vice president George R. Dietz, who was hoping for clearance early in 1995.

The Isomedix irradiation facilities use gamma rays produced by radioactive cobalt-60 or cesium-137. The radioactive rods are typically kept in 20-ft. pools of water that absorb the rays when out of use; the rods are raised to treat products.

The AMI is also backing research into the irradiation of meat using electron beams, instead of radioactive rods. A French-made machine of this type at Iowa State University in Ames has been irradiating ground beef patties, pork and other meat cuts since March 1993.

Project director Dennis Olson says the emphasis of the experiment is to preserve the quality of the meat patties. He says irradiation initially triggers an unusual odor, but taste is unaffected.

"We came across a similar situation when we first started vacuum-packing 25 years ago," says Olson. "You got an odor that dissipates quickly."

AMI also has been negotiating with Sandia National Laboratories in Albuquerque to adapt the labs' Repetitive High Energy Pulsed Power (RHEPP) electron-beam accelerator—originally created to test the radiation-resistance of components in nuclear missiles—as an irradiation device. Sandia senior researcher Ronald J. Kaye says commercial application "could be two to three years away."

The AMI sees a variety of advantages in electron-beam accelerators, which can be used to produce X-rays by slamming the electrons into plates of metal such as tungsten. Unlike the cobalt-60 devices, the electron beams can be switched on and off, and could be placed right on the meat-processing line.

And perhaps most significantly, an electronic device is much easier to sell to the public than a radioactive one. As AMI spokesperson James Marsden puts it: "It has much less emotional baggage."

The big difference between Iowa State's machine and Sandia's version is that the latter emits powerful pulses—up to 120 a second—instead of a continuous stream of electrons. The RHEPP's high power is useful in the inherently inefficient process of converting the electron beam to X-rays—which are necessary for the effective irradiation of products in boxes or on pallets.

About 40 cobalt-60 irradiation plants already exist in the country and are mostly used for sterilizing medical products. However, Andrew Welt, vice president of a New Jersey accelerator-design company, Alpha Omega Technology Inc., points out that most existing plants are already operating near capacity and could not handle the increase in volume that could come with the sudden mass irradiation of food. Alpha Omega is one of two companies petitioning the FDA for approval to irradiate fish.

Welt also says that the existing plants are not all that adaptable. Many are designed to punch high doses of radiation into things like cotton balls and cosmetics at close range, perhaps a few centimeters. Doses for food would have to be much smaller, with delivery at ranges of up to 15 feet.

The cost of opening an irradiation plant, whether electronic or radioactive, runs about $4 million, says Welt. On top of that, the cobalt-60 has to be replenished: In a typical plant, an initial 2 million curies (a measure of radioactivity) at $1.65 a curie decays at 12.3% a year—more than $400,000 worth—and delivers progressively less irradiation.

On the other hand, electron-beam plants run up some hefty costs in the form of heavy utility bills. These economic factors stand in the way of any rush to irradiate food on a mass scale.

As for existing projects, Mulberry, Fla.'s Food TECHnology Service Inc. irradiated its first product —strawberries, to extend shelf life—three years ago and has since added other produce, seafood and chicken. The company uses a cobalt-60 source but is exploring the use of electron-beam machines, which is one reason the firm changed its name from Vindicator, says safety director Fred Harris.

In operation, the plant's procedures are as varied as the products it contracts to handle. While much of the fruit and vegetables it irradiates are for the U.S. market, Harris says, the seafood—notably shrimp—is for export only, pending government clearance for domestic sales.

THE ADDED COST FOR IRRADIATED FOOD, HE says, is only pennies per pound. "As far as the consumer is concerned, we think the average serving" of irradiated chicken "in a fast-food restaurant is going to cost one-quarter cent more," Harris says. "That cost may be negligible because of the benefit they're going to derive from having a safer product," thus avoiding potential medical bills for consumers and food spoilage for restaurants.

Harris says his company is discussing plans for new plants in the Midwest, "closer to the beef and poultry producers." If they go ahead, he says, "our plant here [in Florida] would be more of a training site."

A number of restaurant chains have promised customers or shareholders that they would not serve irradiated food. McDonald's, for instance, was pressured to take the vow by some institutional investors.

Proponents say the cost of irradiating a fast-food chicken sandwich should be well below a penny

And even if they wanted to do so, irradiated products are not currently available in sufficient quantities. "Our plant is the only USDA-approved facility [for chicken] at this point," Harris says.

But Food TECHnology has found no problem with public acceptance of irradiated products, he says. A frozen chicken irradiated by the concern goes to a variety of outlets, including the Carrot Top produce market in McDonald's hometown of Oak Brook, Ill. Irradiated chicken is the only type that the store currently carries.

"The product is selling very well," says Carrot Top owner James Corrigan. But, he adds, customers clearly prefer fresh chicken to frozen.

Corrigan says he's negotiating with his neighbor for possible expansion of his 5,000-sq.-ft. store. And he's in talks with Isomedix to have locally produced chicken processed at its nearby Martin Grove irradiation facility for sale fresh, not frozen. Although FDA approval would be needed, he says, local chicken producers are solidly behind him.

Meanwhile, irradiation is getting a boost from other quarters. Irradiation of fruits and vegetables, in use since 1986 to control insects and ripening, is in line for expansion. Methyl bromide, used for years to fumigate warehoused produce, has been ordered phased out by the year 2000 because it contributes to ozone depletion. Something is going to have to take its place, and irradiation is a prime prospect.

Meanwhile, the FDA is examining two petitions for irradiation of seafood. Alpha Omega submitted one in late 1990, according to Welt. And United States Harvest Technologies Inc. of Baltimore was cleared to submit its petition in April 1991 and has been working on it since, according to chairman and CEO William L. Robinson Jr.

"We would like to see both petitions adopted by the FDA," says the National Fisheries Institute's Martin. "But we think it will take a while."

The FDA's interest in the proposals is whetted by the current concern over contamination of shellfish from the Gulf of Mexico, especially by an organism called vibrio vunificus. The microbe could be eliminated with irradiation.

But foes of irradiation remain active. Organizations such as the Center for Science in the Public Interest, the International Organization of Consumer Unions and Food and Water Inc. oppose the technology on several grounds—ranging from the possible danger associated with the transportation of radioactive cobalt, to concern that irradiation can reduce the nutritional value of food, to fears that the process will create disease-causing or carcinogenic agents within the treated products.

Even STOP—Safe Tables Our Priority, a food-safety group created in the wake of fast-food hamburger deaths by parents and acquaintances of the school-aged victims—opposes irradiation. It worries that the meat industry will use it as a substitute for safe meat-handling practices.

And the opponents have achieved results: Some 30 countries have laws against selling irradiated food, as do the states of New York and Maine.

Yet irradiation proponents can count some heavyweights within their ranks: Close to 40 countries permit food irradiation with France, the Netherlands and South Africa making extensive use of it. The practice also has the strong support of the World Health Organization, not to mention the American Medical Association.

Other domestic powerhouses are clearly warming to the idea. "The science that we've seen does not support concern about irradiation," says Jerry Redding, national communication coordinator of the USDA.

Even some locales that initially opposed irradiation are now reconsidering its use. New Jersey, for example, allowed its moratorium on the sale of irradiated food to expire a couple of years ago.

And New York's legislature is taking a new look at the law that currently bans sale of all irradiated foods except spices and special sterilized diet items for certain hospital patients.

Yet the bill's author, state Sen. William Sears, also introduced a bill that would consider ramifications of the law's repeal in view of what a spokesman called "a lot of evidence on both sides."

Among those watching the development is the Institute of Food Technologists, whose official stance on irradiation sums up the ongoing battle:

"Extension of the ban of food irradiation in New York State is not justified on any scientific basis nor is it in the public's best interest," the Institute says. "When provided factual information about the process, consumers will choose irradiated foods with confidence."

Not enough processing facilities are open in the U.S. to meet the demand for widespread irradiation of food

Health Claims

Quackery has no such friend as credulity.

—C. Simmons

In ancient Rome, Cato the elder prescribed cabbages to cure "everything that ails you" and continued to do so even though his wife died from the "fevers." London pharmacists, in 1632, believed that bananas were so important to health that only trained druggists should administer them. Early in the history of this country, Elisha Perkins promoted vinegar as the cure for yellow fever, yet he died of this disease. All were sincere but wrong. Yet, almost any product, device, or regimen that promises the moon and 5 miles more will develop a following of users and believers.

Quackery is misinformation about health, according to the Food and Drug Administration (FDA). Certain fallacious statements have been made repeatedly by promoters for years, among them: "The American food supply is worthless because it is grown on depleted soil," "Everybody needs vitamin supplements for insurance," "Sugar from honey is healthier than table sugar," and "Natural is better." Such misinformation may be easier to find than facts. For example, popular talk show hosts provide a good promotional forum for misinformation, since their need to capture a large audience draws sensationalism. Nutritionists often have despaired of counteracting the exaggerated and blatantly false information frequently distributed through the popular information media.

But we can assume that anyone interested enough to read *this* book, much less take a nutrition course, is also able to avoid being taken in by misinformation and quackery. Right? Probably not! Will Rogers said, "Everybody is ignorant, only on different subjects," and it takes a great deal of knowledge and consciousness to effectively counteract promoters. Perpetrators of quackery have changed with the times, but their characteristics and goals are the same. At one time or another, most of us—perhaps all of us—have been victims. For this reason, it is critical to understand how manipulators adroitly influence the buying of both ideas and products. Only then will consumers be armed to defend themselves. Toward that end the articles in this unit were chosen.

The first article, "How Quackery Sells," will help you understand the strategies of promoters who have fine-tuned the art of selling to an exquisitely high level. They know how to influence the emotions of the vulnerable, easily convinced customer so that he or she will buy even though some small inner voice advises against it.

The next three articles are concerned with accurate reporting in the media, an important issue since surveys have shown the media to be the primary source of nutrition and food-safety information. In "Confessions of a Former Women's Magazine Writer," Marilynn Larkin, describes how a long-time writer of nutrition articles wrote mainly to make advertisers happy, conscientiously avoiding the use of any information unflattering to the advertisers. By the time she had also manipulated content to conform to the art director's specifications and had ensured (following the publisher's directives) that the reader would not be intellectually challenged, little of substance was left. It is good news, then, that the American Council on Science and Health (ACSH) reports improvement in the quality of nutrition articles found in 20 popular magazines. Nutrition experts rated these magazines for accuracy, presentation style, and recommendations offered. Only minor errors were found in *Better Homes and Gardens, Consumer Reports,* and *Parents,* resulting in very high scores. Twelve others were rated as "good," and *Cosmopolitan* alone was found to be "very poor."

Many of us are relying more and more on the Internet for answers to our questions. Here, too we must be watchful—perhaps even more so, for Web sites and e-mail capabilities allow the easy and rapid promotion of virtually anything. Guidelines for recognizing and avoiding unreliable sites are suggested in the article on spotting a "quacky" Web site. This article comes from a reliable Web site itself and is one of those sites suggested as a new feature of this *Annual Edition.*

When nutrition advice seems to be constantly changing and contradictory, it may also confuse and discourage the consumer. "Why Do These #&*?@! 'Experts' Keep Changing Their Minds?" deals with this issue, explaining that finding the truth is a process, not an event. Thus, recommendations will forever be altered as science becomes more sophisticated and increasingly able to build on prior knowledge. It pays to remain somewhat skeptical, and it certainly pays to wait for general acceptance of theories and information by the experts before jumping on a bandwagon.

Several articles on supplements are included in this edition. In 1994, with the passage of the Dietary Supplement Health and Education Act (DSHEA), Congress made it easier for the large cadre of dedicated vitamin pushers and

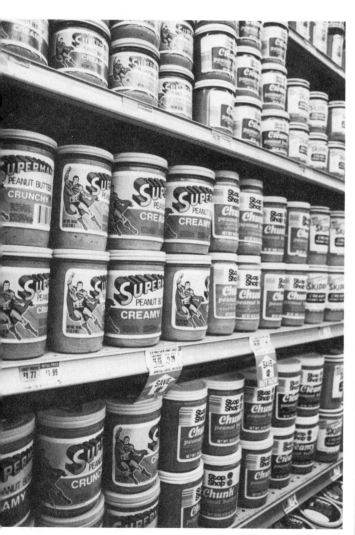

ment is unsafe before it can be removed from the market. Proof of effectiveness is not required to enter or remain on the market.

In a similar vein, advertising now tries to convince lots of us that we need the same specialty products originally developed for use by the weak and the ill in nursing homes and hospitals. It can be argued that, appropriately used, they are a good addition to the choices available. However, as insurance against deficiencies, they make little sense for most of us and may promote the notion that a complete and healthful diet is unlikely or impossible. This is simply untrue.

The final topic, a discussion of athletes and supplements, is included in this unit because athletes typically are searching for a competitive edge and are extremely vulnerable to supplement promotionals. The assortment of promoted products ranges from amino acids for building muscle and creatine for a speedier recovery to products claiming to energize the liver or burn fat. However, athletes should look to a good diet and within themselves, not in a bottle or box.

Victor Herbert has said that consumers with misinformation about nutrition typically fall into two categories: the deceived and the deluded. The deceived, he says, will respond to education, while the deluded are adamant—even fanatical—about their beliefs and will refuse to consider good scientific data or a logical presentation. This unit is offered to readers who are either already informed or are among the deceived searching for answers.

Looking Ahead: Challenge Questions

Why do you think people are so vulnerable to quackery? When have you been a victim?

Identify three current fallacies that you believe are the most dangerous to nutritional health? Why are they fallacies?

Make a list of characteristics you would look for in a *reliable* information source. Use them to evaluate nutrition articles in your local newspaper or a nutrition-oriented talk show.

What provisions would you change or add to the Dietary Supplement Health and Education Act of 1994 to increase its effectiveness?

Explore a variety of Web sites for nutrition information and decide if they offer reliable information.

supplement promoters to expand their sales to a $6 billion a year enterprise, selling in stores, spas, offices, or from door to door. At the same time it became more difficult for the FDA to protect consumers. Well-orchestrated by the supplement industry, passage of this bill expanded the definition of "dietary supplements" to include many additional products. This precludes effectively regulating supplements as drugs, which require the manufacturer's proof of safety and efficacy before they can be sold. By contrast, the FDA must now prove that a dietary supple-

HOW QUACKERY SELLS

William T. Jarvis, Ph.D.
Stephen Barrett, M.D.

Dr. Jarvis is a professor in the Department of Preventive Medicine at Loma Linda University and president of the National Council Against Health Fraud.

Dr. Barrett, who practices psychiatry in Allentown, Pennsylvania, is a board member of the National Council Against Health Fraud. In 1984 he received the FDA Commissioner's Special Citation Award for Public Service in fighting nutrition quackery.

Modern health quacks are supersalesmen. They play on fear. They cater to hope. And once they have you, they'll keep you coming back for more . . . and more . . . and more. Seldom do their victims realize how often or how skillfully they are cheated. Does the mother who feels good as she hands her child a vitamin think to ask herself whether he really needs it? Do subscribers to "health food" publications realize that articles are slanted to stimulate business for their advertisers? Not usually.

Most people think that quackery is easy to spot, but it is not. Its promoters wear the cloak of science. They use scientific terms and quote (or misquote) scientific references. On talk shows, they may be introduced as "scientists ahead of their time." The very word "quack" helps their camouflage by making us think of an outlandish character selling snake oil from the back of a covered wagon—and, of course, no intelligent people would buy snake oil nowadays, would they?

Well, maybe snake oil isn't selling so well, lately. But acupuncture? "Organic" foods? Mouthwash? Hair analysis? The latest diet book? Megavitamins? "Stress" formulas? Cholesterol-lowering teas? Homeopathic remedies? Nutritional "cures" for AIDS? Or shots to pep you up? Business is booming for health quacks. Their annual take is in the *billions!* Spot reducers, "immune boosters," water purifiers, "ergogenic aids," systems to "balance body chemistry," special diets for arthritis. Their product list is endless.

What sells is not the quality of their products but their ability to influence their audience. To those in pain, they promise relief. To the incurable, they offer hope. To the nutrition-conscious, they say, "Make sure you have enough." To a public worried about pollution, they say, "Buy natural." To one and all, they promise better health and a longer life. Modern quacks can reach people emotionally, on the level that counts the most. This article shows how they do it.

Appeals to Vanity

An attractive young airline stewardess once told a physician that she was taking more than 20 vitamin pills a day. "I used to feel run-down all the time," she said, "but now I feel really great!"

"Yes," the doctor replied, "but there is no scientific evidence that extra vitamins can do that. Why not take the pills one month on, one month off, to see whether they really help you or whether it's just a coincidence. After all, $300 a year is a lot of money to be wasting."

"Look, doctor," she said. "I don't care what you say. I KNOW the pills are helping me."

How was this bright young woman converted into a true believer? First, an appeal to her curiosity persuaded her to try and see. Then an appeal to her vanity convinced her to disregard scientific evidence in favor of personal experience—to *think for herself.* Supplementation is encouraged by a distorted concept of *biochemical individuality*—that everyone is unique enough to disregard the Recommended Dietary Allowances (RDAs). Quacks will not tell you that scientists deliberately set the RDAs high enough to allow for individual differences. A more dangerous appeal of this type is the suggestion that although a remedy for a serious disease has not been shown to work for other people, *it still might work for you. (You are extraordinary!)*

A more subtle appeal to your vanity underlies the message of the TV ad quack: *Do it yourself—be your own doctor.* "Anyone out there have 'tired blood'?" he used to wonder. (Don't bother to find out what's wrong with you, however. Just try my tonic.) "Troubled with irregularity?" he asks. (Pay no attention to the doctors who say you don't need a daily movement. Just use my laxative.) "Want to kill germs on contact?" (Never mind that mouthwash doesn't prevent colds.) "Trouble sleeping?" (Don't bother to solve the underlying problem. Just try my sedative.)

Turning Customers Into Salespeople

Most people who think they have been helped by an unorthodox method enjoy sharing their success stories with their

Reprinted with permission from *Nutrition Forum*, March/April 1991, pp. 9-13. © 1991 by Prometheus Books, 59 John Glenn Drive, Amherst, NY 14228.

friends. People who give such *testimonials* are usually motivated by a sincere wish to *help their fellow humans.* Rarely do they realize how difficult it is to evaluate a "health" product on the basis of personal experience. Like the airline stewardess, the average person who feels better after taking a product will not be able to rule out coincidence— or the placebo effect (feeling better because he thinks he has taken a positive step). Since we tend to believe what others tell us of personal experiences, testimonials can be powerful persuaders. Despite their unreliability, they are the cornerstone of the quack's success.

Multilevel companies that sell nutritional products systematically turn their customers into salespeople. "When you share our products," says the sales manual of one such company, "you're not just selling. You're passing on news about products you believe in to people you care about. Make a list of people you know; you'll be surprised how long it will be. This list is your first source of potential customers." A sales leader from another company suggests, "Answer all objections with *testimonials.* That's the secret to *motivating* people!"

Don't be surprised if one of your friends or neighbors tries to sell you vitamins. More than a million Americans have signed up as multilevel distributors. Like many drug addicts, they become suppliers to support their habit. A typical sales pitch goes like this: "How would you like to look better, feel better and have more energy? Try my vitamins for a few weeks." People normally have ups and downs, and a friend's interest or suggestion, or the thought of taking a positive step, may actually make a person feel better. Many who try the vitamins will mistakenly think they have been helped—and continue to buy them, usually at inflated prices.

Faked endorsements are being used to promote anti-aging products and other nostrums sold by mail. The literature, which resembles a newspaper page with an ad on one side and news on the other, contains what appears to be a handwritten note from a friend (identified by first initial). "Dear Anne," it might say, "This really works. Try it! B." Although both the product and the "newspaper page" are fakes, many recipients wonder who among their acquaintances might have signed the note.

The Use of Fear

The sale of vitamins has become so profitable that some otherwise reputable manufacturers are promoting them with misleading claims. For example, for many years, Lederle Laboratories (makers of *Stresstabs*) and Hoffmann-La Roche advertised in major magazines that stress "robs" the body of vitamins and creates significant danger of vitamin deficiencies. Another slick way for quackery to attract customers is the *invented disease.* Virtually everyone has symptoms of one sort or another—minor aches or pains, reactions to stress or hormone variations, effects of aging, etc. Labeling these ups and downs of life as symptoms of disease enables the quack to provide "treatment."

Reactive hypoglycemia" is one such diagnosis. For decades, talk show "experts" and misguided physicians have preached that anxiety, headaches, weakness, dizziness, stomach upset, and other common reactions are often caused by "low blood sugar." But the facts are otherwise. Hypoglycemia is rare. Proper administration of blood sugar tests is required to make the

diagnosis. A study of people who thought they had hypoglycemia showed that half of them had symptoms during a glucose tolerance test even though their blood sugar levels remained normal.

"Yeast allergy" is another favorite quack diagnosis. Here the symptoms are blamed on a "hidden" infection that is treated with antifungal drugs, special diets, and vitamin concoctions.

Food safety and environmental protection are important issues in our society. But rather than approach them logically, the food quacks exaggerate and oversimplify. To promote "organic" foods, they lump all additives into one class and attack them as "poisonous." They never mention that natural toxicants are prevented or destroyed by modern food technology. Nor do they let on that many additives are naturally occurring substances.

Sugar has been subject to particularly vicious attacks, being (falsely) blamed for most of the world's ailments. But quacks do more than warn about imaginary ailments. They sell "antidotes" for real ones. Care for some vitamin C to reduce the danger of smoking? Or some vitamin E to combat air pollutants? See your local supersalesman.

Quackery's most serious form of fear-mongering has been its attack on water fluoridation. Although fluoridation's safety is established beyond scientific doubt, well-planned scare campaigns have persuaded thousands of communities not to adjust the fluoride content of their water to prevent cavities. Millions of innocent children have suffered as a result.

Hope for Sale

Since ancient times, people have sought at least four different magic potions: the love potion, the fountain of youth, the cure-all, and the athletic superpill. Quackery always has been willing to cater to these desires. It used to offer unicorn horn, special elixirs, amulets, and magical brews. Today's products are vitamins, bee pollen, ginseng, *Gerovital,* "glandular extracts," and many more. Even reputable products are promoted as though they are potions. Toothpastes and colognes will improve our love life. Hair preparations and skin products will make us look "younger than our years." And Olympic athletes tell us that breakfast cereals will make us champions.

False hope for the seriously ill is the cruelest form of quackery because it can lure victims away from effective treatment. Even when death is inevitable, however, false hope can do great damage. Experts who study the dying process tell us that while the initial reaction is shock and disbelief, most terminally ill patients will adjust very well as long as they do not feel abandoned. People who accept the reality of their fate not only die psychologically prepared, but also can put their affairs in order. On the other hand, those who buy false hope can get stuck in an attitude of denial. They waste financial resources and, worse yet, their remaining time.

The choice offered by the quack is not between hope and despair but between false hope and a chance to adjust to reality. Yet hope springs eternal. The late Jerry Walsh was a severe arthritic who crusaded coast-to-coast debunking arthritis quackery on behalf of the Arthritis Foundation. After a television appearance early in his career, he received 5,700 letters. One hundred congratulated him for blasting the quacks, but 4,500 were from arthritis victims who asked where they could obtain the very fakes he was exposing!

Clinical Tricks

The most important characteristic to which the success of quacks can be attributed is probably their ability to exude confidence. Even when they admit that a method is unproven, they can attempt to minimize this by mentioning how difficult and expensive it is to get something proven to the satisfaction of the FDA these days. If they exude *self-confidence* and enthusiasm, it is likely to be contagious and spread to patients and their loved ones.

Because people like the idea of making choices, quacks often refer to their methods as *"alternatives."* Correctly used, it can refer to aspirin and Tylenol as alternatives for the treatment of minor aches and pains. Both are proven safe and effective for the same purpose. Lumpectomy can be an alternative to radical mastectomy for breast cancer. Both have verifiable records of safety and effectiveness from which judgments can be drawn. Can a method that is unsafe, ineffective or unproven be a genuine alternative to one that is proven? Obviously not.

Quacks don't always limit themselves to phony treatment. Sometimes they offer legitimate treatment as well—the quackery is promoted as *something extra.* One example is the "ortho-molecular" treatment of mental disorders with high dosages of vitamins in addition to orthodox forms of treatment. Patients who receive the "extra" treatment often become convinced that they need to take vitamins for the rest of their life. Such an outcome is inconsistent with the goal of good medical care, which should be to discourage unnecessary treatment.

The *one-sided coin* is a related ploy. When patients on combined (orthodox and quack) treatment improve, the quack remedy (e.g., laetrile) gets the credit. If things go badly, the patient is told that he arrived too late, and conventional treatment gets the blame. Some quacks who mix proven and unproven treatment call their approach *complementary therapy.*

Quacks also capitalize on the natural healing powers of the body by *taking credit* whenever possible for improvement in a patient's condition. One multilevel company—anxious to avoid legal difficulty in marketing its herbal concoction—makes no health claims whatsoever. "You take the product," a spokesperson suggests on the company's introductory videotape, "and tell me what it does for you." An opposite tack—*shifting blame*—is used by many cancer quacks. If their treatment doesn't work, it's because radiation and/or chemotherapy have "knocked out the immune system."

To promote their ideas, quacks often use a trick where they bypass an all-important basic question and *ask a second question* which, by itself, is not valid. An example of a "second question" is "Why don't the people of Hunza get cancer?" The quack's answer is "because they eat apricot pits" (or some other claim). The first question should have been "Do the people of Hunza get cancer?" The answer is "Yes!" Every group of people on earth gets cancer. So do all animals (vegetarians and meat-eaters alike) and plants. Another common gambit is the question, "Do you believe in vitamins?" The real question should be, "Does the average person eating a well balanced diet need to take supplements?" The answer is no.

Another selling trick is the use of *weasel words.* Quacks often use this technique in suggesting that one or more items on a list is reason to suspect that you *may* have a vitamin deficiency, a yeast infection, or whatever else they are offering to fix.

The *money-back guarantee* is a favorite trick of mail-order quacks. Most have no intention of returning any money—but even those who are willing know that few people will bother to return the product.

Another powerful persuader—*something for nothing*—is standard in advertisements promising effortless weight loss. It is also the hook of the telemarketer who promises a "valuable free prize" as a bonus for buying a water purifier, a 6-month supply of vitamins, or some other health or nutrition product. Those who bite receive either nothing or items worth far less than their cost. Credit card customers may also find unauthorized charges to their account.

The willingness to believe that a stranger can supply unique and valuable "inside" information—such as a tip on a horse race or the stock market—seems to be a universal human quirk. Quacks take full advantage of this trait in their promotion of *secret cures.* True scientists don't keep their breakthroughs secret. They share them with all mankind. If this were not so, we would still be going to private clinics for the vaccines and other medications used to conquer smallpox, polio, tuberculosis, and many other serious diseases.

Seductive Tactics

The practice of healing involves both art and science. The art includes all that is done for the patient psychologically. The science involves what is done about the disease itself. If a disease is psychosomatic, art may be all that is needed. The old-time doctor did not have much science in his little black bag, so he relied more upon the art (called his "bedside manner") and everyone loved him. Today, there is a great deal of science in the bag, but the art has been relatively neglected.

In a contest for patient satisfaction, art will beat science nearly every time. Quacks are masters at the art of delivering health care. The secret to this art is to make the patient believe that he is cared about as a person. To do this, quacks *lather love lavishly.* One way this is done is by having receptionists make notes on the patients' interests and concerns in order to recall them during future visits. This makes each patient feel special in a very personal sort of way. Some quacks even send birthday cards to every patient. Although seductive tactics may give patients a powerful psychological lift, they may also encourage over-reliance on an inappropriate therapy.

Handling the Opposition

Quacks are involved in a constant struggle with legitimate health care providers, mainstream scientists, government regulatory agencies, and consumer protection groups. Despite the strength of this orthodox opposition, quackery manages to flourish. To maintain their credibility, quacks use a variety of clever propaganda ploys. Here are some favorites:

"They persecuted Galileo!" The history of science is laced with instances where great pioneers and their discoveries were met with resistance. Harvey (nature of blood circulation), Lister (antiseptic technique), and Pasteur (germ theory) are notable examples. Today's quack boldly asserts that he is another

example of someone ahead of his time. Close examination, however, will show how unlikely this is. First of all, the early pioneers who were persecuted lived during times that were much less scientific. In some cases, opposition to their ideas stemmed from religious forces. Second, it is a basic principle of the scientific method that the burden of proof belongs to the proponent of a claim. The ideas of Galileo, Harvey, Lister, and Pasteur overcame their opposition because their soundness could be demonstrated.

A related ploy, which is a favorite with cancer quacks, is the charge of "*conspiracy.*" How can we be sure that the AMA, the FDA, the American Cancer Society, and others are not involved in some monstrous plot to withhold a cancer cure from the public? To begin with, history reveals no such practice in the past. The elimination of serious diseases is not a threat to the medical profession—doctors prosper by curing diseases, not by keeping people sick. It should also be apparent that modern medical technology has not altered the zeal of scientists to eliminate disease. When polio was conquered, iron lungs became virtually obsolete, but nobody resisted this advancement because it would force hospitals to change. Neither will medical scientists mourn the eventual defeat of cancer.

Moreover, how could a conspiracy to withhold a cancer cure hope to be successful? Many physicians die of cancer each year. Do you believe that the vast majority of doctors would conspire to withhold a cure for a disease that affects them, their colleagues, and their loved ones? To be effective, a conspiracy would have to be worldwide. If laetrile, for example, really worked, many other nations' scientists would soon realize it.

Organized quackery poses its opposition to medical science as a philosophical conflict rather than a conflict about proven versus unproven or fraudulent methods. This creates the illusion of a "holy war" rather than a conflict that could be resolved by examining the facts.

Quacks like to charge that "*Science doesn't have all the answers.*" That's true, but it doesn't claim to have them. Rather, it is a rational and responsible process that can answer many questions—including whether procedures are safe and effective for their intended purpose. It is quackery that constantly claims to have answers for incurable diseases. The idea that people should turn to quack remedies when frustrated by science's inability to control a disease is irrational. Science may not have all the answers, but quackery has no answers at all! It will take your money and break your heart.

Many treatments advanced by the scientific community are later shown to be unsafe or worthless. Such failures become grist for organized quackery's public relations mill in its ongoing attack on science. Actually, "failures" reflect a key element of science: its willingness to test its methods and beliefs and abandon those shown to be invalid. True medical scientists have no philosophical commitment to particular treatment approaches, only a commitment to develop and use methods that are safe and effective for an intended purpose.

When a quack remedy flunks a scientific test, its proponents merely reject the test. Science writer John J. Fried provides a classic description of this in his book, *Vitamin Politics:*

Because vitamin enthusiasts believe in publicity more than they believe in accurate scientific investigation, they use the media to perpetuate their faulty ideas without ever having to face up to the fallacies of their nonsensical theories. They announce to the world that horse manure, liberally rubbed into the scalp, will

cure, oh, brain tumors. Researchers from the establishment side, under pressure to verify the claims, will run experiments and find that the claim is wrong. The enthusiasts will not retire to their laboratories to rethink their position. Not at all. They will announce to the world that the establishment wasn't using enough horse manure, or that it didn't use the horse manure long enough, or that it used horse manure from the wrong kind of horses. The process is never-ending. . . . The public is the ultimate loser in this charade.

Promoters of laetrile were notorious for shifting their claims. First they claimed that laetrile could cure cancer. Then they said it could not cure but could prevent or control cancer. Then they claimed laetrile was a vitamin and that cancer was a disease caused by a vitamin deficiency. Today they say that laetrile alone is not enough—it is part of "metabolic therapy," which includes special diet, supplement concoctions, and other modalities that vary from practitioner to practitioner.

The *disclaimer* is a related tactic. Instead of promising to cure your specific disease, some quacks will offer to "cleanse" or "detoxify" your body, balance its chemistry, release its "nerve energy," bring it in harmony with nature, or do other things to "help the body to heal itself." This type of disclaimer serves two purposes. Since it is impossible to measure the processes the quack describes, it is difficult to prove him wrong. In addition, if the quack is not a physician, the use of nonmedical terminology may help to avoid prosecution for practicing medicine without a license.

Books espousing unscientific practices typically suggest that the reader consult a doctor before following their advice. This disclaimer is intended to protect the author and publisher from legal responsibility for any dangerous ideas contained in the book. Both author and publisher know full well, however, that most people will not ask their doctor. If they wanted their doctor's advice, they probably would not be reading the book in the first place. Sometimes the quack will say, "You may have come to me too late, but I will try my best to help you." That way, if the treatment fails, you have only yourself to blame. Patients who see the light and abandon quack treatment may also be blamed for stopping too soon.

"Health Freedom"

If quacks cannot win by playing according to the rules, they try to change the rules by switching from the scientific to the political arena. In science, a medical claim is treated as false until proven beyond a reasonable doubt. But in politics, a medical claim may be accepted until proven false or harmful beyond a reasonable doubt. This is why proponents of laetrile, chiropractic, orthomolecular psychiatry, chelation therapy, and the like, take their case to legislators rather than to scientific groups.

Quacks use the concept of "*health freedom*" to divert attention away from themselves and toward victims of disease with whom we are naturally sympathetic. "These poor folks should have the freedom to choose whatever treatments they want," cry the quacks—with crocodile tears. They want us to overlook two things. First, no one wants to be cheated, especially in matters of life and health. Victims of disease do not demand quack treatments because they want to exercise their "rights," but because they have been deceived into thinking that they offer hope. Second, the laws against worthless nostrums are not directed against the victims of disease but at the promoters who attempt to exploit them.

Any threat to freedom strikes deeply into American cultural values. But we must also realize that complete freedom is appropriate only in a society in which everyone is perfectly trustworthy—and no such society exists. Experience has taught us that quackery can even lead people to poison themselves, their children, and their friends.

It is because of the vulnerability of the desperately ill that consumer protection laws have been passed. These laws simply require that products offered in the health marketplace be both safe and effective. If only safety were required, any substance that would not kill you on the spot could be hawked to the gullible.

Some people claim we have too much government regulation. But the issue should be one of quality, not quantity. We can always use good regulatory laws. Our opposition should be toward bad regulations that stifle our economy or cramp our lifestyles unnecessarily. Consumer protection laws need to be preserved.

Unfortunately, some politicians seem oblivious to these basic principles and expound the "health freedom" concept as though they are doing their constituents a favor. In reality, "health freedom" constitutes a hunting license for quackery, with open season declared on the sick, the frightened, the alienated, and the desperate. It represents a return to the law of the jungle in which the strong feed upon the weak.

How to Avoid Being Tricked

The best way to avoid being tricked is to stay away from tricksters. Unfortunately, in health matters, this is no simple task. Quackery is not sold with a warning label. Moreover, the dividing line between what is quackery and what is not is by no means sharp. A product that is effective in one situation may be part of a quack scheme in another. (Quackery lies in the promise, not the product). Practitioners who use effective methods may also use ineffective ones. For example, they may mix valuable advice to stop smoking with unsound advice to take vitamins. Even outright quacks may relieve some psychosomatic ailments with their reassuring manner.

This article illustrates how adept quacks are at selling themselves. Sad to say, in most contests between quacks and ordinary people, the quacks still are likely to win.

CONFESSIONS OF A FORMER WOMEN'S MAGAZINE WRITER

Marilynn Larkin

Ms. Larkin is a freelance writer in New York City. In 1985, she received a first-place award for consumer journalism from the National Press Club. Her most recent work is *What You Can Do About Anemia* [Dell Publishing, 1993].

Writing about "hot" nutrition topics still has impact. During the decade or so that I wrote for women's magazines, I received much positive feedback from readers.

In 1989, at the height of oat bran's popularity as a panacea to lower cholesterol, the president and chief operating officer of a leading cereal manufacturer estimated that sales of oat-bran cereals would grow to nearly $600 million annually. I wrote five oat-bran stories that year for various women's magazines. A year later, when a study called oat bran's health-promoting properties into question, sales plummeted 50 percent within a week; at that point, I couldn't give away an article on oat bran.

I also covered other "hot" nutrition topics. But although they appeared on the nutrition page, these articles tended to be either "food-of-the-month" stories (the grapefruit diet, carrot power) or quasi-entertainment pieces that positioned foods as medicine: to fight cancer, strengthen the immune system, lower blood pressure, cut cholesterol, stave off heart attacks, prevent osteoporosis, reduce stress, or improve your sex life.

Earning a living this way was quick, easy, and—for a while at least—fun. I readily recycled material from publication to publication, since all were prone to hopping on the same bandwagons. And editors who saw my work in one magazine often asked me to "do a story like this for *our* audience." It never dawned on me that I might be misleading the public by promoting "food-as-magic-bullet" mythology. I labored under the illusion that by carefully executing assignments according to the editors' parameters, I was informing the public and being a good writer.

What I was really doing was helping to sell magazines by presenting a lopsided point of view: the world according to women's magazine editors. Their world (and my assignments) was shaped primarily by two considerations: providing a "nice environment" for advertisers and making sure readers were not challenged by anything more than simple tips for healthy living.

(The word *healthful* does not exist in women's magazine stylesheets.)

Elizabeth Whelan, Sc.D., M.P.H., president of the American Council on Science and Health, thinks women's magazines are shirking responsibility by focusing on trivia and ignoring the devastating effects of cigarette smoking. In a recent op-ed piece in *The New York Times,* she said, "What advice do the magazines offer on how to stay healthy? Here is a sampling: Eat lots of broccoli to ward off cancer . . . take vitamins E and C and beta-carotene; eat garlic to fight colds and flu . . . and eat active-culture yogurt to live longer."

Conflicting views are seldom presented in women's magazines. After all, the "logic" goes, readers might become confused if they actually have to weigh more than one side of a story. Instead, editors usually decide in advance what readers should think, infantilizing readers in the process. This condescending philosophy was a major reason why I decided to get out of the whole business and into writing for physicians. Today, more than two years after making the transition, I savor the fact that I am writing for grown-ups.

How Articles Evolve

One reason why trivial and/or incorrect nutrition advice appear so often is the desire to please the magazines' lifeline: advertisers. Most marketing executives view women's magazines as "products" or "vehicles" that are part of a "marketing package" for their wares. That's where the "nice environment" comes in. Before agreeing to buy space, advertisers want to know what kinds of articles will appear in the magazine—and, particularly, what copy will appear near the ad. "Negative" stories—topics that may upset readers or otherwise interfere with a "feel-good" atmosphere—are routinely rejected. Unfortunately, this means that manuscripts that tell the truth (for example, that the link between specific foods and specific health effects is largely hype) seldom get published.

"Women's magazines are controlled by advertisers in ways that other magazines aren't," *Ms.* co-founder Gloria Steinem told a gathering of writers from the American Society of Journal-

Reprinted with permission from *Nutrition Forum,* May/June 1993, pp. 17-20. © 1993 by Prometheus Books, 59 John Glenn Drive, Amherst, NY 14228.

ists and Authors in 1991. She described how women's magazines began as catalogs, with short stories woven in between the ads. The link between advertising and editorial has remained, she said, creating a situation wherein "85 percent of women's magazine copy is really 'unmarked advertorial.'" A few months later, co-founder Patricia Carbine talked about "Advertising and Editorial—The Uneasy Coexistence" to a group of advertising, marketing, and public relations professionals attending a forum on business ethics. "Advertisers are insisting on concessions from women's service magazines that they wouldn't insist on from *Time* or *Newsweek*," she said. According to Ms. Carbine, declining circulation has put even greater pressure on women's publications to continually cross the line between advertising and editorial. Examples include presenting a certain number of recipes that use soup as an ingredient to satisfy a soup advertiser, or refusing to run results of "taste tests" that could offend an advertiser whose product appears at the bottom of the heap.

When I wrote regular nutrition columns for women's magazines, my topics were determined in most cases by advertisements already commissioned or those the publication hoped to bring in. "[A major cereal manufacturer] is advertising in September. Why don't you do a fiber story for that issue?" one editor suggested. "We'd love to get an ad from [a leading manufacturer of lowfat dairy products]. We want you to do a story on foods that are low in fat and high in calcium," said another.

Michael Hoyt, associate editor of *Columbia Journalism Review*, has expressed concern about the blurred boundaries between advertising and editorial content. In the March/April 1990 issue, in an article called "When The Walls Come Tumbling Down," he stated:

> From a reader's perspective this confluence of advertising and editorial is confusing: Where does the sales pitch end? Where does the editor take over? ... Magazines of all stripes are suddenly competing to give advertisers something extra—"value added" in ad-world lingo—in return for their business. Many of these extras are perfectly legitimate and have little or nothing to do with editorial content; others fall into a gray and foggy area; still others involve the selling of pieces of editorial integrity, from slivers to chunks to truckloads.

When it comes to nutrition information, the "confusion" Hoyt alludes to is rampant. In a recent interview (*not* for a women's magazine), Richard Rivlin, M.D., of New York Hospital told me: "The public is enormously confused. They need a better understanding of the role nutrition plays with respect to disease. We haven't been doing a very good job of putting things in perspective." Writing in the *Journal of the American Medical Association*, Dr. Rivlin stressed that it is more realistic to think that good nutrition can help delay the onset or reduce the effects of such illnesses as heart disease, stroke, cancer, and diabetes—not that nutrition can prevent or eliminate these disorders entirely. He added that proper nutrition won't do much to protect an individual who continues to smoke cigarettes, drinks excessively, or leads a sedentary lifestyle.

But that type of moderate message seldom makes its way into magazines where "food as medicine" themes are regarded as an essential editorial ingredient. During my tenure as a health and nutrition writer, I wrote everything from the "diet that can save your life" to the "fertility diet" and the "brain power diet." I also wrote about diets to calm your kids, boost their I.Q., and keep them from becoming overweight adults.

The Ingredients of a "Good" Nutrition Article

The other force that drives the editorial content of women's magazines is the desire to grab attention to boost sales. The quickest, surest way to sell article ideas to a women's magazine is to come up with a great cover line. Once I learned this secret, getting assignments was a snap. Whereas some writers labored long and hard over query letters, I would think up titles and bullet them on a page, fleshing out the "story" with one or two sentences. Examples include: "16 Great Food Finds," "20 Hunger-Fighting Foods," "6 Myths That Keep You Fat," and "What Your Snacks Say About You." At least 75% of the topics I proposed in this way ended up as assignments.

Of course, the process also worked in reverse. Editors would call me and say, "We want such-and-such story (naming a provocative headline). You figure out what to put in the article." Although all this smacks of deception, I did have scruples. Despite the jazzy-sounding titles, in most instances I merely repackaged basic nutrition advice into my articles, slipping in qualifiers ("there's no proof as yet") for spurious speculations and liberally peppering my articles with "may" and "they speculate." Does this excuse me? Not really. What astounds me in retrospect is how many "experts" were willing to go along with this charade.

Another essential ingredient in good articles is the voice of authority. As a women's magazine writer, I needed "experts" to validate my editor's point of view. Many "experts" who regularly appear in women's magazines are willing to trade scientific credibility for the opportunity to have their name in print. Some would give me quotes even when the premise of a story made little sense. For example, one women's magazine editor asked me to do a feature article called "Ten Foods to Make You Prettier." I balked, saying that unless an "expert" would corroborate that such a story could include some substance, I wouldn't do it. I was given the name of an "authority" at the school of public health of a major university. *She* convinced *me* it could be done and provided me with additional sources. I not only wrote the article but recycled it to other women's publications under such titles as "Eat Your Way to Perfect Skin" and "Beauty Is More Than Skin Deep."

Some "experts" I had quoted once were only too pleased to appear in subsequent articles—but not just the spinoffs. In some cases, they "trusted me" to put quotes in their mouths without even doing another interview or clearing the information with them. At one point, I had a psychiatrist, a psychologist, several nutritionists, an eating disorder specialist, and a dietitian that I could pull out of my hat (by making up quotes based on past interviews) whenever an editor wanted a particular viewpoint point substantiated. In other words, I had "instant sources."

I won't speculate on the reasons why people with M.D.s and Ph.D.s (the ones most coveted as sources by women's magazines), who presumably know better, permit themselves to be used in that way. The fact is, many do. Of course, not all have been manipulated. But I'll bet that most are not challenged, either by the writer who interviews them or by others who are quoted.

"Hiring" of Writers

A little-publicized, unethical practice that is more common than writers would like to admit can directly affect what "expert" information gets into a women's magazine and what doesn't. On several occasions, people from public relations agencies representing weight-loss centers and other clients have called me with a proposition. They would "hire" me to write a nutrition story that quoted their client if I would "place" it in a women's magazine. (I was never asked to place a piece in a more "reputable" type of magazine. I guess it was assumed that only women's magazines, and their writers, could be bought.) For an unscrupulous writer, this is an opportunity to be paid twice for the same article. I have consistently refused such work, telling callers that if their client's views were appropriate for something I am writing, they would be used without charge.

In another typical women's magazine scenario, the writer is required to skip attribution altogether—the rationale being that "we want the magazine to be the authority." The result of this abuse of power is that the magazine gives itself a free hand to say whatever it wants, merely by having the writer pepper the article with convenient phrases such as "experts agree," "scientists have found," and "experts say." What experts? The writer and editor, of course.

Style over Substance

Another practice that makes it easier for writers to write for women's magazines than for many other publications—and that has the potential of leaving readers seriously misinformed—is lack of fact-checking. Although some women's magazines call sources to check quotes for accuracy and require writers to provide backup material for statistics, many (I would venture to guess most) don't. I wrote weekly nutrition columns for one women's magazine that preferred to be the authority (in other words, no experts were to be quoted). In more than a year and a half, no one on the magazine's staff ever asked where I got my information. Each column was composed of an article that provided a good headline, a Q&A that I had made up (including a name and city for the supposed writer), and a "fast fact" pertaining to nutrition (for example, that 40% of consumers eat vanilla ice cream). No one ever asked where my "fast facts" came from. [*Editor's note:* Fact-checking can improve accuracy, but does not guarantee it. When checkers limit their contact to people mentioned in the article, errors originating from inaccurate or misleading sources may go undetected. The only way to ensure accuracy is expert prepublication review—a process few media outlets utilize.]

In addition to a catchy headline and good sources, the article must "lay out well" on the page. Typically this means using sidebars and boxes, with cute little quizzes ("What's Your Nutrition IQ?"; "Are You An Emotional Eater?"), fascinating facts ("Did You Know..."), or 2-day "starter menus" for special diet stories. It's a plus if the article itself can be done up in an easy-to-swallow format, such as "Your A-Z Guide To Fighting Fat," "Seven Secrets Every Thin Person Knows," or "Nutrition Myths That Keep You Fat." Editors seem to assume that straightforward stories won't be read, that readers must be entertained, and that "text-heavy" pages will intimidate them.

The women's magazine writer must also understand an editor's mandate to "work with the art director." In many cases, this means the writer must include points in the text to validate the accompanying photos. For example, if the art director thinks a story on summer fruit would "look great" accompanied by a photo of bananas, grapefruit, and kiwi fruit, then the writer must make sure these fruits are mentioned in the article. Sometimes the photography is planned or even executed before the article is written.

The power of the art director was carried *ad absurdum* in one article I wrote on eating "mini-meals." I had paid a registered dietitian to plan meals that would meet all the Recommended Dietary Allowances for adult women. Imagine my shock when my editor called to demand that a meal be changed to include the foods that the art director thought would "look good on the page." "Luscious strawberries" and "juicy orange slices" would have to replace raisins and bananas!

The final ingredient in a "good" nutrition story is the writing style. Three tones are permitted:

1. Bouncy two-year-old: "Don't wait! Start now on our power-packed, energy-boosting diet."

2. Concerned parent: "Eclairs are tempting, so have one—very occasionally . . . If you do have one, make it your only indulgence that day"; "If you must use white sauce, remember: the thinner the sauce, the thinner *you'll* stay."

3. Pseudosophisticated "friend": "Of course you can diet and lose weight. You've done it before . . . and before that . . . but each time the pounds you shed creep back, causing you to groan with disappointment when you step on the scale. Yet we all know women whose weight rarely fluctuates more than a pound or two and former fatties who managed to lose weight and *keep it off* for good . . . Now, we bring you the *real* secrets behind their success."

Once a writer has these chatty tones down pat, she simply asks which style the editor wants, and bingo! Another successful assignment!

No Journalistic Skills Required

What probably helped me most in becoming a successful women's magazine writer was the fact that I had no journalism training whatsoever. I have never taken a writing course in my life.

In 1980, I went into business for myself as a freelance public relations person for various agencies in New York City. The skills I acquired made it easy to shift from press kits into women's magazine writing. These included: (1) the ability to write headlines and opening paragraphs that were punchy and attention-grabbing; (2) an unquestioning attitude towards "experts"; and (3) the ability to produce unfailingly upbeat, inoffensive copy.

Writing press kits for new diet pills, migraine medi-cines, and blood pressure drugs, for example, required me to digest complex information and spew it back in easy-to-swallow, bite-size pieces, rarely using words of more than one syllable and remaining as one-dimensional as possible (sound famil-iar?). Snappy headlines and subheads were more important than hard information—after all, my primary responsibility was to help ensure that our material wasn't hurled immediately into the "circular file."

I made my first women's magazine contacts when pitching editors with story ideas that would include whatever clients I happened to be handling at the time. If the editors wanted more, I would send a press kit or bulleted list of article ideas that could be built around the client. Some of the "low-end" women's magazines willingly take articles provided by public relations firms, which I promptly produced for them. Several even gave me bylines—a joy to someone starting out in the field.

These assignments, paid for by the public relations agencies I worked for, provided me with "clips" which I then used to approach larger publications. Soon editors of women's magazines were asking me to write for them on assignment. Within a year, I had so much magazine work that I stopped doing public relations work altogether.

After a number of years playing at this kind of writing, I grew incredibly bored. Women's magazines like to pigeonhole writers (e.g., "health writer," "travel writer," "money writer"). Even though I managed somewhat to defy definition by writing in all three of these categories, editors who gave me "regular work" really wanted me to write the same stories issue after issue, year after year: How to shed five pounds in five days; Think yourself thin; De-stress yourself; Eat right over the holidays; Get in shape for summer; How to stick to your diet while eating out; Why your food diary is your best friend, etc, etc. These are women's magazine "staples"—the stories read-ers presumably want to read over and over.

Perhaps it's true. Maybe all those women out there really do want to read that stuff. But if that's the case, at least I have the satisfaction of knowing I no longer contribute to the propaganda that feeds such a mindset. And I can't help but believe that women's magazine readers are capable of taking in a healthy dose of hard information, meaningful speculation, and controversy—about food, nutrition, health, life—if their favor-ite magazines would only make the effort, and take the risk, of presenting them.

This article is based on my experiences in writing for more than a dozen women's magazines and talking with fellow journalists. There is no question that some women's magazines have more editorial "depth" than others. Those that cater to "educated" women generally offer less simplistic-sounding articles than those catering to "the secretary in Middle America." And magazines with bigger editorial budgets are apt to subject articles to more scrutiny than those with small budgets and little money for editorial content. Nevertheless, all operate under pressure from the market forces I have described.

FOOD FOR THOUGHT: CAN YOU TRUST YOUR FAVORITE MAGAZINE TO TELL YOU WHAT TO EAT?

DIANE WOZNICKI AND DR. RUTH KAVA

Popular magazines—*Reader's Digest, Good Housekeeping, McCall's* and the like—used to be America's number-one source of nutrition information. Today, magazines take a back seat to TV; but according to the American Dietetics Association, a solid 39 percent of the American public still gets most of its nutrition news from magazines. Those readers need to know that the information they get from their favorite magazines is both accurate and reliable.

Since 1982 the American Council on Science and Health has been conducting a biennial survey of the nutrition coverage in popular magazines. ACSH recently wrapped up its sixth such survey, and there's good news: Fifteen of the 20 magazines studied were found to be "excellent" or "good" sources of nutrition information. Furthermore, for the first time in the 14-

For the first time in the 14-year history of the survey, a strong majority . . . of the magazines reviewed earned ratings in the top two categories.

year history of the survey, a strong majority—75 percent—of the magazines reviewed earned ratings in the top two categories. This reflects a heartening new trend—a trend toward real quality—in magazine nutrition reporting.

Three magazines—*Consumer Reports, Better Homes and Gardens* and *Parents*—were rated as "excellent" sources of nutrition information. Twelve magazines—*Cooking Light, Glamour, Reader's Digest, Mademoiselle, American Health, Prevention, Self, Woman's Day, Good Housekeeping, McCall's, Redbook* and *Health*— were rated as "good." Four magazines—*Men's Health, New Woman, Vogue* and *Runner's World*— were rated as "fair." Only one magazine— *Cosmopolitan*—was rated as a "poor" source of nutrition information.

How the Survey Was Conducted

Using *Advertising Age* circulation figures, ACSH

identified 20 best-selling American magazines that regularly feature nutrition articles. We chose magazines whose target audiences differed in order to sample articles aimed at a variety of consumers. Eight articles per magazine were randomly selected for evaluation; to prevent judging bias, the selected articles were scanned and reset in a uniform format with magazine and author names deleted.

Four experts in nutrition and food science judged each article's accuracy in three areas: providing factual information, presenting information objectively and making sound recommendations. For each article, the judges were presented with comments such as, "The article documented the source of the information," "The headline was an accurate reflection of the article's content" and, "The recommendations were supported by information from the article."

The judges were instructed to say whether they "strongly agreed," "somewhat agreed," "were neutral," "somewhat disagreed" or "strongly disagreed" with the sample comments. These response categories corresponded to numerical scores ranging from a high of five ("strongly agreed") to a low of one ("strongly disagreed"). A composite score for each article was determined by averaging the judges' scores; the overall score for each magazine was derived by averaging the composite scores of each magazine's articles.

An independent statistician tabulated the results and ranked the magazines. The highest rating was set at 100 percent, and categories were assigned as follows: "excellent," 90% to 100%; "good," 80% to 89%; "fair," 70% to 79%; and "poor," below 70%.

Using the composite score for each article, the statistician evaluated individual article performance with respect to factual accuracy, presentation style and recommendations. Generally, articles with high composite scores were found to reflect consistently good scores in all three categories; similarly, articles with poor composites were found deficient in all three categories. The "excellent" and "good" magazines had many articles earning high composite scores, but no single magazine lacked articles whose composite scores were either mediocre or low. Thus, even in the best ranked magazines room was found for improvement.

The 'Excellent' Three

Articles in *Consumer Reports*, *Better Homes and Gardens* and *Parents* were consistently reliable (some minor errors resulted in small point losses).

Consumer Reports' high-scoring, hallmark product-analysis articles provided readers with factual overviews of their subject matter. Data were translated into easy-to-grasp concepts, and specific foods were not labeled "bad" or "good." Instead, *CR*'s authors recommended reasonable alternatives.

Better Homes and Gardens articles promoted lifestyle change rather than food restriction and suggested novel substitutions—such as halving the number of walnuts in a Waldorf salad but toasting them first to enhance their flavor—to lower a meal's fat content. *Better Homes and Gardens* lost a few points for articles such as "Our Food Police," which overstated the role of advocacy groups in monitoring the nation's food supply.

Parents magazine handled new research smoothly. The magazine used well-documented sources, and its recommendations echoed expert scientific opinion. According to one judge, a *Parents* article on milk did a good job of explaining why people are hearing so much controversy over milk, but the judge also noted that the article's implication that consumers are being served antibiotic-tainted milk from treated cows was an overstatement.

There's a Good Deal of 'Good' Out There

Cooking Light led the "good" category. One article cautioned against restricting calories in the high-growth adolescent years. But another piece recommended eating 100 grams of carbohydrate after heavy exercise and following that up with an additional 100 grams every two to four hours. A judge who is also a sports nutritionist noted that that quantity is appropriate for a 200-pound person—and is about double what the average female would need.

Glamour also received a rating. One judge commented that a *Glamour* piece on caffeine presented "the latest on a complex issue" and "did an excellent job of documenting the source and identifying researchers doing the work on caffeine." Overall, *Glamour*'s discussions were balanced, its sources were recognizably expert and the magazine was not afraid to tackle new research; it didn't just stay on safe ground rehashing the same old stuff.

In an article on food poisoning, "good" *Reader's Digest* advised its readers to make sure their meat is cooked beyond the pink stage. It also told restaurant patrons to request a new plate when returning

undercooked meat, since raw meat juices contaminate. A piece called "Attacked by a Killer Egg Roll" satirized low-fat mania, but that article lost points for labeling eggs, mayonnaise and other foods "bad."

Mademoiselle's "Before You Go on Another Diet, Read This" sensibly quoted a variety of experts to point out mainstream thinking on weight issues. An article on herbal products (called "Natural Wonders?") was basically sound, but while it started with an overview of the dangers of herbal products marketed as diet aids, it ended by saying, "It's

> One . . . article, "Fantastic Folic Acid," received a nearly perfect score from the judges. The article served to educate a vulnerable segment of the population and exemplified nutrition reporting at its finest.

up to you to decide if the risk is really worth the weight loss," thus implying that herbal aids are effective. The judges would have preferred a strong condemnation of these unproved products.

American Health is a magazine known for addressing new research. One *American Health* article, "Fantastic Folic Acid," received a nearly perfect score from the judges. The article served to educate a vulnerable segment of the population and exemplified nutrition reporting at its finest. But a piece on antioxidants relied on the unconventional views of a medical researcher who offered unreasonable criticism of both the Recommended Dietary Allowances (RDA) and the Food and Drug Administration (FDA)'s ruling prohibiting antioxidant health claims on product labels. And an article on "Safer Supplements" cited a supplement trade association, whose representatives downplayed the risk of hepatitis from the use of chaparral as a sleep aid and said that the FDA is biased against supplements. The judges noted that quoting a critic of "establishment" nutrition is certainly acceptable, but not providing a counter quote from the FDA presents an unbalanced picture.

On the whole, *Prevention*'s efforts to maintain objectivity were commendable; they earned it its "good." But *Prevention* ran an article on beta-carotene whose title suggested that science already knows this nutrient will provide protection against skin cancer, while the article itself presented the research as preliminary, not proved. An article on "40-Plus Eating" stated that fats should not exceed 25 percent of calorie intake, but the statement wasn't illustrated in a way that would allow the reader to follow through. The article also stated that "Fat calories are the primary source of calories in most people's diets"; according to the United States Department of Agriculture, however, carbohydrates currently contribute the majority of the calories in the average diet.

Self earned its "good" rating with high-scoring articles like "From Twinkies to Tofu," a piece about eating trends. But major point loss occurred with an article that falsely attributed long-known behavior modification techniques to someone with a Ph.D. in psychology but no apparent credentials in nutrition. The article's "me" versus "them" summary of what works to shed pounds lacked objectivity, and the article did not acknowledge that many of the behavioral principles espoused by the profiled practitioner are part of other modern weight-loss strategies.

Woman's Day articles written by nutrition experts contributed to that magazine's "good" rating. *Woman's Day's* "Best Ever One Week Diet" made expert use of the Food Guide Pyramid. A few articles lost minor points for saying "according to experts" instead of documenting their sources, and a "No Time to Diet Diet" failed to provide enough calories.

Good Housekeeping's nutrition coverage, while rated "good" overall, was uneven. An article on frozen yogurt did a competent job of comparing the nutrient profiles of yogurt products, but a September '93 "Eating Right" column sacrificed accuracy for brevity. A reader asked, "Is breast milk really better for my newborn?"; and a physician responded that although breast milk is optimal, "you aren't putting her at any risk by choosing formula." The judges felt that this brief answer failed to provide a complete picture of breast-feeding's benefits.

Redbook's "Hottest Diet Advice in America" was actually based on long-known information, as repackaged by a popular diet guru. The judges found nothing wrong with the article's advice (exercise and eat well), but they didn't find it particularly new or "hot." A piece entitled "The Morning After Diet" explained the physiology of weight loss using experts' quotes. But breakfasts of pancakes, eggs and bacon and chicken and biscuits were called high-carbohydrate meals when in fact both are high in fat.

McCall's well-rated "25 Ways to Eat Chocolate and Not Gain Weight" gave readers permission to indulge as long as portion size was respected. But

in "Lose Three Pounds in One Weekend!" a health spa worker with no nutrition credentials made two statements—"Holiday weight is mostly caused by water retention" and "Avoid alcohol . . . [it] weakens your diet resolve"—that are not necessarily true. Also, the article erroneously referred to olives and hummus as being "low fat."

Health was one of the lower rated magazines in the "good" group. One article, "The Bran News About Rice," was particularly well rated; but when it came to scientific interpretation, *Health* occasionally struggled to present balanced reports.

The 'Fair' Four

On the whole, *New Woman's* message seems rather inconsistent. "Have Yourself a Fat Christmas" erred in its throw-in-the-towel, holiday-weight-gain-is-inevitable stance. But *New Woman* had previously run an article ("Getting Over Overeating") with a conflicting message. The earlier piece was an interesting take on emotional connections to overeating and according to one judge was as objective and balanced as preliminary-research reporting can be. It lost credibility only for implying that sugar was a mood-altering culprit for all individuals.

Men's Health's "Burn Fat Faster" was a summary of fat-burning techniques that work. It was generally balanced and thorough but lost points for failing to document its sources. A piece that purported to be a "Guide to Vitamin and Mineral Supplements" recommended antioxidant supplements to prevent wrinkles and disease, advice the scientific consensus does not support for all individuals.

Vogue ran a well-researched report on "The Death of Dieting" that included the author's own personal testimonial about the shortcomings of commercial weight-loss programs. The article received an almost flawless rating. But Vogue's "Dieting to Extremes: Tipping the Scales" was a major source of point loss. The low-carbohydrate diet described in the article was based on unproved assumptions such as, "Eat all you want but only the right foods and in the right combinations," and, "Exercise is irrelevant."

Runner's World was plagued by problems of oversimplification of complex issues and failure to cite sources. The magazine also singled out certain foods and promoted nutrient supplementation as keys to running faster and living longer. One article said that eating guava lowers cholesterol levels. How much guava, what other dietary or lifestyle changes were necessary and the source of the research were all undocumented.

'Poor' Cosmo!

Cosmopolitan was the only magazine ranked as "poor." While *Cosmo* seemed to run fewer fad diets than in previous years, no other magazine was as conspicuously lax about its credibility quotient. An article called "Do You or Don't You Need Vitamins and Minerals?" was blatantly unscientific; it was written by a physician to promote nutrient cure-alls. The author admonished readers to supplement 15 different vitamins and minerals, stating that young, active women "need them all." The article's misguided advice to take 100 milligrams of vitamin B_6 daily to alleviate PMS has not been clinically proved—and that amount could even be toxic if taken over long periods of time. *Cosmopolitan's* articles, consistently poorly rated as they were, suggest a strong need for real improvement under the magazine's new editor.

How the Magazines Stack Up by Target Audience

As a group, the "consumer-focused" *Consumer Reports, Parents* and *Reader's Digest* scored highest, racking up a 91 percent score overall. ACSH concluded that these magazines' factual approach triumphed over the fluffier approaches common to the lower scoring titles.

The second-highest rated group—the "home-focused" magazines—consisted of *Better Homes and Gardens, Cooking Light* and *Good Housekeeping.* Their group score was 88. Within this group, however, the first two outscored *Good Housekeeping* to a statistically significant extent.

"Health-focused" and "women's" magazines, taken as groups, were significantly less accurate from a statistical standpoint than either the consumer-focused or home-focused groups.

American Health and *Prevention* led the health-focused magazines with similar ratings; they were statistically better than the health-focused *Health, Men's Health* and *Runner's World.* On the whole, the magazines in this group (which scored 82 overall) tended to publish the highest volume of nutrition information.

Glamour was the highest scoring women's magazine, followed by *Mademoiselle, Self, Woman's Day, Redbook* and *McCall's.* According to the survey's statistician, the low-ranking *New Woman, Vogue* and *Cosmopolitan* scored significantly worse than any of the other women's titles and so pulled the women's magazines down as a group. The group score was 82.

Some Advice to the Magazines—and to Consumers

This latest survey found that the accuracy of nutrition reporting in magazines has definitely improved. Dr. Manfred Kroger has served as a judge in every ACSH survey so far, and he attributes the improvement to the fact that "Reporters, writers and editors [are] doing a better job because they recognize [that] ACSH and the public are watching them and their work." Dr. Kroger adds that "The media are increasingly relying on experts to scrutinize their output before going public, a welcome trend."

On the whole, the nutrition reporting in popular magazines is becoming increasingly sophisticated. Outlandish claims, endorsements of fad diets and gross misinterpretations of scientific research —all commonly seen in earlier surveys—have for the most part been replaced by balanced, science-based reports designed to promote nutrition literacy. New research findings are showing up, and the magazines are moving toward providing more hands-on information. Writers are telling readers how to fix poor eating habits and how to make needed lifestyle changes in accord with public health policy.

ACSH commends those magazines whose nutrition reporting was rated "excellent" or "good" and encourages the editors at those magazines rated "fair" or "poor" to assign nutrition topics to writers and researchers who understand science. All magazines should strive to achieve better consistency and better quality in their nutrition articles, with the ultimate goal of educating their readers and stemming the spread of misinformation.

DIANE WOZNICKI, M.S., R.D., IS AN ADJUNCT NUTRITION INSTRUCTOR AT THE UNIVERSITY OF PENNSYLVANIA. RUTH KAVA, PH.D., R.D., IS DIRECTOR OF NUTRITION AT THE AMERICAN COUNCIL ON SCIENCE AND HEALTH. THE ARTICLES FOR THE *SPECIAL REPORT* WERE COMPILED BY RENA SELYA, M.A., A RESEARCH INTERN AT ACSH.

THE SURVEY WAS JUDGED BY:
IRENE BERMAN-LEVINE, PH.D., R.D., ADJUNCT NUTRITION INSTRUCTOR AT THE UNIVERSITY OF PENNSYLVANIA AND NUTRITION CONSULTANT IN PRIVATE PRACTICE IN HARRISBURG, PA.

F.J. FRANCIS, PH.D., PROFESSOR OF FOOD SCIENCE, UNIVERSITY OF MASSACHUSETTS, AMHERST.

KATHRYN M. KOLASA, PH.D., R.D., L.D./N., SECTION HEAD AND PROFESSOR OF NUTRITION, DEPARTMENT OF FAMILY MEDICINE, EAST CAROLINA UNIVERSITY, GREENVILLE, NC.

MANFRED KROGER, PH.D., PROFESSOR OF FOOD SCIENCE AND PROFESSOR OF SCIENCE, TECHNOLOGY AND SOCIETY, THE PENNSYLVANIA STATE UNIVERSITY, UNIVERSITY PARK, PA.

STATISTICAL ANALYSIS BY:
JEROME LEE, PH.D., ASSOCIATE PROFESSOR OF PSYCHOLOGY, ALBRIGHT COLLEGE, READING, PA.

How to Spot a "Quacky" Web Site

Stephen Barrett, M.D.

The best way to avoid being quacked is to reject quackery's promoters. Each item listed below signifies that a web site is not a trustworthy information source.

General Characteristics

- Any site used to market herbs or dietary supplements. Although some are useful I do not believe it is possible to run a profitable business selling them without some form of deception. Deception includes: (1) lack of full disclosure of the facts, (2) promotion or sale of products that lack a rational use, or (3) failure to provide advice indicating who should not use the products. During the past 25 years, I have never encountered a seller who did not do at least one of the three things.
- Any site used to market or promote homeopathic products. No such products have been proven effective.
- Any site that generally promotes "alternative" methods. There are more than a thousand "alternative" methods. The vast majority are worthless.

False Statements about Nutrition

- Everyone should take vitamins.
- Vitamins are effective against stress.
- Taking vitamins makes people more energetic.
- Organic foods are safer and/or more nutritious than ordinary foods.
- Losing weight is easy.
- Special diets can cure cancer.
- Diet is the princip[a]l cause of hyperactivity.

False Statements about "Alternative" Methods

- Acupuncture is effective against a long list of diseases.
- Chelation therapy is an effective substitute for by-pass surgery.
- Chiropractic treatment is effective against a large number of diseases.
- Herbs are generally superior to prescription drugs.
- Homeopathic products are effective remedies.
- Spines should be checked and adjusted regularly by a chiropractor.

False Statements about Dental Care

- Fluoridation is dangerous.
- Mercury-amalgam ("silver") filings should be removed because they make people sick.
- All teeth with root canals should be removed because they make people sick.

Editor's Note: For further explanations on these statements, access *http://www.quackwatch.com/* and connect to the hyperlinks listed there.

Why do those #&*?@! "experts" keep changing their minds?

Let's say that for the last five years you've been paying close attention to health news as reported on TV and in newspapers. Perhaps you learned about antioxidants (notably vitamins E and C and beta carotene), which you can get both from foods and supplements. These antioxidants may help lower the risk of heart disease, cancer, cataracts, and other ills. The scientist who had told you this on the *Today* show was a handsome fellow in a good-looking suit (no rumpled Einstein he). He had led the groundbreaking study that had just appeared in *The Impeccable Journal of Medicine*. Not only was the evidence "very exciting," but he was taking hefty amounts of antioxidant supplements himself. So you started taking the pills. Next thing, you read that a study conducted in Finland showed that not only was beta carotene *not* protective against lung cancer, it actually seemed to increase the risk of getting it. Feeling deceived, you stopped taking your supplements and even gave up your daily carrot. You were tired of carrots anyway.

You may have seen something similar happen with oat bran (good one week, outmoded the next), margarine (you switched to this supposed health food a few years ago, and now it's been tagged as an artery-clogger), DDT and breast cancer (first linked, then not), hot dogs and childhood leukemia (a headline-maker that soon pooped out, since even the researchers had a hard time explaining their findings), and household electricity (cancer again—but by then you had gotten bored). Do these folks just not know what they are talking about?

In fact, the experts don't change their minds as often as it may seem. This newsletter, for example, never told you that margarine was a health food or that oat bran would solve your cholesterol problems. Both these foods were hyped by the media and by manufacturers—but most nutritionists never thought or said there was anything magic about them. A few researchers and journalists eagerly spread the idea that your power line and your electric toaster and clock could give you cancer. Most experts thought all along that the evidence was pretty thin. Headline writers change their minds more often than scientists.

Science is a process, not a product, a work in progress rather than a book of rules. Scientific evidence accumulates bit by bit. This doesn't mean scientists are bumblers (though perhaps a few are), but that they are trying to accumulate enough data to get at the truth, which is always a difficult job. Within the circle of qualified, well-informed scientists, there is bound to be disagreement, too. The same data look different to different people. A good scientist is often his/her own severest critic.

The search for truth in a democracy is also complicated by

- Intense public interest in health
- Hunger for quick solutions
- Journalists trying to make a routine story sound exciting
- Publishers and TV producers looking for audiences
- Scientists looking for fame and grants
- Medical journals thirsting for prestige
- Entrepreneurs thirsting for profits.

It pays to keep your wits about you as you listen, watch, and read.

The search for evidence

In general, there are three ways to look for evidence about health:

Basic research is conducted in a laboratory, involving "test tube" or "in vitro" (within glass) experiments, or experiments with animals such as mice. Such work is vital for many reasons. For one, it can confirm observations or hunches and provide what scientists call plausible mechanisms for a theory. If a link between heart disease and smoking is suspected, laboratory experiments might show how nicotine affects blood vessels.

The beauty of lab research is that it can be tightly controlled. Its limitation is that what happens in a test tube or a laboratory rat may not happen in a free-living human being.

Clinical or interventional trials are founded on observation and treatment of human beings. As with basic research, the "gold standard" clinical trial can and must be rigorously controlled. There'll be an experimental group or groups (receiving a bona-fide drug or treatment) and a control group (receiving a placebo, or dummy, treatment). A valid experiment must also be "blinded," meaning that no subject knows whether he/she is in the experimental or the control group. In a double-blind trial, the researchers don't know either.

But clinical trials have their limitations, too. The researchers must not knowingly endanger human life and health—there are ethics committees these days to make sure of this. Also, selection criteria must be set up. If the research is about heart disease, maybe the researchers will include only men, since middle-aged men are more prone to heart disease than women the same age. Or maybe they'll include only nurses, because nurses can be reliably tracked and are also good reporters. But these groups are not representative of the whole population. It may or may not be possible to generalize the findings. The study that determined aspirin's efficacy against heart attacks, for instance, was a well-designed interventional trial. But, for various reasons, nearly all the participants were middle-aged white men. No one is sure that aspirin works the same way for other people.

■ **Epidemiologic studies.** These generate the most news because so many of them have potential public appeal. An indispensable arm of research, epidemiology looks at the distribution of disease ("epidemics") and risk factors for disease in a human population in an attempt to find disease determinants. Compared with clinical trials or basic research, epidemiology is beset with pitfalls. That's because it deals with people in the real world and with situations that are hard to control.

The two most common types of epidemiologic research are:

Case control studies. Let's say you're studying lung cancer. You select a group of lung cancer patients and match them (by age, gender, and other criteria) with a group of healthy people. You try to identify which factors distinguish the healthy subjects (the "controls") from those who got sick.

Cohort studies. You select a group and question them about their habits, exposures, nutritional intake, and so forth. Then you see how many of your subjects actually develop lung cancer (or whatever you are studying) over the years, and you try to identify the factors associated with lung cancer.

Pitfalls and dead ends

Epidemiologic studies cannot usually prove cause and effect, but can identify associations and risk factors. Furthermore, epidemiology is best at identifying very powerful risk factors—smoking for lung cancer, for example. It is less good at risk assessment when associations are weak—between radon gas in homes and lung cancer, for example.

No matter how well done, any epidemiologic study may be open to criticism. Here are just a few of the problems:

■ People may not reliably report their eating and exercise habits. (How many carrots did you eat each month as an adolescent? How many last month? Few of us could say.) People aware of the benefits of eating vegetables may unconsciously exaggerate their vegetable consumption on a questionnaire. That's known as "recall bias."

■ Hidden variables or "confounders" may cloud results. A study might indicate that eating broccoli reduces the risk of heart disease. But broccoli eaters may be health-conscious and get a lot of exercise. Was it the broccoli or the exercise?

■ Those included in a study may seem to be a randomly selected, unbiased sample and then turn out not to be. For example, searching for a control group in one study, a re-

---

> ## Words for the wise
> ✓ **"May"**: does *not* mean "will."
> ✓ **"Contributes to," "is linked to,"** or **"is associated with"**: does *not* mean "causes."
> ✓ **"Proves"**: scientific studies gather evidence in a systematic way, but one study, taken alone, seldom proves anything.
> ✓ **"Breakthrough"**: this happens only now and then—for example, the discovery of penicillin or the polio vaccine. But today the word is so overworked as to be meaningless.
> ✓ **"Doubles the risk"** or **"triples the risk"**: may or may not be meaningful. Do you know what the risk was in the first place? If the risk was 1 in a million, and you double it, that's still only 1 in 500,000. If the risk was 1 in 100 and doubles, that's a big increase.
> ✓ **"Significant"**: a result is "statistically significant" when the association between two factors has been found to be greater than might occur at random (this is worked out by a mathematical formula). But people often take "significant" to mean "major" or "important."

---

searcher picked numbers out of the telephone book at random and called his subjects in the daytime. But people who stay home during the day may not be a representative sample. Those at home in the daytime might tend to be very young or very old, ill, or recovering from illness.

> ## Some commonsense pointers
> ✓ **Don't jump to conclusions.** A single study is no reason for changing your health habits. Distinguish between an interesting finding and a broad-based public health recommendation.
> ✓ **Always look for context.** A good reporter—and a responsible scientist—will always place findings in the context of other research. Yet the typical news report seldom alludes to other scientific work.
> ✓ **If it was an animal study or some other kind of lab study, be cautious about generalizing.** Years ago lab studies suggested that saccharin caused cancer in rats, but epidemiologic studies later showed it didn't cause cancer in humans.
> ✓ **Beware of press conferences** and other hype. Scientists, not to mention the editors of medical journals, love to make the front page of major newspapers and hear their studies mentioned on the evening news. The fact that the study in question may have been flawed or inconclusive or old news may not seem worth mentioning. This doesn't mean you shouldn't believe anything. Truth, too, may be accompanied by hype.
> ✓ **Notice the number of study participants and the study's length.** The smaller the number of subjects and the shorter the time, the greater the possibility that the findings are erroneous.
> ✓ **Perhaps the most blatantly hyped research of late has been genetic.** But the treatment of human illness by altering human genes is still at a very early stage.

■ Health effects, especially where cancer is concerned, may take 20 years or more to show up. It's not always financially or humanly possible to keep a study running that long.

Reading health news in an imperfect world

And this is only the half of it. Sometimes the flaws lie in the study, sometimes in the way it has been promoted and reported. Science reporters may be deluged with data. Many are expected to cover all science, from physics and astronomy to the health effects of hair dyes. Sometimes health reporters may not even have read the studies in question or may not understand the statistics.

Many medical organizations issue press releases. Some of these are excellent, and some aren't. Some deliberately try to manipulate the press, overstating the case, failing to provide context, and so forth. Researchers, institutions, and corporations often hire public relations people to promote their work. These people may actually know less than the enterprising reporter who calls to interview them.

Finally, people tend to draw their own conclusions, no matter what the article says.

However, the bottom line is pretty good…

None of this means epidemiology doesn't work. *One study may not prove anything, but a body of research, in which evidence accumulates bit by bit, can uncover the truth.* Research into human health has made enormous strides and is still making them. There may be no such thing as a perfect study, but here is only the briefest list of discoveries that came out of epidemiologic research:

■ Smoking is the leading cause of premature death in developed countries.

■ High blood cholesterol is a major cause of coronary artery disease and heart attack.

■ Exercise is important for good health.

■ Good nutrition offers protection against cancer; or, conversely, poor nutrition is a factor in the development of cancer.

■ Obesity is a risk factor for heart disease, cancer, and diabetes.

The list could go on and on. We suggest that you retain a spirit of inquiry and a healthy skepticism, but not lapse into cynicism. *The "flip-flops" you perceive are often not flip-flops at all, except in the mind of some headline writer.*

There is a great deal of good reporting, and it's an interesting challenge to follow health news. You don't believe everything you read or see on TV about politics, business, or foreign relations, so it's no surprise that you shouldn't believe some health news. Luckily, there are many sources for health news—none infallible, but some a lot better than others.

Vitamin and nutritional supplements

Sorting out fact from fiction amid a storm of controversy

"The most powerful nutritional force in the universe, a super-powered, full-spectrum liquid organic supplement with 72 bioelectrical minerals, 16 vitamins, and 18 amino acids."

You've seen advertisements like these in magazines and health food stores. The hype is unavoidable — white oak helps you live longer, melatonin prevents cancer, magnesium eases migraines, and essence of flowers can reverse hot flashes.

Since 1994, when Congress changed Food and Drug Administration (FDA) regulation of "nutritional" supplements, there's been an explosion of "health-enhancing" megavitamins, magic pills and potions. Almost every mall in America has a health food store, shelves lined with products that promise to relieve pain, help you sleep better and give your health, vitality and virility a boost.

It's a $6 billion-a-year business, and it's booming as people search for a fast fix — an easy way to feel better and stay healthy. One-quarter to one-third of Americans now take daily vitamin supplements. Seventy percent take nutritional supplements at least occasionally, and one in three people with chronic disease looks to herbal remedies for help.

Now, more than ever, people are focusing on nutrition to help them remain healthy and active. That's good. But do you need supplements? Do they work? And perhaps most important, are they safe?

The answers to these questions are not always clear-cut. There's disagreement, even within the medical community, as researchers continue to uncover new information about how nutrition affects your health. Further clouding the issue is an almost daily barrage of media reports on new studies — some suggesting benefits from supplements, others indicating harm. And then there are those advertisements, promising health in a capsule or in a steaming herbal brew.

So how do you sort out fact from fiction from outright fantasy amid the swirl of information about vitamin and nutritional supplements? We hope this essay will help. In it, we'll discuss what's known about supplements and what's not. We'll talk about who may need a supplement and who doesn't. And, we'll address critical safety issues surrounding what has become a largely unregulated industry.

From *Mayo Clinic Health Letter,* June 1997, pp. 1-3, 6, 8. © 1997 by the Mayo Foundation for Medical Education and Research, Rochester, MN 55905. Reprinted by permission.

Choosing a vitamin and mineral supplement

Supplements are not substitutes. They can't replace the hundreds of nutrients in whole foods needed for a balanced diet. But if you do decide to take a vitamin supplement, here are things to consider:

■ *Stick to the Daily Value* — Choose a vitamin-mineral combination limited to 100 percent DV or less. Take no more than the recommended dose. The higher the dose, the more likely you are to have side effects.

■ *Don't waste dollars* — Synthetic vitamins are the same as so-called "natural" vitamins. Generic brands and synthetic vitamins are generally less expensive and equally effective. Don't be tempted by added herbs, enzymes or amino acids — they add nothing but cost.

■ *Read the label* — Supplements can lose potency over time so check the expiration date on the label. Also look for the initials USP (for the testing organization U.S. Pharmacopeia) or words such as "release assured" or "proven release," indicating that the supplement is easily dissolved and absorbed by your body.

■ *Store them in a safe place* — Iron supplements are the most common cause of poisoning deaths among children.

■ *Don't self-prescribe* — See your doctor if you have a health problem. Tell him or her about any supplement you're taking. Supplements may interfere with medications.

What is a vitamin?

For centuries, sailors on long voyages battled not only the high seas, but a disease that can cause bones to become brittle, gums to bleed and even death. That disease is scurvy.

It had long been suspected there might be a relationship between the lack of fresh food and the development of scurvy, but it wasn't until 1747 that a carefully planned trial showed that lemons and oranges would prevent the disease. It took until 1928, when the science of chemistry was more advanced, for a researcher to identify the substance in lemons and oranges (and many other fruits and vegetables) that prevents or cures scurvy. The substance was given the name "vitamin C."

Most vitamins and minerals were discovered this way — scientists identifying substances you need because a shortage causes a health problem.

Vitamins and essential minerals are substances required in tiny amounts to promote essential biochemical reactions in your cells. Together, vitamins and minerals are called micronutrients. Lack of a micronutrient for a prolonged period causes a specific disease or condition, which can usually be reversed when the micronutrient is resupplied.

Your body can't make most vitamins and minerals. They must come from food or supplements.

Vitamin and mineral ABCs

There are 13 vitamins. Four — vitamins A, D, E and K — are stored in your body's fat (they're called fat-soluble vitamins). Nine are water-soluble and are not stored in your body in appreciable amounts. They are vitamin C and the eight B vitamins: thiamin (B-1), riboflavin (B-2), niacin, vitamin B-6, pantothenic acid, vitamin B-12, biotin and folic acid (folate).

Vitamins in the right amounts are needed for normal growth, digestion, mental alertness and resistance to infection. They enable your body to use carbohydrates, fats and proteins. They also act as catalysts in your body, initiating or speeding up a chemical reaction. However, you don't "burn" vitamins, so you can't get energy (calories) directly from them.

Your body strives to maintain an optimal level of each vitamin and keep the amount circulating in your bloodstream constant. Surplus water-soluble vitamins are excreted in urine. Surplus fat-soluble vitamins are stored in body tissue. Because they're stored, excess fat-soluble vitamins can accumulate in your body and become toxic. Your body is especially sensitive to too much vitamin A and vitamin D.

Therefore, whether you're taking water-soluble or fat-soluble vitamin supplements, more is not necessarily better and can even be harmful.

Your body also needs 15 minerals that help regulate cell function and provide structure for cells. Major minerals include calcium, phosphorus and magnesium. In addition, your body needs smaller amounts of chromium, copper, fluoride, iodine, iron, manganese, molybdenum, selenium, zinc, chloride, potassium and sodium.

Do you need a vitamin-mineral supplement?

Vitamin hucksters spend millions planting the fear, "Are you getting enough vitamins?" They recommend vitamin, mineral and nutri-

Buyer beware — there's no guarantee dietary supplements are safe

When you buy a product in a store, particularly something you eat, you naturally assume it's safe. Some government agency has checked to make sure it's not harmful, right?

Not any more. In 1994, Congress passed and President Clinton signed the Dietary Supplement Health and Education Act. That act removed dietary supplements from premarket safety evaluations required of food ingredients and drugs.

Drugs and food ingredients still undergo lengthy FDA safety review before they can be marketed. Drugs are also tested for effectiveness. But the 1994 legislation eliminated the FDA's authority to regulate the safety of nutritional supplements before they're on the market. Now, the FDA can intervene only after an illness or injury occurs.

The FDA can still restrict the sale of an unsafe dietary supplement when there's evidence the product presents a significant or unreasonable safety concern. But now the agency must wait for complaints about a product before acting.

Consumers can report problems through a "consumer complaint coordinator" at FDA district offices in cities across the country (listed in the "government" pages of your phone book).

But even after complaints are received, the FDA is required to prove the supplement caused harm when taken "as directed" on the label before a product can be restricted. Harm is usually difficult to prove because people may not take supplements as directed. They often exceed the recommended dose and take different types of supplements simultaneously.

Since passage of the legislation three years ago, the FDA hasn't been able to "prove" harm in a single case, despite reports of illness and even death from supplements.

The 1994 legislation also changed guidelines for marketing supplements. Marketing representatives can make unproven claims, such as saying a product "cures" cancer, as long as they're not selling the product at the same time.

And, while it's illegal to make false or misleading health or nutritional claims on a product label, government agencies lack resources to pursue the multitude of dubious claims that have swept the marketplace.

In addition, since the nutritional supplement industry is now largely unregulated, you can't be sure of product purity or the amount of active ingredient in a supplement — even from one package to the next of the same product.

What all this means for you is that you can't automatically assume the safety and effectiveness of any of the nutritional supplements sold today. If you have questions about a supplement, talk to your doctor or registered dietitian. Or, call the American Dietetic Association's consumer hotline at 1-800-366-1655.

Use DVs as a guide

You've no doubt seen "% Daily Value" listings on food labels.

Daily Values (DV) have their origin in the Recommended Dietary Allowances (RDA) that tell how much of each vitamin and mineral you need, on average, each day to maintain health. The % DV tells you what percent of the DV one serving of a food or supplement supplies. Use it to compare the nutritional value of products.

tional supplements as "vitamin insurance." But there's no need for most people to bank on vitamin insurance. The American Dietetic Association, the National Academy of Sciences, the National Research Council and other major medical societies all agree that you should get the vitamins and minerals you need through a well-balanced diet. Although certain high-risk groups may benefit from a vitamin-mineral supplement, healthy adults can get all necessary nutrients from food.

Experts favor food, rather than supplements, because food contains hundreds of additional nutrients, including phytochemicals. Phytochemicals are compounds that occur naturally in foods and may contain important health benefits. Scientists have yet to learn exactly what role phytochemicals play in nutrition, and there's no RDA established for them. However, if you depend on supplements rather than trying to eat a variety of whole foods, you miss out on possible health benefits from phytochemicals.

In addition, only long-term, well-designed studies can sort out which

Clues to quackery

Even well-informed consumers can be duped by health quackery. Here are some tips to help you sort out dubious claims:

■ *Be cautious about claims to treat diseases* — Vitamins can treat a few rare diseases caused by a vitamin deficiency. In addition, the B vitamin niacin is used to treat high cholesterol levels in some people. But studies show that vitamin and nutritional supplements can't cure diseases such as cancer and arthritis.

■ *Beware of testimonials* — One person's story can't help you distinguish a true benefit from chance or a "placebo effect." In one study of vitamin C, people who thought they were given vitamin C but had been given a placebo, reported that they felt unusually well.

■ *Avoid "tests" that can determine your body's overall nutritional status* — There's no single test that can measure your nutritional well-being and overall health.

■ *Don't assume all advertising is truthful* — The Federal Trade Commission (FTC), doesn't have resources to halt much fraudulent advertising. Be suspicious of words such as "miraculous," "amazing" and "powerful," or products that claim to "strengthen," "rebuild" or "rejuvenate."

■ *Be cautious about buying a nutritional supplement by phone or mail order* — These products are often very expensive and frequently a waste of money. Sometimes promotions are a scam.

nutrients in food are beneficial and whether taking them in pill form provides the same benefit. In the meantime, it's best to concentrate on getting your nutrients from food, not supplements.

However, many people don't get all the nutrients they need from their diets because they don't eat properly. For example, only one person in 10 regularly consumes the recommended five servings a day of fruits and vegetables. Skipping meals, dieting and eating meals high in sugar and fat all contribute to poor nutrition. For these people, taking supplemental vitamins would be reasonable, although the best course of action would be to adopt better eating habits.

Vitamin-mineral supplements shouldn't substitute for a healthful diet. However, there's probably no harm in taking a multiple vitamin-mineral supplement with dose levels no higher the 100 percent of the Daily Value (see "Choosing a vitamin and mineral supplement," and "Use DVs as a guide"). Doses above that don't give extra protection, but do increase your risk of encountering toxic side effects.

For example, taking large amounts of vitamin D can indirectly cause kidney damage, while large amounts of vitamin A can cause liver damage. Even modest increases in some minerals can lead to imbalances that limit your body's ability to use other minerals. And supplements of iron, zinc, chromium and selenium can be toxic at just five times the RDA. Virtually all nutrient toxicities stem from high-dose supplements.

When you may need a supplement

Although most people can get all the vitamins and minerals they need from a balanced diet, there are situations where a supplement may be appropriate. Even if you don't have a documented deficiency, your doctor or dietitian may recommend a vitamin-mineral supplement if:

■ *You're older* — Lack of appetite, loss of taste and smell, and denture problems can all contribute to a poor diet. If you eat alone or are depressed, you also may not eat enough to get all the nutrients you need from food.

In addition, if you're age 65 or older, you may need to increase your intake of vitamin B-6, vitamin B-12 and vitamin D because your body may not be able to absorb these as well. And women, especially those not taking estrogen, may need to increase their intake of calcium and vitamin D to protect against osteoporosis.

There's also evidence that a multivitamin may improve your immune function and decrease your risk for some infections if you're older.

■ *You're on a strict weight-loss diet* — If you eat less than 1,000 calories a day, or your diet has limited variety due to intolerance or allergy, you may benefit from a vitamin-mineral supplement.

■ *You have a disease of your digestive tract* — Diseases of your liver, gallbladder, intestine and pancreas, or previous surgery on your digestive tract, may interfere with your normal digestion and absorption of nutrients. If you have one of these conditions, your doctor may advise you to supplement your diet with vitamins and minerals.

■ *You smoke* — Smoking reduces vitamin C levels and causes production of harmful free radicals. The RDA for vitamin C for smokers is higher—100 milligrams (mg) compared to 60 mg for nonsmokers. Still, you can easily get this much by eating foods rich in vitamin

Nonherbal supplements

Not all supplements come from herbs or vitamins and minerals. Here are three that have been widely promoted:

■ *DHEA (dehydroepiandrosterone)* — Banned before 1994, DHEA is a hormone. It's been promoted as a treatment for everything from heart disease to cancer and Alzheimer's disease. But none of these claims has been proven. Side effects may include acne, increased facial hair and deepened voice in women, and, theoretically, increased risk of breast and prostate cancer.

■ *DMSO* — Dimethyl sulfoxide is an industrial solvent not approved by the FDA for human use. It may relieve pain from sore muscles when rubbed on skin, but it's no more effective than products like BenGay or Mentho-Rub. Taken internally, DMSO can lead to cataracts.

■ *Melatonin* — Melatonin is a hormone produced in your brain. It's thought to set your body's sleep cycle. Supplements may reduce effects of jet lag when taken for short periods. There's less evidence to support claims it will increase immune function and aid sleep.

Claims that melatonin lowers cholesterol and prevents breast cancer are unproven. Melatonin prevents ovulation, so don't use it if you want to become pregnant. Avoid it if you have severe allergies or immune disease, and don't give it to children.

C. If you smoke, try to stop. And don't depend on high-potency supplements to provide necessary nutrients. Two studies of beta carotene have shown an increased risk of lung cancer in smokers who take these supplements.

■ *You drink alcoholic beverages to excess* — If you regularly consume alcohol to excess, you may not get enough vitamins due to poor nutrition and alcohol's effect on the absorption, metabolism and excretion of vitamins.

■ *You're pregnant or breast-feeding* — If you're pregnant or breast-feeding, you need more of certain nutrients, especially folic acid, iron and calcium. Your doctor can recommend a supplement.

■ *You're in another high-risk group* — Vegetarians who eliminate all animal products from their diets may need additional vitamin B-12. And if you have limited milk intake and limited exposure to the sun, you may need to supplement your diet with calcium and vitamin D.

Supplement safety

For the millions of healthy Americans who want to take a daily multivitamin supplement with no more than 100 percent of the Daily Value, the risks of side effects are probably small. But if you're tempted to take high-dose vitamins, thinking that "more is better," think again. High doses of some vitamins can have serious side effects.

And if you're considering herbal and other types of supplements, be particularly cautious (see "Clues to quackery," page 6). Quality and dose potency may not be well-regulated.

For example, in 1989, a sudden illness outbreak that affected more than 1,500 people and caused 38 deaths was linked to L-tryptophan, an amino acid sold as an over-the-counter dietary supplement to treat insomnia. The supplements, manufactured by a foreign pharmaceutical company, were contaminated during the manufacturing process.

Today, experts are concerned about reported health problems linked to popular herbal supplements containing ephedrine. Although the FDA has linked the supplements to more than 600 reports of adverse events and 15 deaths since 1993, they're still on the market (see "Buyer beware — there's no guarantee dietary supplements are safe," page 3, and "Herbs can have many health effects," page 7).

Reported side effects have included abnormal heart rhythm, seizure, stroke, psychosis, heart attack, hepatitis and death. The FDA is considering a ban on ephedrine-containing supplements because no safe level has been identified for its use in dietary supplements.

Play it safe with your diet and your health

The L-tryptophan and ephedrine deaths are tragic consequences of the largely unregulated health-supplement industry and our desire for easy ways to feel better, boost energy, reduce stress, lose weight and stave off disease. But despite the dangers, supplements are proliferating.

If you want to improve your nutritional health, look first to a well-balanced diet. In most cases, making changes in your diet has a far greater chance of promoting health than taking supplements.

Nutrition Shortcut in a Can?

THE STORY

A recent barrage of advertising implies that we could all use a Boost to Ensure we're getting our dietary ReSources or meeting our daily Nutri-Needs. According to the high-profile ads, meals in a can with names like these will help keep us healthy and active and, by improving nutrition, will help ward off the ravages of aging. Here's an example: "Sustacal can't add years to your life, but it may add life to your years." Ads for Boost show fit fortysomethings drinking nutritional supplements to "fill in the blanks" because they skipped a meal or are working too hard.

Ensure, the granddaddy of nutrient supplements, was originally developed for use in hospitals and nursing homes for people who were too sick or too weak to eat. But thanks to an aggressive marketing campaign, it is now being sold in grocery stores and pharmacies. Skyrocketing demand has spawned a bevy of competitors. The *Wall Street Journal* reports that sales of these canned nutritional supplements grew 49 percent in both 1994 and 1995, topping $400 million last year.

Just what can you get from downing one of these supplements? As the table shows, they all contain protein, carbohydrates, vitamins, and minerals, and most contain some fat. A single can costs between $1 and $2. Drinking three cans of Ensure a day (that's what its label suggests) would cost about $1,500 per year.

We asked the chief of surgical nutrition at the New England Deaconess Hospital to discuss the pluses and minuses of meals in a can and to describe who really needs them.

— *The Editors*

THE PHYSICIAN'S PERSPECTIVE

George Blackburn, MD

Thirty years ago, it was not uncommon for cancer patients or people who had undergone surgery to starve to death in hospitals, either because they could not eat or because their illnesses obliterated their appetites. Medical researchers across the country were trying to determine the special nutritional needs of these patients, and whether it was best to deliver nutrients intravenously — into the bloodstream — or through small tubes directly into the stomach or intestines.

Back in 1974, some colleagues and I wrote an article for the *Journal of the American Medical Association* on the causes of malnutrition in hospitalized patients and the critical need for new treatments. Soon after it was published, I was invited to speak on this topic at Ross Laboratories, a leading baby-food maker. Ross researchers were then trying to make a complete "formula" for sick adults. They ultimately came up with Ensure. A person could drink it, or it could be delivered to the digestive system via a small tube.

Because this product was sold as a specialty food, it did not have to go through the extensive and expensive testing process the Food and Drug Administration requires for drugs. And it could also be marketed directly to consumers without the fine print that accompanies ads for prescription drugs.

In the beginning, Ensure and its competitors were sold primarily to hospitals and nursing homes. For people who could

WHAT'S IN THOSE CANS?					
	Boost	Sustacal HP	ReSource	Ensure	NutraStart
Calories	240	240	180	250	210
Total fat	4 g (6%)	6 g (9%)	0	9 g (14%)	2.5 g (4%)
Saturated fat	0.5 g (3%)	1 g (5%)	0	1.5 g (8%)	0.5 g (3%)
Sodium	130 mg (5%)	220 mg (9%)	55 mg (2%)	200 mg (8%)	350 mg (15%)
Total carbohydrates	40 g (13%)	33 g (11%)	36 g (12%)	34 g (11%)	38 g (13%)
Fiber	0	<1 g (<4%)	0	<1 g (<4%)	5 g (20%)
Protein	10 g (20%)	15 g (30%)	9 g (18%)	9 g (18%)	10 g (20%)
Vitamin A	15%	20%	15%	15%	50%
Vitamin C	100%	20%	60%	60%	100%
Vitamin D	25%	20%	15%	15%	25%
Vitamin E	100%	20%	20%	20%	100%
Folate	35%	20%	15%	25%	25%
Iron	20%	20%	15%	15%	20%
Calcium	30%	20%	15%	15%	50%

% = % of Recommended Dietary Allowance

not eat, these products were a godsend and saved thousands of lives. But, as hospital stays shortened, and more people began receiving medical care as outpatients or at home, the makers of nutritional supplements began selling them over the counter. People with AIDS turned to meal replacements in an effort to counter the severe wasting that accompanies this disease. In fact, the meal replacement called Advera is specially designed for people who are HIV positive.

In an effort to broaden their market, manufacturers are no longer limiting their sales pitch to people who are ill or who cannot eat. They are now targeting everyone from frail senior citizens to fit, healthy baby boomers.

Some people can clearly benefit from meal replacements:

◆ People over age 50 who have a chronic illness accompanied by weight loss, weakness, and fatigue, and who are eating fewer than three meals a day.

◆ People who have trouble swallowing or chewing.

◆ People eager to recover from an illness and regain their strength and stamina so they can get back to work or to their normal activities.

◆ People who eat alone, and thus often eat poorly, or those who don't have the money to buy the healthy food they need.

What about people who aren't sick? According to several national surveys, five out of six Americans do not eat three meals a day, and nine out of 10 don't eat breakfast. These meal replacement products actually do represent a reasonable choice for people on the go who skip meals or eat junk food in place of a healthy meal.

Spending $1.50 for a breakfast consisting of a canned meal replacement certainly makes better nutritional sense than spending $2.00 for a cafe latte. A can of Ensure offers 250 calories, nine grams of protein, nine grams of fat, and a dozen or so vitamins and minerals. The best thing is that it requires no preparation. To get the nutritional equivalent of a can of Ensure from food, you would have to eat a bowl of cereal with fruit and low-fat milk, plus a piece of toast, or a cup of yogurt with a piece of fruit and a whole-grain muffin. In each case, you'd have to take a multivitamin tablet too.

But real food has benefits the meal replacements just can't offer. Most don't include any fiber, which is known to help prevent colorectal cancer and may lower cholesterol levels (see *HN*, February 13 and March 26). And despite being fortified with several vitamins and minerals, meal replacements don't contain micronutrients such as isoflavones, carotenoids, and other plant-derived compounds that maintain health and prevent disease.

Certainly, drinking a canned supplement in place of the occasional skipped meal is better than eating junk food or fat-saturated fast food. But in the long run, there are no shortcuts to healthful eating – a can a day won't keep the doctor away. The smart consumer will design his or her own prescription for a healthy, realistic lifestyle, ideally in concert with a registered dietitian or certified nutritionist. In addition to a healthy diet, this lifestyle will include plenty of physical activity and several different strategies for managing stress.

Dr. Blackburn is director of nutrition support services at New England Deaconess Hospital and vice president-elect of the North American Society for the Study of Obesity.

The 'Dietary Supplement' Mess
Commission Report Issued

by Stephen Barrett, MD

In the early 1990s, Congress began considering two bills to greatly strengthen the ability of federal agencies to combat health frauds. One would have increased the FDA's enforcement powers as well as the penalties for violating the Food, Drug, and Cosmetic Act. The other would have amended the Federal Trade Commission Act to make it illegal to advertise nutritional or therapeutic claims that would not be permissible on supplement labels. During the same period, the FDA was considering tighter regulations for these labels.

> *The end result was a law that greatly weakened the FDA's ability to protect consumers.*

Alarmed by these developments, the health-food industry and its allies urged Congress to "preserve the consumer's freedom to choose dietary supplements." To whip up their troops, industry leaders warned retailers that they would be put out of business. Consumers were told that unless they took action, the FDA would take away their right to buy vitamins. These claims, although bogus, generated an avalanche of communications to Congress.

The end result was a law that greatly weakened the FDA's ability to protect consumers. Called the Dietary Supplement Health and Education Act (DSHEA) of 1994, it defined "dietary supplements" as a separate regulatory category and liberalized what information could be distributed by their sellers.

It also created an NIH Office of Dietary Supplements and directed the President to appoint a Commission on Dietary Supplement Labels to recommend ways to implement the act. The Commission's recommendations were released on June 24, 1997. (See "Recommendations from the Dietary Supplement Commission.")

Expanded Definition

The Food, Drug, and Cosmetic Act defines "drug" as any article (except devices) "intended for use in the diagnosis, cure, mitigation, treatment, or prevention of disease" and "articles (other than food) intended to affect the structure or function of the body." These words permit the FDA to stop the marketing of products with unsubstantiated "drug" claims on their labels.

To evade the law's intent, the supplement industry is organized to ensure that the public learns of "medicinal" uses that are not stated on product labels. This is done mainly by promoting the ingredients of the products in books, magazines, newsletters, booklets, lectures, radio and television broadcasts, and oral claims made by retailers.

DSHEA worsened this situation by increasing the amount of misinformation that can be directly transmitted to prospective customers. It also expanded the types of products that could be marketed as "supplements." The most logical definition of "dietary supplement" would be something that supplies one or more essential nutrients missing from the diet. DSHEA went far beyond this to include vitamins; minerals; herbs or other botanicals; amino acids; other dietary substances to supplement the diet by increasing dietary intake; and any concentrate, metabolite, constituent, extract, or combination of any such ingredients. Although

many such products (particularly herbs) are marketed for their alleged preventive or therapeutic effects, DSHEA has made it difficult or impossible for the FDA to regulate them as drugs. Since its passage, even hormones, such as DHEA and melatonin, are being hawked as supplements. DSHEA also prohibits the FDA from banning dubious supplement ingredients as "unapproved food additives." The FDA considered this strategy more efficient than taking action against individual manufacturers who made illegal drug claims. Since DSHEA's passage, the only way to banish an ingredient is to prove it is unsafe. Ingredients that are useless but harmless are protected.

'Nutritional Support' Statements

DSHEA allows dietary supplements to bear "statements of support" that: (1) claim a benefit related to classical nutrient deficiency disease, (2) describe how ingredients affect the structure or function of the human body, (3) characterize the documented mechanism by which the ingredients act to maintain structure or function, or (4) describe general well-being from consumption of the ingredients. The statement "calcium builds strong bones and teeth" is said to be a classic example of an allowable structure/function statement for a food. What constitutes an allowable statement for a supplement has not been specified either by law or by regulation.

To be legal, a "nutritional support" statement must not be a "drug" claim. In other words, it should not suggest that the product or ingredient is intended for prevention or treatment of disease.

The Dietary Supplement Commission expressed concern that "some statements of nutritional support are in fact akin to drug claims." Some members be-

Major Recommendations from the Dietary Supplement Commission

Safety

- Safety of supplement products must be assured.
- The FDA, the supplement industry, scientific groups, and consumer groups should work together to expand and improve postmarketing surveillance, including adverse reporting systems.
- Product information should include appropriate warnings.
- The FDA should take swift enforcement action to address safety issues, such as those posed by ephedra-containing products. The agency should be given additional resources to do this.

Health Claims

- The approval process for health claims should be the same for dietary supplements and conventional foods.
- The standard of "significant scientific agreement" is appropriate but should not require unanimous or near unanimous support.
- To determine whether significant scientific agreement exists for particular claims, the FDA should obtain broad input and use appropriate outside expert panels.

Statements of Nutritional Support

- Statements of nutritional support should provide useful information about the product's intended use.
- Statements of nutritional support should be supported by scientifically valid evidence substantiating that the statements are truthful and not misleading
- Structure/function statements should not suggest disease prevention or treatment.
- Statements that mention a body system, organ, or function affected by a supplement using such terms as "stimulate," "maintain," "support," "regulate," or "promote" can be appropriate when the statements do not suggest disease prevention or treat-

ment or use for a serious health condition beyond the ability of the consumer to evaluate.

- Statements should not be made for products to "restore" normal or "correct" abnormal function where the abnormality implies the presence of disease. (For example, a claim to "restore" normal blood pressure when the abnormality implies hypertension.)
- Statements of nutritional support are not to be drug claims. They should not refer to specific diseases, disorders, or classes of diseases and should not use such drug-related terms as "diagnose," "treat," "prevent," "cure," or "mitigate."

Substantiation of Nutritional Support Statements

- The Dietary Supplement Health and Education Act (DSHEA) requires manufacturers marketing supplements labeled for "nutritional support" to notify the Secretary of Health and Human Services within 30 days after marketing of a product bearing such a statement. To satisfy this requirement, the notice should include: (1) the identity of the ingredient(s) for which the statement is made, (2) the product's intended use, including recommended dosage, (3) appropriate contraindications or warnings, (4) a brief summary of the evidence and conclusions about safety and effectiveness of the stated dosage, and (5) a consumer version of the evidence on which any claim is made.
- DSHEA requires manufacturers marketing supplements labeled for "nutritional support" to have substantiation. To satisfy that requirement, the manufacturer's substantiation files should contain: (1) a copy of the notification letter, (2) key evidence, including an interpretive summary by a qualified individual, (3) the identity and quantity of the pertinent dietary ingredients, (4) evidence substantiating the

ingredient's safety, (5) assurance that good manufacturing practices were followed, and (6) the qualifications of the individual(s) who reviewed the evidence for safety and effectiveness. A consumer version of the evidence should be made available to the public for each product bearing a statement of nutritional support. This version should not state or imply use for preventing or treating disease.

Publications Connected to Sales

- Articles provided to consumers must be balanced and truthful. The FDA should promptly issue warnings or undertake enforcement action if it becomes aware of violations.
- The FDA should monitor practices in this area and issue guidelines as needed.

Botanical Products

- The FDA should establish an OTC review panel to review botanical products intended for preventive or therapeutic use.
- For products unable to meet FDA review requirements, creation of an alternative approval system should be considered.

Assessment of Consumer Education

- Research should be done to determine whether consumers want and can use information required by existing FDA regulations, DSHEA requirements, and Dietary Supplement Commission recommendations. This would include statements of nutritional support as well as point-of-sale literature.

Expert Evaluation

- The dietary supplement industry should consider establishing an expert advisory committee to provide scientific review of label statements and claims and guidance on safety and appropriate labeling. Such a committee might be supported by one or more trade associations or might be established as an independent entity funded by grants and/or fees for services.

lieve that claims related to organs (such as "supports the eyes" or "supports the cardiovascular system") are really drug claims and that DSHEA has created a loophole for such claims. Some members are particularly concerned about statements that mention an acute effect on the structure or function of a major system (such as "reduces heart rate").

Actually, few statements about the biochemical or physiologic properties of nutrients have practical value for consumers. By definition, every essential nutrient is important to proper body function. Simple statements about nutrient function are more likely to be misleading than helpful. A statement such as "vitamin A is essential to good eye function" could suggest: (1) people need to take special steps to be sure they get enough, (2) extra vitamin A may enhance eyesight, and (3) common eye problems may be caused by vitamin A deficiency or remedied by taking supplements. To be completely truthful, a "nutritional support" statement about vitamin A would have to counter all three misconceptions and indicate that people eating sensibly don't need to worry about whether their vitamin A intake is adequate. In other words, truthful statements about nutrient supplements would have to indicate who doesn't need them. No vitamin manufacturer has ever done this or ever will.

Since herbs are not nutrients, the concept of "nutritional support" statements for herbs is absurd. The Dietary Supplement Commission noted: "Many botanicals now are being marketed with statements of nutritional support that suggest only indirectly the type of therapeutic use that is traditional for the product. . . . Most Commissioners believe direct therapeutic statements . . . may be more informative." The Commission's report urges the FDA to develop a review process that could enable herbs that have substantiated therapeutic use to be marketed as over-the-counter drugs.

A recent ad in *Veggie Life* magazine illustrates the absurdities that DSHEA has spawned. The headline states: "IT PROTECTS YOUR HEART THE WAY FORT KNOX PROTECTS GOLD." The body of the ad states: "MaxiLIFE Cardio Protector nutritionally supports healthy cardiovascular function on a whole new level of potency.* That's because it's no ordinary formula, but a nutritional all-star team of cardioprotective agents." The asterisk refers to the disclaimer that DSHEA requires with "support" statements: "This statement has not been evaluated by the Food and Drug Administration. The product is not intended to diagnose, treat, cure or prevent any disease." The Fort Knox analogy, which suggests complete cardioprotection, is printed in half-inch type. The disclaimer is in 4-point type, which is barely visible.

Under some circumstances, some ingredients in Cardio Protector might help protect a person's heart. Its B vitamins, for example, could lower elevated blood homocysteine levels, which are a risk factor for coronary artery disease. However, there is no reason for people whose homocysteine level is normal to use this product. The dozen or so other ingredients have little or no proven value for cardioprotection. People really interested in protecting their heart should follow an individually designed program based on risk-factor analysis. For these reasons, I believe that Cardio Protector has no rational use. Its manufacturer, Twin Laboratories of Ronkonkema, New York, also markets Prostate Protector and Brain Protector.

Under DSHEA, manufacturers who make statements of "nutritional support" must have substantiation that such statements are truthful and not misleading. The law also requires that the Secretary of Health and Human Services be notified no later than 30 days after the first marketing of a supplement for which the statement is being made. The law does not define substantiation.

Publications Connected to Sales

Historically, the FDA has considered literature used directly in connection with the sale of a product to be "labeling" for the product. DSHEA exempts publications from "labeling" if they: (1) are not false or misleading, (2) do not promote a particular manufacturer or brand, (3) present a "balanced" view of pertinent scientific information, and (4) are physically separated from the items discussed. However, since most "dietary supplements" are either useless, irrationally formulated, and/or overpriced, the supplement industry has little reason to provide literature that is not misleading.

The Dietary Supplement Commission concluded that the criteria listed above would be difficult to apply, particularly the requirement for balance. "Balance" is difficult or impossible to define, and standards, if they are developed, would be difficult to enforce. Moreover, no federal agency has the resources to regulate what individual retailers do in their stores.

Further Weakening Proposed

The Nutrition Labeling and Education Act of 1990 prohibits misleading health claims on foods. It requires such claims to be supported by "significant scientific agreement" and be cleared by the FDA before use in the marketplace. Section 618 of the FDA Modernization and Accountability Act (S. 830) would eliminate preclearance and enable claims to be based on statements by any federal agency, even if the agency's position is counter to the prevailing scientific view or fails to take overall diet into account. (Currently, for example, even though some agencies have recommended eating a low-fat diet, the FDA does not permit health claims to be made for low-fat foods that are very high in sodium.) The Food and Nutrition Labeling Group, a 21-member coalition of prominent professional and consumer organizations, has vigorously objected to Section 618.

The Bottom Line

The FDA has never had enough resources to cope with the enormous amount of deception in the supplement and health-food marketplace. DSHEA has made the problem worse. If I were FDA Commissioner, I would drop any pretense of being able to protect the public. Instead, I would announce that unless Congress provides an adequate law, the FDA cannot protect the public from the deceptive marketing of what DSHEA calls "dietary supplements."

See Addendum.

*Stephen Barrett, MD, a retired psychiatrist, is a board member of the National Council Against Health Fraud and webmaster of Quackwatch (**http://www.quackwatch. com**), a guide to quackery, health frauds, and intelligent decision making.*

ADDENDUM

Table 1

Innovations in DSHEA Compared to Prior Law (NLEA and FDCA)

Issue	Provisions Under Prior Law	DSHEA
Definition of dietary supplement.	Only essential nutrients such as vitamins, minerals, and proteins considered.	Adds amino acids, herbs, botanicals, or similar substances or mixtures intended to supplement the diet, and concentrates, metabolites, constituents, extracts or combinations thereof, designed to increase total daily intake in pill, capsule, tablet, powder, or liquid form.
Regulatory framework for assuring safety of products.	More; FDA had more authority to regulate products such as herbs or certain dietary supplements that might be harmful. They could be classified as "food additives" of "new drugs" under the FDCA which required premarket approval. New ingredients in dietary supplements were regulated under the 1958 Food Additive Amendments to the FDCA.	Less; dietary supplements are no longer subject to premarket safety evaluations required of new food or for new uses of old ingredients. Also, regulatory avenues are more circumscribed by the new law for these products. Other safety provisions of the FDCA must be met.
Guidelines for literature now displayed where label and supplements are sold.	Publications such as articles, book chapters, or abstracts of peer reviewed scientific papers were considered labeling and regulated as such when provided in connection with the sale of dietary supplements.	Such information not considered part of the label and is not regulated as such as long as the publications are not false and misleading, do not promote a particular brand or manufacturer and are displayed so as to present a balanced view of the relevant scientific information, physically separate from the dietary supplement.
Use of claims and supporting nutritional statements.	Only appropriate health claims authorized by the FDA allowed for products qualified to bear the health claim.	Nutritional statements allowed without prior approval by FDA. Statements about classical nutrient deficiency disease allowed if the prevalence of the disease in the U.S. is disclosed. Supplement's effects on the structure or function of the body or well-being achieved by consumption of the dietary ingredient are allowed if manufacturer can substantiate that the statements are true and not misleading, and the product label bears the disclaimer that the statement has not been evaluated by FDA, and that the product is not intended to diagnose, treat, cure or prevent any disease. (Note: Structure function claims are not considered health claims.)

Source: *Nutrition & the M.D.*, May 1997, p. 3.

Table 2

**Comparisons of Labeling and Health Claims for Foods
Under NLEA and for Dietary Supplements Under DSHEA**

Issue	NLEA	DSHEA
Definitions	"High potency" not permitted under proposed regulations on foods. Antioxidant content claims permissible on both foods and supplements.	Regulations to define such terms as "high potency" (100% or more the RDI for vitamins and minerals or 100% of the DRV for protein or fiber for at least two-thirds of the nutrients present in the product). Definitions of "antioxidant" (vitamins C, E, beta carotene) provided.
Claims permitted	Certain preapproved disease prevention claims permitted on food packages, when nutrient-disease relationship supported by significant scientific agreement.	Includes all NLEA health claims, a benefit related to "classical nutrient deficiency disease" and discloses its prevalence in U.S.: • Describes role of nutrient/dietary ingredient intended to affect structure or function in humans (that is a statement of how nutrition is supported). • Characterizes the documented mechanism by which nutrient acts to maintain structure or function. • Describes general well-being from consuming supplement.
Ingredient labeling	Required on most food products.	Ingredients not marketed in U.S. before passage of DSHEA permitted unless they contain substances that have not been present in the food supply as a material used for food in a form, or they are in a form that has been chemically altered. If there is evidence that the supplement will reasonably be expected to be safe when used as directed, and the manufacturer provides the FDA with information on which the manufacturer has concluded that the dietary supplement is expected to be safe, it will be permitted.
Reference daily intakes (RDIs)	RDI's are new food label reference values for nutrients, replacing the USRDA's. They did not exist until 1997.	More nutrients have RDIs and % DV can now be stated when present. RDI's may appear on nutrition facts panel as % of Daily Value (DV) for protein and 26 vitamins and minerals. Recently added K, selenium, manganese, chromium, molybdenum, and chloride. No RDI for fluoride.
Nutrient labeling for non-nutrient ingredients	Not allowed	Dietary ingredients that are not nutrients can be displayed prominently on the label following nutrient ingredients.
Nutrition labeling	Information on dietary ingredients for which reference daily intakes (RDI) are available or daily reference values (DRV). RDI that are not available appear only in the ingredient label, not within the nutrition facts panel.	Supplements must bear supplement facts with dietary ingredients for which FDA has established DVs listed first. DSHEA also permits the label to include information on substances that are not nutrients listed next. For example, herbal substances may now be listed on the label panel, and the source of the substance may also be listed.

Source: *Nutrition & the M.D.*, May, 1997, p. 5.

Dead doctors don't lie, but people who sell minerals...

Last year people started sending us copies—dozens of copies—of *Dead Doctors Don't Lie,* a taped lecture by a veterinarian/naturopath named Joel Wallach, which promotes a "colloidal mineral" elixir. "Should we buy this stuff?" our readers asked. It's sold by dozens of companies under names such as Mineral Solutions, Clark's Mineral Formula, Mineral Toddy, Micro-Min, Colloidal Silver, Essential Minerals. Testimonials have flooded the Internet. *The warning signs were clear right away:*

Uh-oh. The products cure/prevent *everything*: AIDS, cancer, TB, malaria, lupus, syphilis, scarlet fever, herpes, pneumonia, typhoid, tetanus, rheumatism, parasites, chronic fatigue, whooping cough, hemorrhoids, ringworm, candida, bubonic plague, obesity, liver disease, thyroid problems, acne, sunburn, menstrual cramps, memory problems, and on and on. Testimonials are the sole support. Cure-alls seldom cure anything.

Hmm. They are sold primarily via multi-level marketing, which turns customers into salespeople. That is, if you buy the product, you can become a distributor and then sell it, via altruistic pitches, to your friends and relatives, who sell it to their friends, etc., with profits passing up to the top of the pyramid, at least in theory. Such "network marketing" of health-related products should always make you suspicious.

Huh? The promotional materials repeatedly state that we can't get the minerals we need from vegetables, fruits, and grains grown on our "depleted" soil. This is not true (see box at right). The real problem is that Americans simply eat so little produce.

What? Printed on the cassettes was the claim that "the average life-span of an M.D. is only 58 years." That's supposed to prove that doctors don't know much about health. But doctors actually have an above-average life expectancy—more than 75 years.

A prophet brings profits
The story starts in a pseudo-mythic haze. In 1925 Thomas Clark,

Is our soil depleted of minerals?
The claim that American soil has been ruined for growing food is often used to sell nutritional supplements, including colloidal minerals. But, convenient as it may be for salespeople, this idea is a figment of the colloidal imagination. One study by Firman Bear of Rutgers University in 1949 has been relentlessly misquoted in support of this point. The study simply compared the mineral content of several types of vegetables grown in different areas. Because of soil type and fertilizer use, some vegetables had more minerals than others—not a surprise. According to Dr. W. Shaw Reid, director or the Cornell Nutrient Analysis Lab at Cornell University, improved farming methods and fertilizers have made our soil richer than ever. The claim that fertilizers contain synthetic minerals as opposed to the "organic" ones found in colloidal mineral products is also meaningless, since all minerals are inorganic. To a plant, and to the human body, it doesn't matter where the minerals come from.

Plants just won't grow in depleted soil. Vitamins in foods are created by the plants themselves. Minerals—such as phosphorus, potassium, iodine, calcium, copper, iron, selenium, fluoride, molybdenum, and zinc—must come from the soil. If the soil lacks any of these, fertilizers compensate. Climate, weather, amount of sunlight, and other factors also affect overall nutritive value. But if the fruits and vegetables you buy look healthy, you can be certain they contain the nutrients they should.

a rancher in central Utah, finds a legendary spring that Indians claimed had healing powers. Following the spring, he discovers the mineral remains (sometimes called humic shale) of a prehistoric rain forest. He extracts the minerals and passes on the "miracle liquid" to friends and neighbors. This "original" product has spawned a mini-industry, with various companies claiming that their product is the real thing and that the rest are useless, bogus, or dangerous imitations. The elixirs, which often look like muddy water, cost $25 to $50 for a one-month supply. Colloidal minerals are also sold in capsule form.

The array of minerals varies greatly from product to product: silver, arsenic, cadmium, lead, aluminum, lithium, titanium, and dozens of others. The colloidal marketers claim that you absorb only 5% of the minerals you normally consume, while their products allow you to absorb nearly 100%. Their minerals supposedly have a natural negative electrical charge that allows them to enter cells easily, as well as to flush out "toxins" that are attracted to them. (A colloid is, like milk and purées, simply a suspension of particles in a liquid.) Minerals from foods and from ordinary supplements are poorly absorbed, they say, because these have a positive charge and can build up to toxic levels in the body. This results in virtually all the debilitating diseases of today. Says them.

A closer look

All the nutrition experts we spoke with dismissed the claims made for colloidal minerals. According to Dr. C. J. van Oss, a specialist in microbiology, geology, and chemical engineering at SUNY Buffalo Medical School, the charge on a mineral should not affect its absorption. The fact that the minerals are in a colloidal suspension also wouldn't matter. Dr. Sheldon Margen, chairman of our Editorial Board, says that *even if these minerals were better absorbed, that wouldn't necessarily be desirable, since some of them are potentially toxic and many are of no known use to humans.* Moreover, some brands are contaminated by bacteria, according to Dr. Ellen Kamhi of the Corsello Center for Complementary Medicine in New York City. There's no evidence that colloidal silver products, in particular, are safe or can prevent/treat any disease, according to the FDA.

Some of the companies claim that clinical tests have been done on their products, but we have not been able to find a single published study. **The conclusion is clear:** *No one should take colloidal minerals. Fruits and vegetables are the way to go.*

Don't Buy Phony 'Ergogenic Aids'

The real story vs. a mountain of hype

by Stephen Barrett, MD

More than a hundred companies are marketing phony "ergogenic aids," combinations of various vitamins, minerals, amino acids, and other "dietary supplements" claimed to build muscles and/or enhance athletic performance. In 1991, researchers from the U.S. Centers for Disease Control and Prevention surveyed 12 popular health and bodybuilding magazines (one issue each) and found ads for 89 brands and 311 products with a total of 235 unique ingredients. *Health Foods Business* estimates that in 1996, total sales of such products through health-food stores exceeded $204 million. They are also sold through pharmacies and superstores.

The Start of 'Ergogenic' Myths

The notion that massive amounts of protein are necessary during training have evolved from the ancient beliefs that great strength could be obtained by eating the raw meat of lions, tigers, or other animals that displayed great fighting strength. Today, although few athletes consume raw meat, the idea that "you are what you eat" is still widely promoted by food faddists.

During the 1900s, when muscles were discovered to contain protein, athletes and coaches mistakenly concluded that protein was the principal component. (Actually, it is water.) These protein beliefs were further reinforced during the 1930s by Bob Hoffman (1899–1985) and later by Joe Weider (1923–), both of whom published magazines that catered to bodybuilders and weightlifters. They asserted that athletes have special protein needs, that protein

supplements have special muscle-building and health-giving powers, and that the most efficient way to get enough protein is by using supplements. The scientific facts are otherwise. Muscle-building is not caused by eating extra protein. It is stimulated by increased muscular work. Once basic protein needs have been met, the small additional amount needed during intense training is easily obtainable from a balanced diet. Few Americans fail to consume adequate amounts of protein.

> *Hoffman and Weider asserted that protein supplements have special muscle-building and health-giving powers.*

Hoffman marketed supplement products and bodybuilding equipment through his York Barbell Company of York, Pennsylvania. A prolific writer, he published two magazines and more than 30 books on fitness and nutrition. For many years, York Barbell's nutritional products were promoted with false and misleading claims. In 1960, the company was charged with misbranding its Energol Germ Oil Concentrate because literature accompanying the oil claimed falsely that it could prevent or treat more than 120 diseases and conditions, including epilepsy, gallstones, and arthritis. In 1961, 15 other York Barbell products were seized as misbranded. In 1968, a larger number of products came under at-

tack by the government for similar reasons. In 1972, the FDA seized three types of York Barbell protein supplements, charging that they were misbranded with false and misleading bodybuilding claims. In 1974, the company was again charged with misbranding Energol and protein supplements. The oil had been claimed to be a special source of vigor and energy. False bodybuilding claims had been made for the protein supplements.

Despite his many brushes with the law, Hoffman achieved considerable professional prominence. During his athletic career, first as an oarsman and then as a weightlifter, he received over 600 trophies, certificates, and awards. He was the Olympic weightlifting coach from 1936 to 1968 and was a founding member of the President's Council on Physical Fitness and Sports.

Weider began bodybuilding as a teenager and was 16 when he launched a newsletter called *Your Physique*. A few years later, he started a company that sold bodybuilding equipment and instructional booklets through the mail. In 1946, Joe's brother Ben joined the business, and they set up the International Federation of Bodybuilders, which promotes the sport worldwide and sponsors competitions. According to press reports, their business empire now grosses over $500 million annually.

Weider Health & Fitness is the dominant player in the sports-supplement marketplace. It publishes seven magazines, sells bodybuilding equipment, broadcasts "Muscle Magazine" on ESPN, and sponsors many athletic and aerobic events throughout the year. The magazines are *Muscle & Fitness, Shape, Flex, Living Fit, Men's Fitness, Prime Health & Fitness,* and *Senior*

Reprinted with permission from *Nutrition Forum,* May/June 1997, pp. 17, 19–21, 24. © 1997 by Prometheus Books, 59 John Glenn Drive, Amherst, NY 14228.

Golfer. The supplements include Anabolic Mega-Pak, Dynamic Life Essence, Dynamic Super Stress-End, Dynamic Power Source, Dynamic Driving Force, Dynamic Fat Burners, Dynamic Liver Concentrate Energizer, Dynamic Sustained Endurance, Dynamic Recupe, Dynamic Body Shaper, and Dynamic Muscle Builder. None of these products appears capable of doing what its name suggests, and none contains any nutrients not readily obtainable from a balanced diet.

> *None of these products appears capable of doing what its name suggests.*

In 1984, the FTC charged that ads for Anabolic Mega-Pak (containing amino acids, minerals, vitamins, and herbs) and Dynamic Life Essence (an amino acid product) had been misleading. The FTC complaint was settled in 1985 when Weider and the company agreed not to falsely claim that these products can help build muscles or are effective substitutes for anabolic steroids. They also agreed to pay a minimum of $400,000 in refunds or (if refunds did not reach this figure) to fund research on the relationship of nutrition to muscle development. Although the forbidden claims no longer appear in Weider ads, similar messages appear in articles in the magazines and are implied by endorsements and pictures of muscular athletes as well as by names of the products themselves. False and misleading claims have also appeared in a series of 18 booklets published in 1990 by Weider Health & Fitness and marketed through GNC stores.

The Market Grows

During the 1970s, in addition to protein supplements and assorted vitamins, the main products touted to athletes were wheat germ oil and bee pollen (falsely claimed to boost energy and endurance). In the early 1980s, Weider Health & Fitness introduced an "Olympians" line said to have been developed by working closely with "Olympians and nutritional researchers." Most were sustained-release vitamin concoctions that included an exotic ingredient or two. As public interest in fitness grew, several drug companies began falsely claiming that multivitamin or "stress" supplements were just what active people needed.

Life Extension, by Durk Pearson and Sandy Shaw, was published in 1982 and was followed by appearances by the authors on hundreds of radio and television talk shows. The book claimed that supplements of certain amino acids would cause the body to release growth hormone, which would produce muscle growth and fat loss with little or no effort. These claims were based on faulty extrapolations of experiments in which animals were given large does of these amino acids by injection. Swallowing amino acids does not cause humans to release growth hormone.

> *False and misleading claims have also appeared in a series of 18 booklets published in 1990 by Weider Health & Fitness and marketed through GNC stores.*

But the massive publicity garned by Pearson and Shaw inspired the health-food industry to market hundreds of new products for athletes and would-be dieters. Many of these products are falsely claimed to be "natural steroids" or "steroid substitutes." In the ensuing years, scores of other useless ingredients have been added to "ergogenic aids."

Some manufacturers make no claims in their ads but imply them in product names. Many use pictures of athletes to convey their messages. Some make explicit claims in their ads or product literature, while others use simple puffery. Several have published charts suggesting which products are good for specific purposes. Some even market products for specific sports.

Just the Facts

Athletes who eat a balanced diet don't need extra protein or vitamins. In *The Complete Sports Medicine Book for Women,* sports medicine specialist Gabe Mirkin, MD, and gynecologist Mona Shangold, MD, explain why: "You don't need much extra protein even to enlarge your muscles. For example, 1 pound of muscle contains only about 100 grams of protein, since it is composed of more than 72% water. So if you are gaining 1 pound of muscle every week in an excellent strength training program, you are adding only about 100 grams of protein each week, or about 15 grams of protein each day. Two cups of corn and beans will meet this need—far less than you would expect. In addition, requirements for only four vitamins increase with exercise: thiamin, niacin, riboflavin, and pantothenic acid. These vitamins are used up minimally in the breakdown of carbohydrates and, to a small degree, protein for energy. But you will find them abundantly in food. Furthermore, deficiencies of these vitamins have never been reported in athletes."

What about other products? The most thorough investigation has been conducted by David Lightsey, MD, an exercise physiologist and nutritionist who coordinates the National Council Against Health Fraud's Task Force on Ergogenic Aids. During the past several years, he has telephoned more than 100 companies that market "ergogenic aids." In a recent interview, Lightsey told me: "In each case, I told a company representative that I had been asked to collect data on the company's product(s) and issue a formal report. After they described the alleged benefits, I would ask how data supporting these claims were collected. As my questions became more specific, their responses became more vague. Some said they could not be more specific because they did not wish to reveal trade secrets.

Hot but risky?

Creatine has been described as the "hottest" ergogenic supplement of the decade. It is popular because it can increase endurance and speed recovery from strenuous activities, which can enhance strength training for certain sports. However, a significant percentage of users experience cramps, muscle spasms, and pulled muscles. Scientific studies have shown that depletion of creatine stores may be associated with the onset of muscle fatigue and that supplementation can increase muscle creatine levels after a few days. The increase was greatest among vegetarians who were found to have the lowest stores. It is not known whether people with adequate dietary intake to begin with run the greatest risk of trouble with supplements. The NCAA Committee on Competitive Safeguards and Medical Aspects of Sports has urged that research be done to determine whether long-term use is safe and whether certain individuals might be predisposed to negative side effects.

"I ended each interview with a request for written documentation. Fewer than half sent anything. Most of the studies they sent were poorly designed and proved nothing. The few that were well designed did not support product claims but were taken out of context.

"Some companies claimed that one team or another was using their products. In each such case, I contacted the team management and learned that although one or more players used the company's products, the management had neither endorsed the products nor encouraged their use."

Lightsey believes there are two reasons why many athletes believe that various products have helped them: (1) use of the product often coincides with natural improvement due to training, and (2) increased self-confidence or a placebo effect inspires greater performance. Any such "psychological benefit," however, should be weighed against the dangers of misinformation, wasted money, misplaced faith, and adverse physical effects—both known and unknown—that can result from megadoses of nutrients. Moreover, how many people who are involved in fitness programs or recreational sports need a placebo for inspiration?

Lack of Action

Little government effort has been made to protect consumers from wasting money on "sports nutrient" products. The FTC took the action noted above against Weider Health & Fitness, the market leader. In 1986, the agency acted against A. H. Robins and its subsidiary, the Viobin Corporation, which had been making false claims for wheat germ oil products for more than 15 years. The case was settled with a consent agreement prohibiting representations that the oil could help consumers improve endurance, stamina, vigor, or other aspects of athletic fitness, or that its active ingredient "octacosanol" is related in any way to body reaction time, oxygen uptake, oxygen debt, or athletic performance.

In 1992, the New York City Department of Consumer Affairs (DCA) published a report called "Magic Muscle Pills! Health and Fitness Quackery in Nutrition Supplements." DCA investigators found that manufacturers they contacted for information about their products were unable to provide a single published report from a scientific journal to back the claims that their products could benefit athletes.

Along with its report, DCA issued "Notices of Violation" to six companies whose products it had investigated. It also warned consumers to beware of terms like "fat burner," "fat fighter," "fat metabolizer," "energy enhancer," "performance booster," "strength booster," "ergogenic aid," "anabolic optimizer," and "genetic optimizer." Calling the bodybuilding supplement industry "an economic hoax with unhealthy consequences," DCA officials urged the FDA and FTC to stop the "blatantly drug-like claims" and false advertising used to promote these products.

In 1994, the FTC reached a consent agreement under which General Nutrition, Inc., paid $2.4 million to settle charges that it had falsely advertised 41 products, most of which had been packaged by other manufacturers. The products included Weider's Super Fat Burners, eleven other "muscle builders," and five other phony "ergogenic aids." No action was taken against the other manufacturers. The FTC's staff is well aware that the "sports nutrition" marketplace needs cleaning up, but it lacks the resources to pursue the majority of offenders. A Trade Regulation Rule that would govern the entire industry could make enforcement more efficient, but the agency has expressed no interest in this approach.

The FDA has the legal right to ban claims that the products stimulate hormone activity or alter the body's metabolism. (Claims of this type enable the agency to classify them as drugs and ban unapproved uses.) In 1994, David Lightsey and I petitioned the FDA to ban all ingredients in these products that had not been proven safe and effective for their intended use and to issue a public warning that the FDA does not recognize them as effective. The agency replied that our petition "did not contain scientific evidence that the claims described in the petition were such that products are . . . unapproved new drugs" and that it "did not provide scientific evidence that would allow the FDA to evaluate the validity of the claims."

Dr. Barrett is board chairman of Quackwatch, Inc., and a board member of the National Council Against Health Fraud. His best-known book is The Vitamin Pushers: How the "Health Food" Industry Is Selling America a Bill of Goods (Prometheus, 1994).

Hunger and Global Issues

Why does one-seventh of the world's population face starvation daily—when enough food is produced every year to feed everybody in the world?
—N.G.O Forum, Rome, November 1996.

The World Food Summit met in Rome in November 1996 and was attended by officials from nearly 200 nations. They declared that all people have the right to be free from hunger through access to safe, nutritious, and culturally acceptable food. In making this declaration, officials pledged to work together to provide a political environment within which they could implement economic and social policies capable of delivering this promise. Permeating the discussions was an emphasis on changing world trade policies as the key to improving food access. They did not sign a binding agreement.

Only a few miles away the N.G.O. (nongovernmental organizations) Forum also met, but these attendees represented a variety of secular and religious organizations that work directly with people to increase food security. One reviewer (see "The Hungry Seventh of the World" by Martin M. McLaughlin, *America*, May 3, 1997) summed the contrast between the two conferences this way: "The Summit saw food security as a supply problem, to be solved by controlling the population growth of the South and expanding the capital-intensive agriculture of the North. . . . The Forum, on the other hand, viewed food security as largely a demand problem, to be solved by distributing food more fairly, reducing overconsumption by the relatively affluent North and improving sustainable smallholder agriculture in the South."

There is also disagreement over the extent of global hunger. Current figures from the Food and Agriculture Organization (FAO) of the United Nations report that 14 percent of the world's population, or 800 million people, do not have enough food to meet basic needs. This accounting is consistent with previous reports over the past half century, each of which has indicated that the problem is worsening. Yet, Nicholas Eberstadt from the Harvard Center for Population and Development, in an address to the Summit, says that the problem may actually be considerably smaller, even two-thirds less in some locations. The available data upon which previous conclusions have been reached, he says, are both flawed and inadequate. In many cases, we really do not know what the nutritional needs of people are; nor do we have good information about their health status. Furthermore, dramatic improvements can be seen in infant mortality rates and estimates of life expectancy in developing countries. Part of the reason for this has to be improved nutrition.

The articles in this unit were chosen to represent the current events and current thinking regarding global hunger and malnutrition. The first article reports on events at the Food Summit and describes the state of world hunger in terms with which we are familiar. Then "Will the World Starve? Feast and Famine" addresses our ability to meet the food demands of a population that is growing in numbers and affluence.

In "Running Out of Water, Running Out of Time," a review of the critical water situation is presented. The two articles that follow represent more hopeful signs of progress. See Fred Pearce's essay, "Crop Gurus Sow Some Seeds of Hope" and "New Farm Techniques Spur Ethiopia Rebirth."

The causes of hunger are multiple, and experts acknowledge that their complexity is difficult to analyze and define: natural disasters, such as periodic cycles of droughts and floods, which are particularly devastating in vulnerable economies; overpopulation and environmental degradation; social upheaval and wars; and an absence of commitment on the part of governments. But the lack of purchasing power is ultimately behind the failure to secure food. Most of the world's poor are in semi-subsistence agriculture and are unable to produce cash crops. They will spend half or more of their small incomes to feed themselves and may still eat less than recommended calories or nutrients.

Hunger is also visible at home. Experts say that U.S. hunger differs from hunger in developing countries in that its cause is poverty uncomplicated by natural disasters, war, or an undeveloped economy. The 1995 Department of Agriculture study of eating patterns in the United States determined that about 12 percent of the 100 million households surveyed either experienced hunger or could not afford good diets. Over 200,000 young children suffered severe hunger. Thus, more people go to bed hungry now than did in the mid-1980s, and millions in our country are said to have food insecurity. While they may not be hungry every day, the food available will not stretch over an entire month. They may skip meals, scavenge, or rely on soup kitchens. Quality and ethnic appropriateness of foods are also concerns. Minorities represent a disproportionate number of the poor, with one-third of all African American families and one-quarter of Hispanics living in poverty. Nor has hunger remained within class boundaries. People from all social levels have lost jobs, and there is ample evidence that hunger and malnutrition have spread to the middle class as well.

Federal Food Assistance Programs, such as food stamps, have undergone changes in a new political climate, resulting in reduced resources that many fear will adversely affect the nutritional status of the needy. Food programs that are intended to supplement the family's food budget sometimes become the primary source of food. WIC (an aid program for women, infants, and children) in particular has been documented to be extremely cost-effective, saving $3 in potential medical costs for every dollar spent, according to the General Accounting Office.

Even these programs do not reach all of the needy. Since 1980, private sector emergency feeding programs such as soup kitchens, food pantries, and homeless shelters have multiplied all over the country. Many of them report turning people away or closing temporarily due to increased demand and dwindling resources.

Mark Twain said that hunger is the handmaid of genius. This aphorism notwithstanding, hunger felt or vicariously experienced by millions has certainly aroused intense emotions of survival and compassion. Experts and ordinary citizens have been challenged to find solutions. Their tireless courage and successful efforts will provide the energy from which future victories will come.

Looking Ahead: Challenge Questions

Should more be done about hunger in the United States? Whose responsibility is it, that of the government or of the private sector? How could you help?

What should be the roles of the United States and other developed countries in solving world hunger? To what extent should countries be expected to solve their own problems?

What criteria would you use to decide when to help another country and how much?

Some argue that we should all become vegetarians. Would this solve the hunger problem at home or abroad? What are the implications of changing the Western diet to one based on plants?

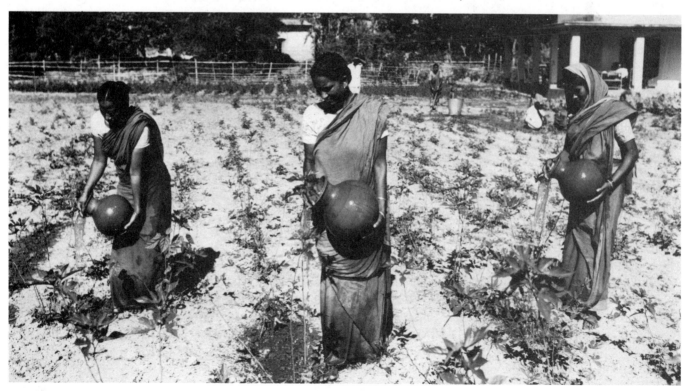

Table Set Thinly as Food Summit Pledges to Halve World Hunger in 20 Years

The Right to Be Free from Hunger

Member States of the United Nations early on identified access to adequate food as a universal human right and collective responsibility. The 1948 Universal Declaration on Human Rights recognized that "everyone has a right to a standard of living adequate for the health and well-being of himself and his family, including food". These concepts were developed more explicitly in the 1966 International Covenant on Economic, Social and Cultural Rights, which stressed the "right of everyone to ... adequate food" and specified that the fundamental right of everyone is to be free from hunger.

O ver the past half century, agricultural production has managed to keep pace with and even outstrip population growth. Yet, there are today some 840 million people worldwide who are chronically undernourished, unable to get enough food to meet their body's energy or nutrient requirements. Over 200 million children under the age of five still suffer from basic protein and energy deficiencies. Millions suffer from diseases and retarded development related to diet deficiencies. And every year, nearly 13 million children die unnecessarily as a direct or indirect result of hunger and malnutrition. *That means that while you read this paragraph, 20 more children have died of hunger and malnutrition.*

By the year 2030, planet Earth is expected to have to nourish 8.7 billion people—up by half from the current 5.7 billion inhabiting this Earth. Just maintaining current levels of food availability will require rapid and sustainable production gains to increase supplies by more than 75 per cent—all without destroying the natural resources on which our survival depends.

It is clear that achieving food security for the world's hungry, who make up 20 per cent of the population of developing countries, means policies that can make it possible for them to grow or buy the food they need today and into the future.

Meeting against this backdrop and in the shadow of the emergency in eastern Zaire, the World Food Summit (13-17 November 1996) concluded in Rome by setting a course for achieving universal food security—"Food for All"—when it adopted by acclamation the Rome Declaration on World Food Security and the World Food Summit Plan of Action. These documents also pledge efforts to halve the number of hungry in the world no later than 2015.

Representatives of 186 countries in the Rome Summit included 41 Presidents, 15 Vice-Presidents and 41 Prime Ministers. A total of 9,863 delegates attended, including repre- sentatives of non-governmental organizations (NGOs), United Nations agencies and other international bodies, journalists and support staff. NGOs, youth, parliamentarians, family farmers associations and the private sector held parallel meetings in Rome and reported back to the Summit on their conclusions.

In the Declaration, Heads of State and Government or their representatives said it was "intolerable" and "unacceptable" that over three quarters of a billion people throughout the world "do not have enough food to meet their basic nutritional needs". Reaffirming that "a peaceful, stable and

From *UN Chronicle,* Vol. 33, No. 4, 1996, pp. 24-28. © 1996 by the United Nations. Reprinted by permission of the United Nations Department of Public Information (DPI).

enabling political, social and economic environment is the essential foundation" to food security, they pledged "actions and support" to implement the Summit Plan of Action.

The Action Plan, which is also intended to help deal effectively in the future with emergencies such as in Zaire, contains seven detailed commitments, including sustainable increases in food production, poverty eradication, access to adequate food, and the contribution of trade to food security.

In the Plan of Action, 186 countries pledged their "political will and common and national commitment" to an ongoing effort to eradicate hunger from the world by ensuring that "all people, at all times, have physical and economic access to sufficient, safe and nutritious food to meet their dietary needs and food preferences for an active and healthy life".

The Rome Declaration and Plan of Action give Governments the prime responsibility for achieving food security, and call on them to actively cooperate in a "Food for All" campaign to be based on the Plan's commitments.

'Race against time'

At the Summit's closing session, Food and Agriculture Organization Director-General Jacques Diouf challenged the world to a "race against time" to achieve the Summit goal of reducing the number of hungry by half by 2015. "This is not a maximum goal; it's a minimum goal", he said. The Summit was only the beginning of the fight to ensure that "babies would not cry of hunger and that mothers will not be looking at children who have no hope". He added: "We have the possibility to do it. We have the knowledge. We have the resources. And with the Rome Declaration and the Plan of Action, we've shown that we have the will."

The need for a Summit, said South African Deputy President

Over three quarters of a billion people do not have enough food to meet their basic nutritional needs

Thabo Mbeki, "surely constitutes a severe rebuke for all of us, that through the ages, we could have given birth to a human civilization, one of whose legacies is dire poverty for hundreds of millions of fellow human beings". The delegates clearly knew what needed to be done; otherwise, "we would not have produced the directives to ourselves" contained in the two documents.

As President of the Council of the European Union, Irish Prime Minister John Bruton endorsed the Rome Declaration and the Plan of Action, saying the Union was convinced that the Plan provided a "sound basis" for moving towards eradicating hunger and providing adequate food for all. Their commitments, he stressed, "must not be empty promises. We have a solemn duty as national and international leaders to ensure that words are matched by actions."

Italian Prime Minister and Summit Chairman Romano Prodi said the agreements were a milestone. "Before the eyes of the world, you made a public commitment", he said, adding: "I hope we will never forget our commitment."

While the Summit opened with the adoption by acclamation of the Declaration and Plan of Action, it closed with unresolved disparities concerning implementation. Although the texts had been approved in advance, after more than two years of negotiations that led to compromise language in contentious areas such as trade, development aid, population, sanctions and women's rights, in a sign of the abiding differences 15 countries, including the world's biggest food aid donor—the United States—lodged reservations or interpretative statements.

Although the United States called the Declaration and Plan of Action "a realistic road map", it said in a written interpretive statement that it had not agreed to a target of spending 0.7 per cent of annual economic wealth on official development assistance. It would, however, continue to provide high quality aid on a case-by-case basis as appropriate. It also believed that the

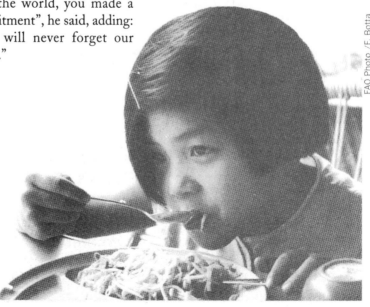

FAO Photo / F. Botta

The Problem

Some 840 million people in developing countries today face chronic undernutrition, and almost 200 million children under the age of five suffer from protein or energy deficiencies. As many as 82 nations fall into the category of low-income food-deficit countries: 41 in sub-Saharan Africa, 19 in Asia and the Pacific, 7 in Latin America and the Caribbean, 6 in the Near East/North Africa, and 9 in Europe/Commonwealth of Independent States. At the same time, commitments of external assistance (bilateral and multilateral) to developing country-agriculture dropped from $18.6 billion in 1982 to $11.7 billion in 1992 (in constant 1990 United States dollars).

Agriculture's share in total official development finance also fell, from 24 to 16 per cent over the same period. To make matters worse, fisheries resources are being over-exploited and forests are being destroyed, with available arable land per caput currently at 0.25 hectare.

The Commitments

In addition to pledging an ongoing effort aimed at "reducing the number of undernourished people to half their present level no later than 2015", the Rome Declaration on World Food Security and the World Food Summit Plan of Action also record seven commitments for national and international action:

◆ Ensure an enabling political, social, and economic environment ... for the eradication of poverty and for durable peace, based on full and equal participation of women and men.

◆ Implement policies aimed at eradicating poverty and inequality and improving physical and economic access by all, at all times, to sufficient, nutritionally adequate and safe food.

◆ Pursue participatory and sustainable food, agriculture, fisheries, forestry and rural development policies and practices ... which are essential to adequate and reliable food supplies ... and combat pests, drought and desertification.

◆ Strive to ensure that food, agricultural trade and overall trade policies are conducive to fostering food security for all through a fair and market-oriented world trade system.

◆ Endeavour to prevent and be prepared for natural disasters and man-made emergencies and to meet transitory and emergency food requirements in ways that encourage recovery, rehabilitation, development and a capacity to satisfy future needs.

◆ Promote optimal allocation and use of public and private investments to foster human resources, sustainable food, agriculture, fisheries and forestry systems, and rural development.

◆ Implement, monitor and follow up this Plan of Action at all levels in cooperation with the international community.

Participatory and sustainable policies are essential for adequate and reliable food supplies

---

attainment of any " 'right to adequate food' or 'fundamental right to be free from hunger' is a goal or aspiration to be realized progressively that does not give rise to any international obligations nor diminish the responsibilities of national Governments toward their citizens".

Maintaining the position it took at the 1994 Cairo Conference on Population and Development and the 1995 Beijing Conference on Women, the Holy See expressed concern over

such terms as "family planning" and "reproductive health care services". Several Islamic countries joined in

those objections. A number of countries, including Iraq, Libya, Burundi and Sudan, expressed reservations regarding economic sanctions, saying these ran counter to the Summit's pledge to alleviate hunger.

The Plan of Action contains seven commitments, which are expected to lead to significant reductions in

---

Twelve per cent of total military spending in developing countries would provide primary health care and safe drinking water for all, eliminate severe malnutrition and cut in half moderate malnutrition

---

Crop Patterns

◆ In the industrialized world, people are consumed by the dangers of weighing too much. In too many parts of the world, people are more concerned about the dangers of weighing too little.

◆ The first recorded famine was in Egypt in 3500 BC.

◆ During the Irish potato famine from 1845 to 1850, more than 1 million people died and at least as many migrated. While the immediate cause may have been failures in the potato crop in successive years due to blight, a variety of social and political factors were also at work, exacerbated by widespread poverty.

◆ In 1943, the Bengal famine claimed between 2 million and 3 million people—not because food was in short supply, but because the price of food was beyond the reach of the poor.

◆ The average daily energy supply has risen from 2,440 calories to 2,720 calories over the last two decades.

◆ Most chronically undernourished people live in over 80 low-income food-deficit countries.

◆ The largest number of chronically undernourished people—512 million or well over half the world's hungry—is in South and Southeast Asia.

◆ Sub-Saharan Africa has the highest proportion of chronically undernourished people: 43 per cent of the population as compared to 20 per cent overall in developing countries.

◆ One in seven people in the world go to bed hungry every night.

◆ For every farmer in the developed world, there are 19 in the developing world.

◆ A gene transferred from a wild rice plant in India has conferred disease resistance to varieties that are now grown across 11 million hectares in Asia.

◆ During the 1980s, more than 15 million hectares of tropical forests were lost each year.

◆ 12 per cent of total military spending in developing countries would provide primary health care for all, including immunization of all children, eliminate severe malnutrition and halve moderate malnutrition, and provide safe drinking water for all.

◆ Three crops—maize, wheat and rice—provide over half the world's calories.

◆ Over 500 species of insect and mite are resistant to pesticides.

◆ Nature needs 3,000 to 12,000 years to build up a layer of soil sufficient to support agriculture.

Rural poverty and food insecurity are closely linked. About 800 million people in developing countries face chronic undernutrition, and almost 200 million children suffer from protein or energy deficiencies. By the year 2030, the world's population will have grown by another 3 billion people, thus further stretching the world's food resources. Ensuring adequate and affordable food supplies, through implementation of the commitments of the 1996 World Food Summit, will be a major challenge facing developing countries and the international community in the twenty-first century.

chronic hunger. These cover: the general conditions for economic and social progress conducive to food security; poverty eradication and access to adequate food; sustainable increases in food production; the contribution of trade to food security; preparedness, prevention and response to food emergencies; optimal investment in human resources, sustainable production capacity and rural development; and cooperation in implementing and monitoring the Action Plan.

Under resolution 51/171 of 16 December, the General Assembly welcomed the outcome of the Food Summit and urged the international community, including international and regional financial institutions, "to cooperate actively in a coordinated manner" in the Plan's implementation. It also recommended that, at next year's special session that will review the implementation of Agenda 21—the action plan that emerged from the 1992 Rio Earth Summit—the Assembly give "due attention" to the Rome results.

WILL THE WORLD STARVE?

Feast and famine

Why should anyone believe today's Malthusian forecasts when earlier ones have been proved wrong?

CROPS come up every year. Forecasts of famine seem to come up about every 20 years. The last time was in the mid-1970s. A giant food conference, held in Rome in 1974, met against a background of soaring food prices, rising population and deep pessimism. Many people worried there would be a world food crisis in the early 21st-century as the unstoppable surge in population overwhelmed mankind's ability to produce food, which was nearing a natural ceiling.

This week thousands of politicians, bureaucrats and lobbyists gathered for the first such meeting since that time, also in Rome, the world food summit held at the headquarters of the United Nation's Food and Agriculture Organisation (FAO). It too is meeting against a background of rising prices and falling stocks. Between June 1993 and May this year, *The Economist's* index of food prices rose by 47% after many years of decline (see chart). The world's grain stocks have fallen to 13% of annual consumption—the lowest ever recorded.

And now, the range of longer-run concerns is even greater than it was. Worries unknown in 1974 have appeared. Global warming threatens to render once-productive lands desolate. Scientists, in their quest for ever-higher yielding crops, are using genetic engineering, a science which many believe to be dangerous.

The older concern—that the world is reaching some sort of natural limit to food—has not gone away, though it is now focused on particular areas, especially the sea: almost everywhere, fish stocks have been plundered to the point of exhaustion.

World population is still rising fast, though the rate of increase has stabilised.

And a backlash is developing against the sorts of policies encouraged during the 1960s and 1970s, which were largely technological solutions to the problem of increasing food supply, such as irrigation and the use of farm chemicals and new high-yielding seed varieties. Across Asia vast areas of irrigated land have become waterlogged. Chemical fertilisers have run off into rivers and lakes causing ugly, slimy blooms of algae. Crop diseases such as late blight in potatoes, the virulent fungus responsible for the Irish famine, appear to be spreading again, having developed resistance to traditional farm chemicals.

Lester Brown, the world's leading modern Malthusian and president of the Worldwatch Institute, an environmental group, argues that the world is entering an era of food scarcity. He reckons that growing demand for grain from China, in particular, could soon overwhelm the capacity of all the world's grain-producing countries. He says that the most important result from the summit would be a one-word letter from the FAO to the United Nations Population Fund: "Help!"

So is population growth beginning to outstrip food production, as Thomas Malthus predicted 200 years ago? Has the "green revolution" run out of steam? Will the expansion of world food supply ruin the environment? The answer to all these questions is a qualified "no"; qualified, because proving the pessimists wrong will not be a simple task.

Why are prices rising?

Consider, first, the recent behaviour of food prices and stocks. Clearly, these are doing damage, especially to the many African countries which are net importers of food. According to the FAO, higher prices last year increased the cost of cereal imports to developing countries by $4 billion.

Equally clearly, these are market signals that some kind of shortage is developing. But what kind? As yet, there is little evidence that the shortage is the result of world food supplies bumping against a natural limit. Rather, it seems to be a consequence of short-term and reversible developments. One of the main reasons for the rise in prices was bad weather in America (its huge maize crop, for example, was hit by a particularly wet May last year). Since 1990 food production has also dropped dramatically in the countries of the former Soviet Union because subsidies were with-

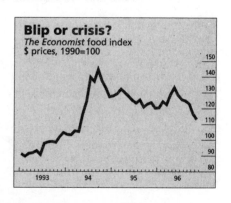

Blip or crisis?
The Economist food index
$ prices, 1990=100

drawn from inefficient state-run farms. If food supplies really were reaching a ceiling, you would expect prices to be rising in the long run as well as the short. But they are not. The current upward movement is a blip in a long-term decline (see chart).

Moreover grain stocks fell partly because of changes in rich countries' farm policies. After surpluses reached embarrassingly high levels in the mid-1980s, politicians in Washington and Brussels started paying farmers to let land lie fallow. Over the past ten years, America, the world's largest grain exporter, has taken out nearly 15m hectares of cropland, 20% of the total, under its Conservation Reserve Programme.

Recently farmers in a host of countries, including America, Argentina and Australia, have responded to higher prices by bringing land back into production. Grain prices have now begun to fall. Barring more bad weather, this year's grain harvest is predicted to be the largest ever. In short, markets are not signalling some sort of impending crisis; they are adjusting to the weather and to various policy decisions—just as you would expect.

Can supply increase?

What about the world food market further into the future? Food analysts at sober organisations such as the World Bank and Washington's International Food Policy Research Institute (IFPRI) praise Lester Brown for shaking common complacency about food security. *Sotto voce*, however, they say that his predictions of impending disaster are "probably nonsense".

Begin with the demand side of the equation. There is little dispute that food demand will grow rapidly, driven both by the absolute number of mouths to feed and by rising expectations about what to eat.

The world's population is expected to exceed 8 billion within 30 years, and to peak at 10 billion-11 billion by about 2050—twice the present level. The rate of population growth has begun to slow, after increasing dramatically in the past 50 years. The increase in numbers from 5 billion to 6 billion will have taken 11 years (ending next year); so will the rise from 6 billion to 7 billion. But the rise from 7 billion to 8 billion will take 12 years, that from 8 billion to 9 billion will take 14 years and that from 9 billion to 10 billion is expected to take 19 years. All that suggests the world may have a little more time to find extra food than had appeared in the 1970s.

In principle, it might be possible to reduce food demand directly by restraining population growth. But experience suggests that this is possible only through massive social intervention (as with China's one-child policy) or through social change that occurs only when countries are relatively rich (as in the West and a few Asian dragons, where population growth has slowed dramatically).

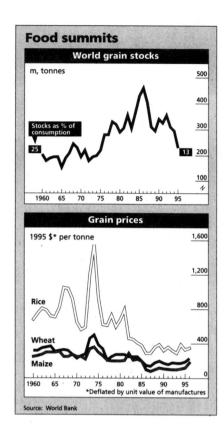

Food summits

World grain stocks

m, tonnes

Stocks as % of consumption

Grain prices

1995 $* per tonne

Rice

Wheat

Maize

*Deflated by unit value of manufactures

Source: World Bank

Anyway, as families lift themselves out of poverty they start to buy meat, which puts greater demands on grain production. You need roughly two kilos of grain, to produce a kilo of chicken; seven kilos of grain for a kilo of beef.

Put those trends together and it appears that the world's supply of grain will, eventually, have to double, at least, by the middle of the next century. It might have to rise considerably more. A recent study by IFPRI predicts that China, for example, will have to boost its grain imports from 16m tonnes in 1995 to 43m tonnes in 2010. Mr Brown suggests even higher numbers.

Can the world grow all that extra grain? Estimates of total capacity vary wildly, influenced by the quantity and quality of land, the impact of technology and future weather patterns. Take the weather first. Assuming global warming is happening (and not all scientists are convinced), its effect on agriculture is anyone's guess. Higher levels of carbon dioxide in the atmosphere should raise the yields of many crops, yet higher temperatures could lead to droughts and the spread of pests. The best guess of scientists working for the United Nations is that climate change will cause dramatic changes across different regions but will not affect total food production.

With or without climate change, there is some scope for expanding food supply simply by ploughing up more land. In spite of the rapid growth of cities in the developing world, there are new areas suitable for

farming both in Latin America and Africa. Farm acreage could increase by 10% over the next 40 years, on one World Bank estimate. Whether that will happen, however, is a different matter. In many cases it would mean destroying forests or other sensitive habitats, so environmentalists might limit the expansion of cultivated land.

In any case, some farm land is likely to disappear at the same time. Mr Brown's prediction that China will overwhelm world food markets by its voracious appetite is based partly on the assumption that the country will lose roughly half its grainland by 2030, as roads, factories and golf courses spread across the countryside. Others, including many Chinese farm experts, think that the loss of land will be much smaller. Whatever the truth of China's particular case, it is clear that, overall, taking more land under cultivation can play only a small part in boosting world food supplies. A much greater part will have to come from squeezing more from existing land—as China's own politicians recognised when they increased government spending on farm research in response to recent food-price rises.

Throughout the world more certainly could be squeezed from existing land. The technologies of the green revolution failed to penetrate much of sub-Saharan Africa. Fertiliser use in Africa is a fifteenth of Chinese levels. Peter Hazell of IFPRI points out that India successfully feeds twice as many people as Africa on 13% of the land area, even though growing conditions in the two regions are roughly comparable.

Even in Asia average crop yields are a mere 40% of the yields achieved by scientists using the best technology now available. In Andhra Pradesh, in India, for example, scientists have boosted yields almost six-fold by planting a double crop of sorghum and chickpea instead of the single cropping method used by local farmers. And at least with rice, a dramatic leap forward is in sight. Researchers at the International Rice Research Institute (IRRI) in the Philippines have recently bred a new strain which invests around 50% of its energy in growing its ear—which contains the edible bits—compared with 30% in older varieties.

Relying on existing technologies, however, will allow food supply to continue to grow only for so long. Already there are signs of diminishing returns: yields of three of the most important crops in developing countries—rice, wheat and maize—have recently been rising at a slower rate than in the 1960s and 1970s. So traditional technological improvements can go part of the way to feeding the world, but not all of it.

The biotech hope

Biotechnology may hold the key to future jumps in yields. For a start, the use of genetic maps and markers allows scientists to breed existing plant species much more efficiently. There are some 250,000 known plant species, although a mere nine supply three-quarters of all human energy intake derived from crops.

Old-style plant breeding involved crossing parent plants which exhibited desirable characteristics, such as resistance to drought or pests. The trouble is that not all the genetic characteristics of a plant are immediately apparent. Some are exposed in the plant's offspring (in the same way that two brown-eyed parents can have a blue-eyed baby). Biotechnology, however, enables scientists to select the best plant by examining its genetic make-up directly.

It also allows genes to be transferred between species. Researchers at the International Institute of Tropical Agriculture, which has a network of stations across Africa, have inserted foreign genes into cowpeas, an important source of protein for millions of West Africans. Their aim is to make the plant resistant to insect pests.

Asian scientists, meanwhile, are working on a strain of rice resistant to a type of caterpillar which bores inside the stem of the plant. This involves inserting a gene from a common soil bacterium, *Bacillus thuringiensis*, which kills caterpillars. Scientists have already inserted the same gene into maize, cotton and potatoes. Biotechnology even promises to revolutionise fishing: researchers have devised a version of the tilapia, a fish farmed in Asia and Africa, which grows much bigger than usual.

Biotechnology, in short, has the capacity to create another green revolution. But it would be wrong to suggest it is on the verge of doing this. Most research and development in genetic engineering is concentrated in medicine, not farming; its cutting edge is the Human Genome Project, not a human green project. Where agricultural R&D is taking place, it is being done by private firms in the West, who make much of their money from tinkering with the qualities of fruit and vegetables for rich markets, not from boosting the sheer quantity of basic grains for the poor.

So either grain prices will have to rise to improve the incentives for bio-engineers, or the whole business will need a push from governments in rich countries, who have paid for most of the research so far. That does not seem likely soon. After steady growth since the 1960s, aid fatigue has set in for farm research. IRRI is now laying off about a third of its 1,500 employees following cuts in its budget.

The trouble is that rich countries are under political pressures from an irresistible combination of budget cutters and greens. Green lobby groups are now campaigning furiously against biotechnology. The opening of the food summit itself, for example, was enlivened by three naked women brandishing slogans at America's agricul-

Just when you thought it was safe

MOST environmental panics about food seem to be just that—panics. On two issues, however, environmentalists' warnings deserve to be taken seriously: fish and water.

According to the FAO, around 70% of the world's fish stocks are being harvested near or beyond what is sustainable. Depleted fish stocks have brought otherwise civilised countries to blows. Last year Canada and Spain battled over who should fish Greenland Halibut. European countries are continually squabbling over their remaining fish.

Ismail Serageldin of the World Bank argues that the wars of the next century will be over water. Worldwide there is more than enough fresh water to meet human needs, but in certain regions, including the Middle East and parts of Africa, supplies are precarious. The main culprit is irrigation, which swallows over two-thirds of the water used by humans. Irrigation in both India's Punjab and across large areas of northern China has led to dramatic falls in water tables.

The problems with both fish and water, however, are as much the result of short-sighted policies as the breaching of any natural limit to production. Few governments have successfully devised

regulations which encourage fishermen to co-operate with each other in sustaining stocks. Left to their own devices, fishermen have an overwhelming incentive to take as much fish as quickly as possible. Moreover, rather than shut down bankrupt fisheries, many governments sustain them with subsidies (the FAO reckons the world's fishing fleets make annual losses of some $50 billion).

In most countries farmers are charged for water at a fraction of the true cost of supply. Little surprise that much of it goes to waste: less than half the water withdrawn in many irrigation schemes actually reaches the crops. Higher prices would encourage farmers to invest in technologies such as drip irrigation, which uses pipes to target small amounts of water directly at the root of plants.

The trouble is that raising water prices is just as politically difficult as allowing quaint fishing communities to go bankrupt. Throughout the world, the farmers which rely most on irrigation tend to be wealthy and politically well-connected, rather than peasant smallholders. No one doubts that feeding the world's growing population will require clever scientists. But it will also demand more of a rarer breed: brave politicians.

ture secretary saying "Ban the Gene Bean"—a reference to a controversial practice of genetically modifying soyabeans. Governments in rich countries—and particularly in Europe—have become reluctant to finance research into genetically-engineered crops for poor countries.

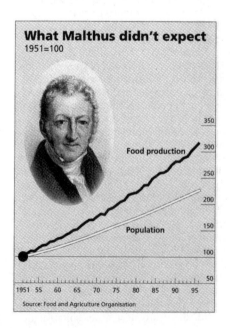

What Malthus didn't expect
1951=100

Food production

Population

350
300
250
200
150
100
50

1951 55 60 65 70 75 80 85 90 95

Source: Food and Agriculture Organisation

The green revolution has certainly caused environmental problems. Millions of hectares of irrigated land have become waterlogged or rendered infertile because the water has left deposits of salt. Many insects and funghi have evolved resistance to farm chemicals. Yet the green revolution has also protected the environment by allowing more food to be produced without a dramatic increase in the area of land under crops. Dennis Avery, a former agricultural analyst at America's Department of State, calculates that 10m square miles (26m square kilometres)—equivalent to the whole of North and Central America—would have been cleared for farming had the green revolution never happened.

In sum, biotechnology may prove the means of closing the last part of the food gap, once more land is brought under cultivation and the impact of traditional green-revolution improvements has diminished. Most scientists reckon that biotechnology, provided it is well regulated, poses negligible risks to the environment. Even if the risks were large, they would still have to be weighed against the loss of human life if food supplies start to fail. And in that basic fear of mass starvation lies a hope: it may be the main reason for thinking the world not only can, but will, be fed.

Running Out of Water, Running Out of Time

By ARUN P. ELHANCE

NEW YORK—Here is something to think about as celebrations to greet the dawn of the new millennium or New Age get going. Before that midnight comes around, 27 million of the world's citizens—currently living and yet to be born—will have died because of water scarcity and water-borne and water-based diseases. At the rate of 25,000 deaths per day, more people, mostly infants and young children, will perish in the next three years than have been killed in all the wars in this century.

Not much will and can be done in the next thousand days to save most of these unfortunates, but international awareness and a concerted global effort, starting today, may be able to save hundreds of millions of other lives in the next century. Ninety percent of all growth in world population in the next century will concentrate in the mostly water-deficient regions in the so-called "Third World." Millions will die prematurely from a lack of drinking water and from diseases caused by contaminated water.

A recent U.N. report warns that some 80 countries—supporting 40 percent of the world's population—already suffer from serious water shortages for personal and household needs. As many as 1.2 billion people suffer physically from shortages of potable water, and 1.8 billion people lack adequate water for sanitation.

About 80 percent of all illnesses and 30 percent of all unnatural deaths in the Third World are due to water-borne diseases and consumption of polluted water. By 2025, some 37 countries are likely to be without enough water for household and agricultural needs, let alone for sustaining fisheries and animal husbandry, industries, energy production, navigation and other societal needs.

By 2000, about 300 million people in Africa alone will be living in an acutely water-scarce environment. Throughout sub-Saharan Africa water-borne and water-based diseases are already endemic. A recent World Bank report states that "diarrheal deaths in Africa are the highest in the world; schistosomiasis affects 28 percent of the population; malaria causes 800,000 deaths every year; and onchocerciasis has caused blindness in up to 25 percent of the population in some villages."

By 2025, Africa's population will exceed 1 billion; by then the number of African countries experiencing acute water stress will have risen to 18 compared to 8 in 1990. This would jeopardize the survival, livelihood and well-being of close to 600 million people.

Women and children in poor rural families suffer the most from water scarcity, since they often have the primary responsibility for fetching water, often highly contaminated water, in some cases from sources as far away as two or three hours of walking time. This can burn off up to 600 calories per day, about one-third of their average daily food intake.

The price of water

Even in the urban areas, scarce water of potable quality is often provided disproportionately to the upper strata of society. The urban poor have to either buy water of questionable quality from private venders, at prices estimated to be 4 to 100 times higher than the piped city water supply, or make do with free but highly contaminated water from other sources. In both rural and urban areas infants and young children are the most vulnerable to water-borne diseases.

The Food and Agricultural Organization has estimated that for the Third World simply to maintain its presently inadequate food supply will require the extension of irrigation to an additional 53 million acres of farmland and delivery of an additional 440 billion cubic meters of water by 2000.

Recent estimates by the World Bank show a need for investing $60 to $70 billion every year over the next decade for irrigation, hydropower, water supply and sanitation in the developing world. However, only about $10 billion per year is currently invested in these countries for water and sanitation systems. Worse still, most developing countries are heavily in debt, and likely to remain so in the foreseeable future. As their populations rise, more and more water-related investments will be needed just to maintain even the currently dismal standard of living and quality of life of hundreds of millions of people.

Rivers currently provide 80 percent of human freshwater needs; many other sources—aquifers, lakes, wetlands and marshes—are also often linked to the catchment and drainage basins of rivers. In many areas of the world, rivers are also the most polluted sources of freshwater because of the dumping of agricultural and industrial chemicals and raw sewage.

To make matters worse, while many river basins are fully contained within the borders of individual countries, more than 200 river basins world-wide are shared by two or more countries, mostly without enforceable water-sharing agreements between them. In the absence of such agreements, unilateral over-exploitation, wastage and degradation of the scarce trans-boundary water resources continue to be the norm.

Almost all remaining exploitable sources of freshwater are in river basins shared by two or more countries. Growing competition for trans-boundary water resources in the next century is bound to greatly accentuate the potential for acute social upheaval and conflict in many regions.

At the very least, poverty alleviation, food security, health maintenance, economic development and preservation of many ecological assets in the Third World will be increasingly contingent upon efficient, equitable and sustainable development and sharing of water resources in these international river basins.

Unfortunately, historical experience shows that negotiations for water-sharing between sovereign states can stretch over decades. Full implementation of signed water agreements also takes many years. Even when the needed cooperation, financial resources and technical expertise are all in place, large water projects can take anywhere from 10 to 20 years to implement.

Thus, even if a concerted global effort to develop inter-state cooperation in all the international river basins in the Third World were begun today, and assuming it were successful, the full benefits of such cooperation might not be forthcoming well into the early part of the next century.

In the meantime, tens of millions would die from thirst and avoidable diseases. The world is fast running out of water for many of its current and future citizens, and running out of time to do something meaningful about this grotesque state of affairs.

Arun P. Elhance, a geographer, is the program director for research on global environmental changes at the Social Science Research Council.

Crop gurus sow some seeds of hope

Fred Pearce

THE scientists who gave the world the "green revolution"—the new crop varieties that have doubled global food output since the mid-1960s—last week promised to repeat the trick over the next 30 years. The promise comes in the run-up to next week's World Food Summit in Rome, and against a backdrop of increased uncertainty about humanity's ability to feed itself.

People left behind by the first revolution will be the focus this time, according to the Consultative Group on International Agricultural Research, which includes research centres, governments and international bodies such as the World Bank. "Scientists are laying the foundations for a second global food production campaign that will exceed in scope the green revolution of the 1960s and 1970s," the CGIAR declared last week at a meeting in Washington DC.

"There is good news," said Donald Winkelmann, chairman of the CGIAR's technical advisory committee. He was speaking during a forum on research priorities, held on the 25th anniversary of the group's formation. "In our judgment there will be adequate food to feed the 8 billion people we expect in the world by 2025. The food will be produced and food prices will continue to fall."

A CGIAR report released to coincide with the meeting promises Africa a "super cassava" that can increase tenfold the yields of this basic, drought-resistant crop. For Asia, it offers a new breed of rice that "can produce 25 per cent more grain on the same amount of land." The new variety, being developed at the International Rice Research Institute in the Philippines, could "help feed an additional 450 million people a year," it says.

Meanwhile, the CGIAR's International Potato Center in Peru is developing a genetically engineered potato that is resistant to tropical bacterial diseases and can be picked within 60 days of planting—a third of the time needed for potatoes to grow in cooler climates. And its International Maize and Wheat Improvement Center, near Mexico City, is promising new varieties of maize genetically engineered to withstand the kind of drought that hit southern Africa last year, and to grow in acidic soils of the kind that cover half of Latin America, for instance.

Some observers say the claims are too good to be true. "Of course there is more research to be done, especially tailored to making the best of local climatic and soil conditions," says Lester Brown of the Worldwatch Institute in Washington DC. "But we shouldn't kid ourselves there is another green revolution coming." Brown argues that there are three natural constraints on further increases in crop yields: shortages of irrigation water and of new land that can be put under the plough, and the limit to how much more plants can benefit from fertilisers.

Gordon Conway, vice-chancellor of the University of Sussex and a leading adviser to the CGIAR, believes there can be a new green revolution, but warns against relying on "miracle varieties" to feed the world. "I think genetic engineering of new varieties will be vital, but only if we tailor the new crops to the needs of poor rural farmers and their families—the people who go hungry even when grain stores are full."

In 1994, Conway published a report for the CGIAR calling for a "super-green revolution" based on protecting the environment and involving small farmers who work on poor soils. Two years on, he says the message is slowly beginning to reach researchers. "There is a real danger that if you go on intensifying farm production you will turn good soils into poor marginal lands. You can see this in the Punjab in India, where water tables are falling, soils are being poisoned by salt and metals, and pests and diseases are spreading."

The chairman of the CGIAR, World Bank official Ismail Serageldin, backs Conway's call to focus on the poorest farmers. "We must bring the best cutting-edge science, the highest technology, to bear on the problems of the poorest farmers," he says.

The forum backed his call for new research collaborations with poor farmers to meet their farming needs and to tap the benefits of traditional farming methods, such as mixing crops with certain trees to keep down pests. "The revolutions in molecular biology and in information technology offer us unprecedented opportunities for harnessing new resources on behalf of the poor," he said. But "the era of research which produces technological innovations without reference to the needs of the producers is behind us."

To meet the needs of poor farmers, government-funded research is essential Conway says. "The private sector won't invest in this area. It is not sufficiently profitable." But the CGIAR report reveals that the proportion of government development aid spent on agriculture has fallen from 20 per cent in 1980 to 14 per cent today. And out of every $100 of development aid, only 5 cents goes into international agricultural research.

New farm techniques spur Ethiopia rebirth

A momentous Live Aid concert in 1985 focused attention on hundreds of thousands of starving Ethiopians and led to unprecedented outpourings of international grief and giving.

But after just a few months, the problem was forgotten except by a few international agencies. Tragically, the underlying issues of **food** security—which include productive land, plentiful **food** and the ability to harvest, process and store **food**—that created the Ethiopian famine are not being addressed. And after decades of work and billions of dollars, chronic hunger is still widespread around the world.

African leaders and individual families are eager to help themselves. With the appropriate technology and the right policies and counsel, a stable *supply* of **food** can be achieved quickly and at relatively low cost. Let me give you an example.

The famine in Ethiopia and surrounding countries prompted a partnership in 1986 among the Japanese-based Sasakawa Africa Association, Nobel Laureate Norman Borlaug and the nonprofit Carter Center. Called Sasakawa-Global 2000 (or SG 2000) this nongovernmental organization began working to improve agricultural production in sub-Saharan Africa.

In Ethiopia and 13 other countries, we've witnessed extremely inefficient farming techniques. Slash-and-burn procedures often are used, where a few plants are grown on a plot without fertilizer. The area then rapidly erodes and is abandoned after one or two growing seasons.

Knowledge about improved practices was available but not flowing from African research centers through government services to small-scale farmers. This bottleneck, coupled with Africa's high birth rate, means the population grows faster than **food** production. We set out to break this logjam, and now more than half-a-million small-farm families have greatly increased their yields. Our strategy is a simple one. We first negotiate an understanding with each president and key Cabinet members, pledging ourselves to a five-year program. We then enroll a few farm families, each working a total of about two acres. The farmer plants half the land in the traditional way and the other half following our prescription. We introduce simple techniques such as seedbed preparation, timely planting in contour rows, improved seed varieties, weeding, moderate use of fertilizer and pesticides, and proper harvesting and storage. Invariably, plots based on our techniques have exceeded traditional yields by 200% to 400%. The farmers and their neighbors rapidly adopt these "new" technologies.

Unlike many other private and international aid programs, we work hand in hand with each country's government, which allows the network to extend from the highest political officials to the individual farmer. The government employs hundreds of extension workers, who are trained by our single adviser.

In 1993, we began working in Ethiopia. The following year, as harvest time approached, I invited Prime Minister Meles Zenawi to visit some of our plots. He suggested that we dress as farmers and spurn the usual motorcade. When we arrived, the farmers at first were unaware that their head of state was examining the crop. They were enthusiastic in describing their experience with our methodology. The next day, the prime minister instructed his minister of agriculture and our representative to introduce this approach throughout Ethiopia. The 1994 harvest, which was being reaped during our field visit, produced 5.4 million tons of grain, far below the nation's needs. A year later, Ethiopian farmers produced an all-time record harvest of 9.7 million tons.

Just last month, the prime minister informed me that, with nearly 400,000 farm families using our method in 1996, the yield was 11.7 million tons. On Jan. 13, the first shipment from the nearly 1 million tons of surplus grain was being exported to Kenya. He hastened to add that Ethiopia still faces many challenges in **food** production. The government and SG 2000 are just beginning to address the lack of adequate storage facilities, transportation systems and marketing mechanisms. Nevertheless, he wrote, "I had always hoped to see Ethiopia producing enough grain to feed its people, but I had never expected it to happen so soon and so fast."

What has happened in Ethiopia demonstrates that a plentiful **food supply** is possible for all nations. But it takes the right mixture of people and resources: the full support of high-level leaders, the dedicated hard work of thousands of farmers and hundreds of extension workers, and modest assistance from international friends with access to the necessary tools.

Organizations such as The Carter Center are ready to help, but our capabilities are limited. What is needed is the political and social will of the developed world to address the root causes of **food** shortages, not just to donate money. With a little help, our Ethiopian neighbors launched a rebirth of their nation. Surely it's worth the effort to help others, too.

Jimmy Carter

Former president Jimmy Carter is the founder of the nonprofit Carter Center in Atlanta, Georgia. The Center seeks to improve global health, prevent and resolve conflict, and enhance freedom and democracy.

Glossary

Absorption The process by which digestive products pass from the gastrointestinal tract into the blood.

Acid/base balance The relationship between acidity and alkalinity in the body fluids.

Amino acids The structural units that make up proteins.

Amylase An enzyme that breaks down starches; a component of saliva.

Amylopectin A component of starch, consisting of many glucose units joined in branching patterns.

Amylose A component of starch, consisting of many glucose units joined in a straight chain, without branching.

Anabolism The synthesis of new materials for cellular growth, maintenance, or repair in the body.

Anemia A deficiency of oxygen-carrying material in the blood.

Anorexia nervosa A disorder in which a person refuses food and loses weight to the point of emaciation and even death.

Antioxidant A substance that prevents or delays the breakdown of other substances by oxygen; often added to food to retard deterioration and rancidity.

Arachidonic acid An essential polyunsaturated fatty acid.

Arteriosclerosis Condition characterized by a thickening and hardening of the walls of the arteries and a resultant loss of elasticity.

Ascorbic Acid Vitamin C.

Atherosclerosis A type of arteriosclerosis in which lipids, especially cholesterol, accumulate in the arteries and obstruct blood flow.

Avidin A substance in raw egg white that acts as an antagonist of biotin, one of the B vitamins.

Basal metabolic rate (BMR) The rate at which the body uses energy for maintaining involuntary functions such as cellular activity, respiration, and heartbeat when at rest.

Basic Four The food plan outlining the milk, meat, fruits and vegetables, and breads and cereals needed in the daily diet to provide the necessary nutrients.

Beriberi A disease resulting from inadequate thiamin in the diet.

Beta-carotene Yellow pigment that is converted to vitamin A in the body.

Biotin One of the B vitamins.

Bomb calorimeter An instrument that oxidizes food samples to measure their energy content.

Buffer A substance that can neutralize both acids and bases to minimize change in the pH of a solution.

Calorie The energy required to raise the temperature of one gram of water one degree Celsius.

Carbohydrate An organic compound composed of carbon, hydrogen, and oxygen in a ratio of 1:2:1.

Carcinogen A cancer-causing substance.

Catabolism The breakdown of complex substances into simpler ones.

Celiac disease A syndrome resulting from intestinal sensitivity to gluten, a protein substance of wheat flour especially and of other grains.

Cellulose An indigestible polysaccharide made of many glucose molecules.

Cheilosis Cracks at the corners of the mouth, due primarily to a deficiency of riboflavin in the diet.

Cholesterol A fat-like alcohol found only in animal products; important in many body functions but also implicated in heart disease.

Choline A substance that prevents the development of a fatty liver; frequently considered one of the B-complex vitamins.

Chylomicron A very small emulsified lipoprotein that transports fat in the blood.

Cobalamin One of the B vitamins (B_{12}).

Coenzyme A component of an enzyme system that facilitates the working of the enzyme.

Collagen Principal protein of connective tissue.

Colostrum The yellowish fluid that precedes breast milk, produced in the first few days of lactation.

Cretinism The physical and mental retardation of a child resulting from severe iodine or thyroid deficiency in the mother during pregnancy.

Dehydration Excessive loss of water from the body.

Dextrin Any of various small soluble polysaccharides found in the leaves of starch-forming plants and in the human alimentary canal as a product of starch digestion.

Diabetes (diabetes mellitus) A metabolic disorder characterized by excess blood sugar and urine sugar.

Digestion The breakdown of ingested foods into particles of a size and chemical composition that can be absorbed by the body.

Diglyceride A lipid containing glycerol and two fatty acids.

Disaccharide A sugar made up of two chemically combined monosaccharides, or simple sugars.

Diuretics Substances that stimulate urination.

Diverticulosis A condition in which the wall of the large intestine weakens and balloons out, forming pouches where fecal matter can be entrapped.

Edema The presence of an abnormally high amount of fluid in the tissues.

Emulsifier A substance that promotes the mixing of foods, such as oil and water in a salad dressing.

Enrichment The addition of nutrients to foods, often to restore what has been lost in processing.

Enzyme A protein that speeds up chemical reactions in the cell.

Epidemiology The study of the factors that contribute to the occurrence of a disease in a population.

Essential amino acid Any of the nine amino acids that the human body cannot manufacture and that must be supplied by the diet as they are necessary for growth and maintenance.

Essential fatty acid A fatty acid that the human body cannot manufacture and that must be supplied by the diet as it is necessary for growth and maintenance.

Fat An organic compound whose molecules contain glycerol and fatty acids; fat insulates the body, protects organs, carries fat-soluble vitamins, is a constituent of cell membranes, and makes food taste good.

Fatty acid A simple lipid—containing only carbon, hydrogen, and oxygen—that is a constituent of fat.

Ferritin A substance in which iron, in combination with protein, is stored in the liver, spleen, and bone marrow.

Fiber Indigestible carbohydrate found primarily in plant foods; high fiber intake is useful in regulating bowel movements, and may lower the incidence of certain types of cancer and other diseases.

Flavoprotein Protein containing riboflavin.

Folic acid (folacin) One of the B vitamins.

Fortification The addition of nutrients to foods to enhance their nutritional values.

Fructose A six-carbon monosaccharide found in many fruits as well as honey and plant saps; one of two monosaccharides forming sucrose, or table sugar.

Galactose A six-carbon monosaccharide, one of the two that make up lactose, or milk sugar.

Gallstones An abnormal formation of gravel or stones, composed of cholesterol and bile salts and sometimes bile pigments, in the gallbladder; they result when substances that normally dissolve in bile precipitate out.

Gastritis Inflammation of the stomach.

Glucagon A hormone produced by the pancreas that works to increase blood glucose concentration.

Glucose A six-carbon monosaccharide found in sucrose, honey, and many fruits and vegetables; the major carbohydrate found in the body.

Glucose tolerance factor (GTF) A hormone-like substance containing chromium, niacin, and protein that helps the body to use glucose.

Glyceride A simple lipid composed of fatty acids and glycerol.

Glycogen The storage form of carbohydrates in the body; composed of glucose molecules.

Goiter Enlargement of the thyroid gland as a result of iodine deficiency.

Goitrogens Substances that induce goiter, often by interfering with the body's utilization of iodine.

Heme A complex iron-containing compound that is a component of hemoglobin.

Hemicellulose Any of various indigestible plant polysaccharides.

Hemochromatosis A disorder of iron metabolism.

Hemoglobin The iron-containing protein in red blood cells that carries oxygen to the tissues.

High-density lipoprotein (HDL) A lipoprotein that acts as a cholesterol carrier in the blood; referred to as "good" cholesterol because relatively high levels of it appear to protect against atherosclerosis.

Hormones Compounds secreted by the endocrine glands that influence the functioning of various organs.

Humectants Substances added to foods to help them maintain moistness.

Hydrogenation The chemical process by which hydrogen is added to unsaturated fatty acids, which saturates them and converts them from a liquid to a solid form.

Hydrolyze To split a chemical compound into smaller molecules by adding water.

Hydroxyapatite The hard mineral portion (the major constituent) of bone, composed of calcium and phosphate.

Hypercalcemia A high level of calcium in the blood.

Hyperglycemia A high level of "sugar" (glucose) in the blood.

Hypocalcemia A low level of calcium in the blood.

Hypoglycemia A low level of "sugar" (glucose) in the blood.

Incomplete protein A protein lacking or deficient in one or more of the essential amino acids.

Inorganic Describes a substance not containing carbon.

Insensible loss Fluid loss, through the skin and from the lungs, that an individual is unaware of.

Insulin A hormone produced by the pancreas that regulates the body's use of glucose.

Intrinsic factor A protein produced by the stomach that makes absorption of B_{12} possible; lack of this protein results in pernicious anemia.

Joule A unit of energy preferred by some professionals instead of the heat energy measurements of the calorie system for calculating food energy; sometimes referred to as "kilojoule."

Keratinization Formation of a protein called keratin, which, in vitamin A deficiency, occurs instead of mucus formation; leads to a drying and hardening of epithelial tissue.

Ketogenic Describes substances that can be converted to ketone bodies during metabolism, such as fatty acids and some amino acids.

Ketone bodies The three chemicals—acetone, acetoacetic acid, and betahydroxybutyrie—that are normally involved in lipid metabolism and accumulate in blood and urine in abnormal amounts in conditions of impaired metabolism (such as diabetes).

Ketosis A condition resulting when fats are the major source of energy and are incompletely oxidized, causing ketone bodies to build up in the bloodstream.

Kilocalorie One thousand calories, or the energy required to raise the temperature of one kilogram of water one degree Celsius; the preferred unit of measurement for food energy.

Kilojoule See Joule.

Kwashiorkor A form of malnutrition resulting from a diet severely deficient in protein but high in carbohydrates.

Lactase A digestive enzyme produced by the small intestine that breaks down lactose.

Lactation Milk production/secretion.

Lacto-ovo-vegetarian A person who does not eat meat, poultry, or fish but does eat milk products and eggs.

Lactose A disaccharide composed of glucose and galactose and found in milk.

Lactose intolerance The inability to digest lactose due to a lack of the enzyme lactase in the intestine.

Lacto-vegetarian A person who does not eat meat, poultry, fish, or eggs but does drink milk and eat milk products.

Laxatives Food or drugs that stimulate bowel movements.

Lignins Certain forms of indigestible carbohydrate in plant foods.

Linoleic acid An essential polyunsaturated fatty acid.

Lipase An enzyme that digests fats.

Lipid Any of various substances in the body or in food that are insoluble in water; a fat or fat-like substance.

Lipoprotein Compound composed of a lipid (fat) and a protein that transports both in the bloodstream.

Low-density lipoprotein (LDL) A lipoprotein that acts as a cholesterol carrier in the blood; referred to as "bad" cholesterol because relatively high levels of it appear to enhance atherosclerosis.

Macrocytic anemia A form of anemia characterized by the presence of abnormally large blood cells.

Macroelements (also macronutrient elements) Those elements present in the body in amounts exceeding 0.005 percent of body weight and required in the diet in amounts exceeding 100 mg/day; include sodium, potassium, calcium, and phosphorus.

Malnutrition A poor state of health resulting from a lack, excess, or imbalance of the nutrients needed by the body.

Maltose A disaccharide whose units are each composed of two glucose molecules, produced by the digestion of starch.

Marasmus Condition resulting from a deficiency of calories and nearly all essential nutrients.

Melanin A dark pigment in the skin, hair, and eyes.

Metabolism The sum of all chemical reactions that take place within the body.

Microelements (also micronutrient elements; trace elements) Those elements present in the body in amounts under 0.005 percent of body weight and required in the diet in amounts under 100 mg/day.

Monoglyceride A lipid containing glycerol and only one fatty acid.

Monosaccharide A single sugar molecule, the simplest form of carbohydrate; examples are glucose, fructose, and galactose.

Monosodium glutamate (MSG) An amino acid used in flavoring foods, which causes allergic reactions in some people.

Monounsaturated fatty acid A fatty acid containing one double bond.

Mutagen A mutation-causing agent.

Negative nitrogen balance Nitrogen output exceeds nitrogen intake.

Niacin (nicotinic acid) One of the B vitamins.

Nitrogen equilibrium (zero nitrogen balance) Nitrogen output equals nitrogen intake.

Nonessential amino acid Any of the 13 amino acids that the body can manufacture in adequate amounts, but which are nonetheless required in the diet in an amount relative to the amount of essential amino acids.

Nutrients Nourishing substances in food that can be digested, absorbed, and metabolized by the body; needed for growth, maintenance, and reproduction.

Nutrition (1) The sum of the processes by which an organism obtains, assimilates, and utilizes food. (2) The scientific study of these processes.

Obesity Condition of being 15 to 20 percent above one's ideal body weight.

Oleic acid A monounsaturated fatty acid.

Organic foods Those foods, especially fruits and vegetables, grown without the use of pesticides, synthetic fertilizers, etc.

Osmosis Passage of a solvent through a semipermeable membrane from an area of higher concentration to an area of lower concentration until the concentration is equal on both sides of the membrane.

Osteomalacia Condition in which a loss of bone mineral leads to a softening of the bones; adult counterpart of rickets.

Osteoporosis Disorder in which the bones degenerate due to a loss of bone mineral, producing porosity and fragility; normally found in older women.

Overweight Body weight exceeding an accepted norm by 10 or 15 percent.

Ovo-vegetarian A person who does not eat meat, poultry, fish, milk, or milk products but does eat eggs.

Oxidation The process by which a substrate takes up oxygen or loses hydrogen; the loss of electrons.

Palmitic acid A saturated fatty acid.

Pantothenic acid One of the B vitamins.

Pellagra The niacin deficiency syndrome, characterized by dementia, diarrhea, and dermatitis.

Pepsin A protein-digesting enzyme produced by the stomach.

Peptic ulcer An open sore or erosion in the lining of the digestive tract, especially in the stomach and duodenum.

Peptide A compound composed of amino acids that are joined together.

Peristalsis Motions of the digestive tract that propel food through the tract.

Pernicious anemia One form of anemia caused by an inability to absorb vitamin B_{12}, owing to the absense of intrinsic factor.

pH A measure of the acidity of a solution, based on a scale from 0 to 14: a pH of 7 is neutral; greater than 7 is alkaline; less than 7 is acidic.

Phenylketonuria (PKU) A genetic disease in which phenylalanine, an essential amino acid, is not properly metabolized, thus accumulating in the blood and causing early brain damage.

Phospholipid A fat containing phosphorus, glycerol, two fatty acids, and any of several other chemical substances.

Polypeptide A molecular chain of amino acids.

Polysaccharide A carbohydrate containing many monosaccharide subunits.

Polyunsaturated fatty acids A fatty acid in which two or more carbon atoms have formed double bonds, with each holding only one hydrogen atom.

Positive nitrogen balance Condition in which nitrogen intake exceeds nitrogen output in the body.

Protein Any of the organic compounds composed of amino acids and containing nitrogen; found in the cells of all living organisms.

Provitamins Precursors of vitamins that can be converted to vitamins in the body (e.g., beta-carotene, from which the body can make vitamin A).

Pyridoxine One of the B vitamins (B_6).

Pull date Date after which food should no longer be sold but still may be edible for several days.

Recommended Daily Allowances (RDAs) Standards for daily intake of specific nutrients established by the Food and Nutrition Board of the National Academy of Sciences; they are the levels thought to be adequate to maintain the good health of most people.

Rhodopsin The visual pigment in the retinal rods of the eyes which allows one to see at night; its formation requires vitamin A.

Riboflavin One of the B vitamins (B_2).

Ribosome The cellular structure in which protein synthesis occurs.

Rickets The vitamin D deficiency disease in children characterized by bone softening and deformities.

Saliva Fluid produced in the mouth that helps food digestion.

Salmonella A bacterium that can cause food poisoning.

Saturated fatty acid A fatty acid in which carbon Is joined with four other atoms; i.e., all carbon atoms are bound to the maximum possible number of hydrogen atoms.

Scurvy A disease characterized by bleeding gums, pain in joints, lethargy, and other problems; caused by a deficiency of vitamin C (ascorbic acid).

Standard of identity A list of specifications for the manufacture of certain foods that stipulates their required contents.

Starch A polysaccharide composed of glucose molecules; the major form in which energy is stored in plants.

Stearic acid A saturated fatty acid.

Sucrose A disaccharide composed of glucose and fructose, often called "table sugar."

Sulfites Agents used as preservatives in foods to eliminate bacteria, preserve freshness, prevent browning, and increase storage life; can cause acute asthma attacks, and even death, in people who are sensitive to them.

Teratogen An agent with the potential of causing birth defects.

Thiamin One of the B vitamins (B_1).

Thyroxine Hormone containing iodine that is secreted by the thyroid gland.

Toxemia A complication of pregnancy characterized by high blood pressure, edema, vomiting, presence of protein in the urine, and other symptoms.

Transferrin A protein compound, the form in which iron is transported in the blood.

Triglyceride A lipid containing glycerol and three fatty acids.

Trypsin A digestive enzyme, produced in the pancreas, that breaks down protein.

Underweight Body weight below an accepted norm by more than 10 percent.

United States Recommended Daily Allowance (USRDA) The highest level of recommended intakes for population groups (except pregnant and lactating women); derived from the RDAs and used in food labeling.

Urea The main nitrogenous component of urine, resulting from the breakdown of amino acids.

Uremia A disease in which urea accumulates in the blood.

Vegan A person who eats nothing derived from an animal; the strictest type of vegetarian.

Vitamin Organic substance required by the body in small amounts to perform numerous functions.

Vitamin B complex All known water-soluble vitamins except C; includes thiamin (B_1), riboflavin (B_2), pyridoxine (B_6), niacin, folic acid, cobalamin (B_{12}), pantothenic acid, and biotin.

Xerophthalmia A disease of the eye resulting from vitamin A deficiency.

Index

Credits/Acknowledgments

Cover design by Charles Vitelli

1. Trends Today and Tomorrow
Facing overview—© 1998 by Cleo Freelance Photography. 12—*FDA Consumer* illustration by Richard Thompson, Jr.

2. Nutrients
Facing overview—Dushkin/McGraw-Hill photo by Nick Zavalishin.

3. Through the Life Span: Diet and Disease
Facing overview—© 1998 by Cleo Freelance Photography. 105-106—*Food Insight* illustration by Alex Kim.

4. Fat and Weight Control
Facing overview—© 1998 by PhotoDisc, Inc.

5. Food Safety
Facing overview—Dushkin/McGraw-Hill photo by Jeremy Brenner.

6. Health Claims
Facing overview—Dushkin/McGraw-Hill photo by Frank Tarsitano.

7. Hunger and Global Issues
Facing overview—World Bank photo by Kay Chernush.

ANNUAL EDITIONS ARTICLE REVIEW FORM

■ NAME: _____ DATE: _____

■ TITLE AND NUMBER OF ARTICLE: _____

■ BRIEFLY STATE THE MAIN IDEA OF THIS ARTICLE: _____

_____

■ LIST THREE IMPORTANT FACTS THAT THE AUTHOR USES TO SUPPORT THE MAIN IDEA:

_____

_____

_____

_____

■ WHAT INFORMATION OR IDEAS DISCUSSED IN THIS ARTICLE ARE ALSO DISCUSSED IN YOUR TEXTBOOK OR OTHER READINGS THAT YOU HAVE DONE? LIST THE TEXTBOOK CHAPTERS AND PAGE NUMBERS:

_____

_____

_____

_____

■ LIST ANY EXAMPLES OF BIAS OR FAULTY REASONING THAT YOU FOUND IN THE ARTICLE:

_____

_____

_____

_____

■ LIST ANY NEW TERMS/CONCEPTS THAT WERE DISCUSSED IN THE ARTICLE, AND WRITE A SHORT DEFINITION:

_____

_____

_____

_____

*Your instructor may require you to use this ANNUAL EDITIONS Article Review Form in any number of ways: for articles that are assigned, for extra credit, as a tool to assist in developing assigned papers, or simply for your own reference. Even if it is not required, we encourage you to photocopy and use this page; you will find that reflecting on the articles will greatly enhance the information from your text.

We Want Your Advice

ANNUAL EDITIONS revisions depend on two major opinion sources: one is our Advisory Board, listed in the front of this volume, which works with us in scanning the thousands of articles published in the public press each year; the other is you—the person actually using the book. Please help us and the users of the next edition by completing the prepaid article rating form on this page and returning it to us. Thank you for your help!

ANNUAL EDITIONS: NUTRITION 98/99
Article Rating Form

Here is an opportunity for you to have direct input into the next revision of this volume. We would like you to rate each of the 57 articles listed below, using the following scale:

1. **Excellent: should definitely be retained**
2. **Above average: should probably be retained**
3. **Below average: should probably be deleted**
4. **Poor: should definitely be deleted**

Your ratings will play a vital part in the next revision. So please mail this prepaid form to us just as soon as you complete it.
Thanks for your help!

Rating	Article	Rating	Article
	1. "What We Eat in America" Survey		31. Three Major U.S. Studies Describe Trends
	2. Fruits & Vegetables: Eating Your Way to 5 a Day		32. The History of Dieting and Its Effectiveness
	3. Health Claims under the Nutrition Labeling and Education Act		33. Diet Pills: Are Millions of Women Playing Russian Roulette with Their Health?
	4. Today's Special Nutrition Information		34. Obesity: No Miracle Cure Yet
	5. Meat Meets Its Match?		35. Diet and Exercise: What Kids Need Today
	6. Phytochemicals: Drugstore in a Salad?		36. Dysfunctional Eating: A New Concept
	7. The Food Police		37. Reduced-Fat Foods: Dieter's Dream or Marketer's Ploy?
	8. High Price of Shelf Space		38. Foodborne Illness: Role of Home Food Handling Practices
	9. The Coming Boom(er) Market		39. For Safety's Sake: Scrub Your Produce
	10. A Type of Fat We May Need More Of		40. New Risks in Ground Beef Revealed
	11. The Facts about Fats		41. How Much Are Pesticides Hurting Your Health?
	12. Should You Be Eating More Protein—or Less?		42. After the Glow
	13. A 'Bran-New' Look at Dietary Fiber		43. How Quackery Sells
	14. Food for Thought about Dietary Supplements		44. Confessions of a Former Women's Magazine Writer
	15. Vitamin C: Is Anyone Right on Dose?		45. Food for Thought: Can You Trust Your Favorite Magazine to Tell You What to Eat?
	16. The Trials of Beta-Carotene: Is the Verdict In?		46. How to Spot a "Quacky" Web Site
	17. Too Little Sun?		47. Why Do Those #&*?@! "Experts" Keep Changing Their Minds?
	18. Fluoridation: A Triumph of Science over Propaganda		48. Vitamin and Nutritional Supplements
	19. Yes, But *Which* Calcium Supplement?		49. Nutrition Shortcut in a Can?
	20. Beating the Odds: Best Bets for Cancer Prevention		50. The 'Dietary Supplement' Mess: Commission Report Issued
	21. Most Frequently Asked Questions . . . about Diet and Cancer		51. Dead Doctors Don't Lie, But People Who Sell Minerals . . . ,
	22. Diet and Hypertension: Progress Towards a Better Understanding		52. Don't Buy Phony 'Ergogenic Aids': The Real Story vs. a Mountain of Hype
	23. Boning Up on Osteoporosis		53. Table Set Thinly as Food Summit Pledges to Halve World Hunger in 20 Years
	24. Heart Disease Handbook—Part 2: Deciphering Blood Cholesterol		54. Will the World Starve? Feast and Famine
	25. Heart Disease Handbook—Part 3: Triglycerides Turn Troublesome		55. Running Out of Water, Running Out of Time
	26. Breast-Feeding Best Bet for Babies		56. Crop Gurus Sow Some Seeds of Hope
	27. Lactose Intolerance		57. New Farm Techniques Spur Ethiopia Rebirth
	28. When Eating Goes Awry: An Update on Eating Disorders		
	29. Nutritional Implications of Ethnic and Cultural Diversity		
	30. Alcohol: Weighing the Benefits and Risks for You		

(Continued on next page)

ABOUT YOU

Name _____ Date _____

Are you a teacher? ❏ Or a student? ❏

Your school name _____

Department _____

Address _____

City _____ State _____ Zip _____

School telephone # _____

YOUR COMMENTS ARE IMPORTANT TO US!

Please fill in the following information:

For which course did you use this book? _____

Did you use a text with this *ANNUAL EDITION*? ❏ yes ❏ no

What was the title of the text? _____

What are your general reactions to the *Annual Editions* concept?

Have you read any particular articles recently that you think should be included in the next edition?

Are there any articles you feel should be replaced in the next edition? Why?

Are there any World Wide Web sites you feel should be included in the next edition? Please annotate.

May we contact you for editorial input?

May we quote your comments?

ANNUAL EDITIONS: NUTRITION 98/99

BUSINESS REPLY MAIL

First Class   Permit No. 84   Guilford, CT

Postage will be paid by addressee

Dushkin/McGraw·Hill
Sluice Dock
Guilford, CT 06437